Commemorative Issue: 15 Years of the Sleep Medicine Clinics Part 2: Medication and Treatment Effect on Sleep Disorders

Editors

ANA C. KRIEGER
TEOFILO LEE-CHIONG

SLEEP MEDICINE CLINICS

www.sleep.theclinics.com

September 2022 • Volume 17 • Number 3

ELSEVIER

1600 John F. Kennedy Boulevard • Suite 1800 • Philadelphia, Pennsylvania, 19103-2899

http://www.theclinics.com

SLEEP MEDICINE CLINICS Volume 17, Number 3
September 2022, ISSN 1556-407X, ISBN-13: 978-0-323-96165-3

Editor: Joanna Collett
Developmental Editor: Axell Ivan Jade M. Purificacion

Sleep Medicine Clinics (ISSN 1556-407X) is published quarterly by Elsevier Inc., 360 Park Avenue South, New York, NY 10010-1710. Months of issue are March, June, September and December. Business and Editorial Offices: 1600 John F. Kennedy Blvd., Ste. 1800, Philadelphia, PA 19103-2899. Customer Service Office: 3251 Riverport Lane, Maryland Heights, MO 63043. Periodicals postage paid at New York, NY and additional mailing offices. Subscription prices are $234.00 per year (US individuals), $100.00 (US and Canadian students), $653.00 (US institutions), $272.00 (Canadian individuals), $267.00 (international individuals) $135.00 (International students), $682.00 (Canadian and International institutions). Foreign air speed delivery is included in all *Clinics* subscription prices. All prices are subject to change without notice. **POSTMASTER:** Send change of address to *Sleep Medicine Clinics*, Elsevier Health Sciences Division, Subscription Customer Service, 3251 Riverport Lane, Maryland Heights, MO 63043. Customer Service: **Tel: 1-800-654-2452 (U.S. and Canada); 314-447-8871 (outside U.S. and Canada). Fax: 314-447-8029. E-mail: journalscustomerservice-usa@elsevier.com (for print support); journalsonline-support-usa@elsevier.com (for online support).**

Reprints. For copies of 100 or more of articles in this publication, please contact the Commercial Reprints Department, Elsevier Inc., 360 Park Avenue South, New York, NY 10010-1710. Tel.: 212-633-3874; Fax: 212-633-3820; E-mail: reprints@elsevier.com.

Sleep Medicine Clinics is covered in *MEDLINE/PubMed (Index Medicus)*.

SLEEP MEDICINE CLINICS

FORTHCOMING ISSUES

December 2022
A review of PAP therapy for the treatment of Obstructive Sleep Apnea
Matthew R. Ebben, *Editor*

March 2023
Adjunct Interventions to Cognitive Behavioral Therapy for Insomnia
Joshua Hyong-Jin Cho, *Editor*

June 2023
Pediatric Sleep Clinics
Haviva Veler, *Editor*

RECENT ISSUES

June 2022
Commemorative Issue: 15 Years Of The Sleep Medicine Clinics - Part 1: Sleep And Sleep Disorders
Ana C. Krieger and Teofilo Lee-Chiong, *Editors*

March 2022
Causes of Sleep Complaints
Keith Romeo A. Aguilera, and Agnes T. Remulla, *Editor*

December 2021
Measuring Sleep
Erna Sif Arnardottir, *Editor*

Contributors

CONSULTING EDITORS

TEOFILO LEE-CHIONG Jr, MD
Professor of Medicine, National Jewish Health, Professor of Medicine, University of Colorado, Denver, Colorado, USA; Chief Medical Liaison, Philips Respironics, Murrysville, Pennsylvania, USA

ANA C. KRIEGER, MD, MPH, FCCP, FAASM
Chief, Division of Sleep Neurology, Medical Director, Weill Cornell Center for Sleep Medicine, Professor of Clinical Medicine, Professor of Medicine in Neurology and Genetic Medicine, Weill Cornell Medical College, Cornell University, New York, New York, USA

EDITORS

ANA C. KRIEGER, MD, MPH, FCCP, FAASM
Chief, Division of Sleep Neurology, Medical Director, Weill Cornell Center for Sleep Medicine, Professor of Clinical Medicine, Professor of Medicine in Neurology and Genetic Medicine, Weill Cornell Medical College, Cornell University, New York, New York, USA

TEOFILO LEE-CHIONG Jr, MD
Professor of Medicine, National Jewish Health, Professor of Medicine, University of Colorado, Denver, Colorado, USA; Chief Medical Liaison, Philips Respironics, Murrysville, Pennsylvania, USA

AUTHORS

GALIA V. ANGUELOVA, MD, MSc, PhD
Center for Sleep and Wake Disorders, Haaglanden Medical Center, The Hague, the Netherlands

ISABELLE ARNULF, MD, PhD
Service des pathologies du sommeil, Sleep Clinic, Pitie-Salpetriere Hospital, Sorbonne University, Paris, France

HELEN J. BURGESS, PhD
Biological Rhythms Research Laboratory, Department of Behavioral Sciences, Rush University Medical Center, Chicago, Illinois, USA

MICHELLE CAO, DO
Divisions of Pulmonary, Allergy, Critical Care Medicine, and Sleep Medicine, Stanford University School of Medicine, Stanford, California, USA

ED DE BRUIN, PhD
Research Institute of Child Development and Education, University of Amsterdam, Amsterdam, the Netherlands

JULIA DEWALD-KAUFMANN, PhD
Department of Psychiatry and Psychotherapy, University Hospital, LMU Munich, Hochschule Fresenius, University of Applied Sciences, Munich, Germany

PAULINE DODET, MD
Service des pathologies du sommeil, Sleep Clinic, Pitie-Salpetriere Hospital, Paris, France

SYLVIE DUJARDIN, MD
Sleep Medicine Center Kempenhaeghe, Heeze, the Netherlands

NICHOLAS-TIBERIO ECONOMOU, MD, PhD
Sleep Study Unit, Department of Psychiatry, University of Athens, Enypnion Sleep-Epilepsy

Center, Bioclinic Hospital Athens, Athens, Greece

JACK D. EDINGER, PhD
Department of Medicine, National Jewish Health, Denver, Colorado, USA

JONATHAN S. EMENS, MD
Department of Psychiatry, Department of Medicine, Oregon Health & Science University, VA Portland Health Care System, Portland, Oregon, USA

LUIGI FERINI-STRAMBI, MD, PhD
Division of Neuroscience, University Vita-Salute San Raffaele, Milan, Italy

SHEILA N. GARLAND, PhD
Department of Psychology, Faculty of Science, Division of Oncology, Faculty of Medicine, Memorial University of Newfoundland, St John's, Newfoundland, Canada

PRIYA GOPALAN, MD
Department of Psychiatry, Western Psychiatric Institute and Clinic, University of Pittsburgh Medical Center, Pittsburgh, Pennsylvania, USA

JAN HEDNER, MD, PhD, FERS
Center for Sleep and Vigilance Disorders, Department of Internal Medicine and Clinical Nutrition, Sahlgrenska Academy, University of Gothenburg, Gothenburg, Sweden

JONATHAN P. HINTZE, MD
Division of Pediatric Sleep Medicine, University of South Carolina School of Medicine-Greenville, Greenville Health System, Greenville, South Carolina, USA

SHAHROKH JAVAHERI, MD
Division of Pulmonary and Sleep Medicine, Bethesda North Hospital, Cincinnati, Ohio, USA; Division of Medicine, The Ohio State University, Columbus, Ohio, USA

VICTORIA A.J. KAVANAGH, BA
Department of Psychology, Faculty of Science, Memorial University of Newfoundland, St John's, Newfoundland, Canada

ARTHUR G.Y. KURVERS, MD
Center for Sleep and Wake Disorders, Haaglanden Medical Center, The Hague, the Netherlands

GERT JAN LAMMERS, MD, PhD
Department of Neurology, Leiden University Medical Center, Leiden, the Netherlands; Sleep-Wake Centers of SEIN, Heemstede, the Netherlands

SMARANDA LEU-SEMENESCU, MD
Service des pathologies du sommeil, Sleep Clinic, Pitie-Salpetriere Hospital, Paris, France

RONEIL G. MALKANI, MD, MS
Associate Professor of Neurology, Division of Sleep Medicine, Department of Neurology, Center for Circadian and Sleep Medicine, Northwestern University Feinberg School of Medicine, Jesse Brown Veterans Affairs Medical Center, Chicago, Illinois, USA

RAFFAELE MANNI, MD
Sleep Medicine and Epilepsy, IRCCS Mondino Foundation, Pavia, Italy

LAURA P. MCLAFFERTY, MD
Psychiatrist, Included Health; Department of Psychiatry and Human Behavior, Thomas Jefferson University, Philadelphia, Pennsylvania, USA

GRADISAR MICHAEL, PhD
School of Psychology, Flinders University, Adelaide, South Australia

SEIJI NISHINO, MD, PhD
Sleep and Circadian Neurobiology Laboratory, Department of Psychiatry and Behavioral Sciences, Stanford University School of Medicine, Palo Alto, California, USA

LINO NOBILI, MD, PhD
Department of Neuroscience, Centre of Sleep Medicine, Centre for Epilepsy Surgery, Niguarda Hospital, Piazza Ospedale Maggiore, Milan, Italy; Department of Neuroscience (DINOGMI), University of Genoa, Child Neuropsychiatry, Gaslini Institute, Via Gerolamo Gaslini, Genoa, Italy

TAISUKE ONO, MD, PhD
Sleep and Circadian Neurobiology Laboratory, Department of Psychiatry and Behavioral Sciences, Stanford University School of Medicine, Palo Alto, California, USA; Department of Geriatric Medicine, Kanazawa Medical University School of Medicine, Ishikawa, Japan

DIRK PEVERNAGIE, MD, PhD
Sleep Medicine Center Kempenhaeghe, Heeze, the Netherlands; Department of Internal Medicine and Paediatrics, Faculty of Medicine and Health Sciences, Ghent University, Ghent, Belgium

ANGELIQUE PIJPERS, MD, PhD
Sleep Medicine Center Kempenhaeghe, Heeze, the Netherlands

PAOLA PROSERPIO, MD
Department of Neuroscience, Centre of Sleep Medicine, Centre for Epilepsy Surgery, Niguarda Hospital, Milan, Italy

JOSHUA A. RASH, PhD
Department of Psychology, Faculty of Science, Memorial University of Newfoundland, St John's, Newfoundland, Canada

ROSELYNE M. RIJSMAN, MD, PhD
Center for Sleep and Wake Disorders, Haaglanden Medical Center, The Hague, the Netherlands

MEREDITH SPADA, MD
Department of Psychiatry, Western Psychiatric Institute and Clinic, University of Pittsburgh Medical Center, Pittsburgh, Pennsylvania, USA

PASCHALIS STEIROPOULOS, MD, PhD, FCCP
Sleep Unit, Department of Pulmonology, Medical School, Democritus University of Thrace, University Campus, Dragana, Alexandroupolis, Greece

SHINICHI TAKENOSHITA, MD, MPH
Sleep and Circadian Neurobiology Laboratory, Department of Psychiatry and Behavioral Sciences, Stanford University School of Medicine, Palo Alto, California, USA

MICHELE TERZAGHI, MD
Sleep Medicine and Epilepsy, IRCCS Mondino Foundation, Pavia, Italy

ANN VAN GASTEL, MD
Multidisciplinary Sleep Disorders Centre and University Department of Psychiatry, Antwerp University Hospital, Faculty of Medicine and Health Sciences, Collaborative Antwerp Psychiatric Research Institute (CAPRI), University of Antwerp (UA), Campus Drie Eiken, Antwerp, Belgium

MONIQUE H.M. VLAK, MD, PhD
Center for Sleep and Wake Disorders, Haaglanden Medical Center, The Hague, the Netherlands

PHYLLIS C. ZEE, MD, PhD
Benjamin and Virginia T. Boshes Professor of Neurology, Division of Sleep Medicine, Department of Neurology, Center for Circadian and Sleep Medicine, Northwestern University Feinberg School of Medicine, Chicago, Illinois, USA

DING ZOU, MD, PhD
Center for Sleep and Vigilance Disorders, Department of Internal Medicine and Clinical Nutrition, Sahlgrenska Academy, University of Gothenburg, Gothenburg, Sweden

Contents

big concern not only from a medical but also from a public health point of view. Patients with EDS have the possibility of falling asleep even when they should wake up and concentrate, for example, when they drive, play sports, or walk outside. In this article, clinical characteristics of common hypersomnia and pharmacologic treatments of each hypersomnia are described.

Brain Stimulation for Improving Sleep and Memory **505**

Roneil G. Malkani and Phyllis C. Zee

Sleep has been increasingly recognized for its importance in many functions, including cognition. Emerging techniques aim to stimulate the brain to enhance sleep, particularly slow wave sleep, and improve memory. Several methods have shown promise, such as transcranial electrical stimulation and transcranial magnetic stimulation. In particular, acoustic stimulation of slow wave sleep shows significant potential to enhance slow wave sleep, sleep spindles, their phase coupling and declarative memory. While these methods may enhance memory non-specifically, targeted memory reactivation uses associated cues to consolidate specific memories. Future research is necessary to determine long-term potential as tools in healthy and clinical populations.

Hypnotic Discontinuation in Chronic Insomnia **523**

Jonathan P. Hintze and Jack D. Edinger

Insomnia disorder is common in adults and children. The estimated prevalence ranges from 9% to 15% in the general population, with higher prevalence in certain subpopulations. Hypnotic medications are those that tend to produce sleep and are frequently used to treat insomnia. Commonly used hypnotics in adults include benzodiazepines (BZDs), BZD receptor agonists, antihistamines, antidepressants, melatonin receptor agonists, orexin receptor antagonists, and antipsychotics. However, hypnotic discontinuation is difficult and often unsuccessful. This article discusses strategies to discontinue hypnotics and evidence supporting their use.

Sleep-Related Drug Therapy in Special Conditions: Children **531**

Nicholas-Tiberio Economou, Luigi Ferini-Strambi, and Paschalis Steiropoulos

Pharmacologic treatment of the most common pediatric sleep disorders lacks evidence, and alternative methods, which have been proved to alleviate the symptoms, are preferred in most cases. The implementation of specific guidelines is of great importance because sleep disorders in children are not rare and they can negatively affect children's development and their cognitive and social skills. This article summarizes the current therapeutic management of sleep disorders in children, bearing in mind the absence of evidence-based guidelines on this topic.

Preface

Sleep Medicine: The Uncertain Future

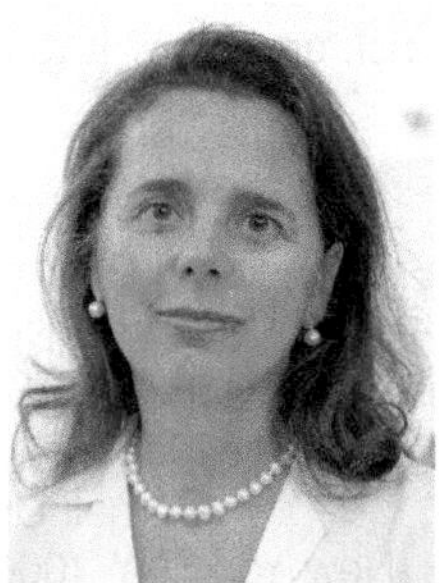

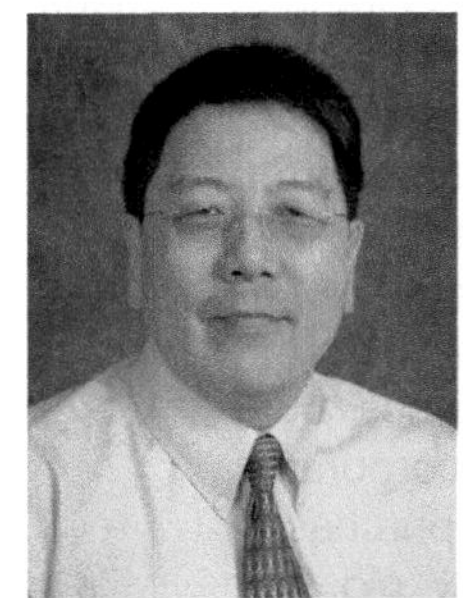

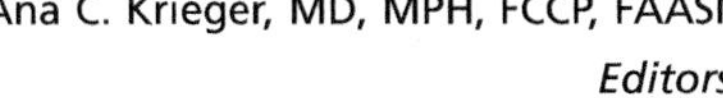

Ana C. Krieger, MD, MPH, FCCP, FAASM   Teofilo Lee-Chiong Jr, MD

Editors

The future of sleep medicine is yet to come. *Today's* perspectives for a bright future will eventually arrive, and the closer we get to that future, the faster it will come to meet us.

It is clear that knowledge in sleep medicine has been gained at a faster pace than ever. There are daily developments and discoveries in the basics of sleep science that will soon be translated into clinical care, including the development and validation of technological innovations to monitor sleep and sleep disorders. These changes are expected to continue into our future at a rapid pace as we integrate and share knowledge in a seamless manner.

It is essential to recognize that the future of sleep medicine is not just about innovations in medications, procedures, or devices. It is much more than the latest articles showing better results or unrecognized dangers. And it is certainly more exciting than having newer companies or centers offering yet unavailable services, which can sometimes be a dangerous journey for patient care. Although new PAP technology, an improved oral appliance, and news regarding a more effective hypnotic or stimulant are important elements to patient care, there are a lot more exciting developments ahead.

The greatest advances in sleep medicine will involve the *way we think*. It is how we use our scientific and clinical findings; these new devices, knowledge, and services; how we replace old technologies and select among the new ones, which ones are valid and should be embraced; how we combine them to advance and facilitate access to patient care; and how we continue to improve them. It is vital that we transform technology from a one-size-fits-all to targeted diagnostics and therapeutics. It is important that we change patient management by trial and error and what everyone else does toward sleep medicine by design, with personalized approaches. Lastly, it is crucial that we stop reflecting upon the way it usually is and allow ourselves to believe in the seemingly endless possibilities of science and health care.

This new way of thinking will have a broad impact in all areas of sleep medicine: education and research, patient care and public health, regulatory policies, reimbursement for products and services, resource allocation, insurance coverage, and medical philosophy and ethics; in short, the way we learn, work, get paid, and feel about health care in sleep medicine.

We cannot simply rely on our knowledge of yesterday and today to forecast the future. When attending conferences, we must avoid getting caught in the light of the latest flashing news and make sure we embrace the experiences and new research developments at large, not just from the keynote talks. An attentive look at the smaller sessions, abstracts, and poster presentations will provide a glimpse of what the keynote topics will be 10 years from now.

There are brewing changes in product development. When searching for sleep products, we should go beyond just comparing devices and drugs that are available today, allowing time to also review new patent applications and technical

Sleep Med Clin 17 (2022) xiii–xiv
https://doi.org/10.1016/j.jsmc.2022.07.001
1556-407X/22/© 2022 Published by Elsevier Inc.

and pharmaceutical journals; these are the inventions that we might be using a decade from today.

This also applies when discussing sleep medicine, by not limiting our conversations with fellow health care providers and scientists. Rather, talking to engineers, information technology specialists, patients and their advocates, insurance providers, and policymakers. Consider mentoring new students or teaching a class; it is from them that you will acquire fresh perspectives, form new ideas, and identify new opportunities.

Preparing for the future of sleep medicine is more than just bending with every new gust of knowledge, test, or treatment that comes our way. We can ill afford to either rapidly incorporate or disregard every new discovery; to purchase every new device and throw out every old; to disdain every new skill and persist in doing every old; or to follow every fad, fancy, or headline. It will take a lot of discipline and perspective to avoid seeing only sensational news and ignoring slowly moving trends.

Our job, as scientists and health care professionals, is not to predict exactly how the future of sleep medicine will unfold, but rather to reduce uncertainties so that we and our patients are not caught unaware and unprepared. Predicting the future of sleep medicine is not a prophesy that everything will get better or that all will be worse. Rather, predicting the future is a conviction that things *will* change, and that, somehow, we can all help to improve it by playing an important role advocating for solid research, having a strong base of knowledge in science and patient care needs, and not losing perspective; otherwise, we may put the future at risk and allow it to become worse.

Ana C. Krieger, MD, MPH, FCCP, FAASM
Division of Sleep Neurology
Weill Cornell Center for Sleep Medicine
Weill Cornell Medical College
Cornell University
New York, NY 10065, USA

Teofilo Lee-Chiong Jr, MD
National Jewish Health
University of Colorado
Denver, CO 80206, USA

Philips Respironics
Murrysville, PA 15668, USA

E-mail addresses:
ack2003@med.cornell.edu (A.C. Krieger)
lee-chiongT@njc.org (T. Lee-Chiong)

Prescription Drugs Used in Insomnia

Sylvie Dujardin, MD[a], Angelique Pijpers, MD, PhD[a], Dirk Pevernagie, MD, PhD[a,b,*]

KEYWORDS

• Chronic insomnia • Prescription drugs • Pharmacotherapy • Sleep-effect

KEY POINTS

- Several prescription drugs are available that at least temporarily improve sleep duration and continuity, objectively and subjectively, with acceptable side effects.
- Prescription drugs used for insomnia promote sleep by a limited number of different mechanisms: enhancing GABAergic neurotransmission, antagonizing receptors for the wake-promoting monoamines, or binding the melatonin receptors. Orexin receptor antagonists comprise a new class of hypnotic drugs.
- The ideal sleeping pill still does not exist.
- Wen available, cognitive behavioral therapy for insomnia remains the first-line therapy for chronic insomnia.

INTRODUCTION

Various studies have shown the efficacy of cognitive behavioral therapy for insomnia (CBT-I) and were recently confirmed by meta-analysis.[1] The American Academy of Sleep Medicine (AASM) clinical practice guideline and the European guideline for the treatment of insomnia state that this nonpharmacologic therapeutic approach is the treatment of choice for chronic insomnia in adults, regardless of age.[2,3] By acting on different sleep mechanisms, CBT-I helps to tilt the delicate neurobiologic balance from wakefulness to sleep.

Prescription of pharmacologic treatment is to be considered when CBT-I is not available or not effective. In the acute phase of CBT-I, adding pharmacotherapy may have a slightly better effect compared with CBT-I alone, provided the medication is discontinued in the maintenance phase of CBT-I.[4] However, pharmacotherapy is not indicated for chronic use and efforts at discontinuation should be made when this is the case.[3] Moreover, discontinuation may improve rather than worsen the effects of CBT-I.[5]

Many studies have been conducted to evaluate the pharmacologic treatment of chronic insomnia. Unfortunately, large randomized controlled trials (RCTs) with representative patient populations are lacking. Studies are often weak from a methodologic point of view and, in addition, difficult to compare because of differences in patient samples, diagnostic and inclusion criteria, and outcome criteria. Finally, many studies are sponsored by the industry, which could lead to publication bias.

It is important to keep in mind that in the treatment of insomnia, whether pharmacologic or behavioral, a substantial placebo effect may confound clinical results. In a meta-analysis, the placebo effect was contended to account for almost two-thirds of the drug effect.[6] A recent meta-analysis comparing placebo with no treatment groups confirms the placebo effect in the subjective but not objective sleep measures.[7]

The authors have no disclosures to report.
Sleep Med Clin 13 (2018) 169-182 https://doi.org/10.1016/j.jsmc.2018.03.001 155-407X/18/

[a] Sleep Medicine Center Kempenhaeghe, PO Box 61, Heeze 5590 AB, the Netherlands; [b] Department of Internal Medicine and Paediatrics, Faculty of Medicine and Health Sciences, Ghent University, Corneel Heymanslaan 10, Ghent 9000, Belgium
* Corresponding author. Sleep Medicine Center Kempenhaeghe, PO Box 61, Heeze 5590 AB, the Netherlands.
E-mail address: pevernagied@kempenhaeghe.nl

Sleep Med Clin 17 (2022) 315–328
https://doi.org/10.1016/j.jsmc.2022.06.001
1556-407X/22/

This article provides an overview of pharmacologic and biologic features of different hypnotic drugs, with a reference to medical practice in adults with chronic insomnia without comorbidities. The focus is on prescription drugs and discussed are benzodiazepines (BZDs), non-BZD BZD receptor agonists (NBBzRAs), melatonin receptor agonists, orexin receptor antagonists, antidepressants, and antipsychotics. Over-the-counter preparations, including antihistamines, are outside the scope of this article. The main characteristics of the reviewed drugs are summarized in **Table 1**.

The reviewed compounds all have an impact on the neurobiologic processes of sleep and may even change its normal macrostructure and microstructure. Because hypnotic drugs act via different pathways within the central nervous system, they have dissimilar neuropharmacologic profiles. Remarkably, these differential properties have not been translated into evidence that would facilitate clinical decision-making based on the pharmacologic signature of the drug.[8]

Practical advice for the optimization of drug treatment is outside the scope of this article. For further study, we refer the reader to other references.[9]

BENZODIAZEPINES

Neuropharmacology

BZD receptor agonists constitute the most important class of drugs prescribed for insomnia and encompass BZDs and NBBzRAs. Both groups intensify g-aminobutyric acid $(GABA)_A$-mediated neurotransmission and are therefore $GABA_A$ agonists.

GABA is the most important and abundant inhibitory neurotransmitter in the nervous system. Stimulating GABAergic action promotes sleep but the exact locations in the brain are not yet fully disclosed.[10] At very high dose, $GABA_A$ agonists suppress c-Fos expression in the entire central nervous system, including the sleep–wake control centers.[11] At lower dose, $GABA_A$ agonists increase c-Fos expression in ventrolateral preoptic area (VLPO) neurons, although less than in natural sleep. The VLPO (and the median preoptic nucleus) contain sleep-active GABAergic neurons that send anatomic projections to the arousal systems, in which GABA release has been shown to increase during sleep.[12] Besides, systemic injection of $GABA_A$ receptor agonists consistently suppressed the expression of c-Fos in the tuberomammillary nucleus (TMN).[11] The VLPO and the TMN mutually inhibit each other.[12] Thus $GABA_A$ agonists might stimulate sleep through reinforcing the relief of the inhibition of the VLPO by theTMN.[11] Microinjections of triazolam into the perifornical hypothalamus containing hypocretin neurons significantly increased sleep.[13] BZDs might thus also act via inhibition of the hypocretin wake-promoting system.

Pharmacologic Properties

BZDs act as positive allosteric modulators of $GABA_A$ receptors: they increase the effect of GABA binding. $GABA_A$ receptors are located postsynaptically and consist of a pentameric complex forming a chloride channel. When the GABA is released in the synaptic cleft, the chloride channel opens. With BZD, the $GABA_A$ receptor increases the frequency of opening of its chloride-channel. By this mechanism, the cellular membrane of the postsynaptic neuron becomes hyperpolarized, thus inhibiting the activation of the neuron.[14]

The $GABA_A$ receptor carrying the α_1 subunit is believed to be the mediator of the sedative and amnesic effects of BZDs. The anxiolytic, myorelaxant, motor-impairing, and ethanol-potentiating effects are attributed to $GABA_A$ receptor, carrying other α subunits (α subunits 2, 3, 5).[15] Currently available BZDs are nonselective for $GABA_A$ receptors with different α subunits.[14]

Clinical Effects

BZDs have a positive effect on objective and subjective sleep parameters of people with insomnia. Recently, a meta-analysis was performed on 2 BZDs: triazolam and temazepam.[2] Two studies including a total of 72 patients addressed subjective sleep latencies (SL) and total sleep time (TST).[16,17] In the second study of 34 patients, objective SL and TST also were assessed.[17] Temazepam, 15 mg, decreased subjective SL by 20 minutes and objective SL by 37 minutes versus placebo. It increased subjective TST by 64 minutes and objective TST by 99 minutes versus placebo. The evidence for efficiency of triazolam is scarce. In a study of only subjective data with triazolam, 0.25 mg, improvements of subjective SL and TST (respectively −9 minutes and −25 minutes vs placebo) were not clinically relevant.[18]

Tolerance to hypnotic effect is a frequent manifestation in chronic use of BZDs. It has been shown that after 24 weeks of chronic BZD intake, the subjective sleep quality drops to a level below baseline. This was observed in BZDs with short and long half-lives (lorazepam and nitrazepam, respectively).[19] Rebound insomnia is the most frequent symptom following acute withdrawal of BZDs, occurring in up to 71% of subjects.[20] Next to tolerance, dependence is of concern. The

Table 1
Prescription drugs used for insomnia: main characteristics

Drug (Class)	Predominant Mode of Action for Sedative Effect	T_{max} (h)	Ti/2 (h)	Recommended Use	Dose[a] (mg)	FDA
			Approved/CSA IV			
BZD						
Triazolam	Nonselective $GABA_A$ agonism	1–2	2–6	Sleep onset insomnia	0.125–0.25	+/+
Temazepam	Nonselective $GABA_A$ agonism	1–2	8–15	Sleep onset and sleep maintenance insomnia	7.5–30	+/+
Quazepam	Nonselective $GABA_A$ agonism	2–3	48–120	Not recommended		+/+
Estazolam	Nonselective $GABA_A$ agonism	1.5–2	8–24	Not recommended		+/+
Flurazepam	Nonselective $GABA_A$ agonism	1.5–4.5	48–120	Not recommended		+/+
NBBzRA						
Zopiclone	$GABA_A$-$\alpha_{1,2,3}$ agonism	1.5–2	5	Sleep onset and sleep maintenance insomnia	3.75–7.5	+/+
Eszopiclone	$GABA_A$-$\alpha_{1,2,3}$ agonism[b,c]	1–1.5	6	Sleep onset and sleep maintenance insomnia	1–3	+/+
Zolpidem	$GABA_A$-α_1 agonism	1–2	2.6	Sleep onset and sleep maintenance insomnia	1.75–10 6.25–12.5 ER	+/+
Zaleplon	$GABA_A$-α_1 agonism	~1	0.7–1.4	Sleep onset insomnia	5–20	+/+
Orexin receptor antagonists						
Suvorexant	OxR1 and OxR2 antagonism	2–3.5	12	Sleep onset and sleep maintenance insomnia	5–20	+/+
Melatonin and melatonin receptor agonists						
Ramelteon	Melatonin receptor agonism	0.75–1	1–2.5	Sleep onset insomnia	8	+/–
Melatonin	Melatonin receptor agonism	~0.75	–0.75	Not recommended		NA
Circadin®	Melatonin receptor agonism	0.75–3	3.5–4	Sleep onset and sleep maintenance insomnia, age >55 y	2	
Drug (Class)	Predominant mode of action for sedative effect	T_{max} (h)	$T_{1/2}$ (h)	Recommended use	Dose[a] (mg)	FDA

Drug (Class)	Predominant Mode of Action for Sedative Effect	T_{max} (h)	T1/2 (h)	Recommended Use	Dose[a] (mg)	FDA
Approved/CSA IV						
Antidepressants						
Doxepin	H_1 antagonism	2–8	20	Sleep maintenance insomnia	3–6	+/–
Amitriptyline	H_1, α_1, M_1 antagonism	2–8	30	Not recommended		–/–
Trazodone	$5HT_{2A}$, α_1 antagonism	1–2	9	Not recommended		–/–
Mirtazapine	H_1, $5HT_{2A/2C}$ antagonism	1–3	25	Not recommended		–/–
Antipsychotics						
Quetiapine	H_1 but also α_I, M_1, 5HT, D_2 antagonism	1–2	6	Not recommended		–/–
Olanzapine	H_1 but also 5HT, M_1, D_2, α_I antagonism	4–6	20–54	Not recommended		–/–

Abbreviations: 5HT, 5-hydroxytryptamine (serotonin); α_I, alpha-1 adrenergic receptor; CSA IV, Controlled Substance Act schedule IV controlled substances; D_2, dopamine receptor D_2; ER, extended release; FDA approved, US Food and Drug Administration approved for the treatment of insomnia; GABA, γ-aminobutyric acid; $GABA_A$ $\alpha_{1,2,3}$, $GABA_A$ receptor alpha subunits 1,2,3; H1, histamine receptor type 1; M1, Muscarinic acetylcholine receptor 1; NA, not applicable; OxR1-2, orexin receptors type 1 and 2.

[a] The lowest effective dose should be used to minimize side effects.

[b] Precise mechanism unknown.

[c] European Medicines Agency approval.

Data from Refs.[26,31,74,77,97–99]

prevalence of misuse and dependency of BZDs and related Z-drugs has been estimated to be 5% in a German population. Approximately 20% of BZD users have a problematic intake. Overall, 50% of BZD users list insomnia as the reason for taking the drug.[20]

Important to highlight is that older adults are especially vulnerable because BZDs increase the risk of cognitive impairment, delirium, falls, fractures, and motor vehicle accidents. Therefore, BZDs of any type should be avoided for the treatment of insomnia, according to the American Geriatrics Society Beers Criteria for Potentially Inappropriate Medication Use in Older Adults.[21] Sleep apnea is a contraindication for BZDs, although the available evidence indicates the effects on respiration are moderate.[22]

BZDs have an effect on the sleep macroarchitecture. Studies on healthy volunteers and those with insomnia have consistently shown that BZDs reduce the percentage of slow wave sleep.[23] Percentage of stage 2 sleep increases, and spectral power of the spindle frequency range (11–14 Hz) is enhanced.[24,25] The effect on rapid eye movement (REM) sleep is variable and less pronounced. In some individuals, a reduction of the amount of REM sleep has been reported.[26]

It seems paradoxic that BZDs improve subjective sleep quality while they decrease slow wave sleep. This paradox can possibly be explained by observations on the microstructure of sleep. In a recent study, the sleep of 6 chronic BZD abusers versus healthy control subjects was compared. The abusers had significantly more awakenings but fewer fast frequency arousals and lower indexes of non-REM (NREM) instability as measured by cyclic alternating pattern rate. It has been hypothesized that chronic BZD use may affect the function of the thalamic filter. In normal subjects, incoming stimuli are able to produce arousals without awakenings. Potentially, the thalamic filter of chronic BZD users is less adaptive: the response to stimuli is either no reaction (no arousal) or a full awakening.[27]

Medical Prescription

Five BZDs are approved by the US Food and Drug Administration (FDA) as prescription insomnia drugs: (1) quazepam, (2) estazolam, (3) flurazepam, (4) triazolam, and (5) temazepam. In Europe, approval varies across countries.

American guidelines support the prescription of triazolam, 0.25 mg, for sleep onset, and temazepam, 15 mg, for sleep onset and sleep maintenance insomnia versus no treatment in adults.[2] Because of lack of data appropriate for statistical analysis, the AASM could not give clinical practice recommendations for the other 3 FDA-approved drugs (quazepam, estazolam, flurazepam). Their long elimination half-life (>15 hours) is not favorable for use in insomnia.

In European guidelines, the use of BZDs is recommended for short-term treatment (less than 4 weeks), if CBT-I is not effective or not available. Shorter half-life drugs are favored and intermittent dosing is strongly recommended. Long-term treatment of insomnia with BZDs is not recommended because of lack of evidence, side effects, and risks of tolerance and dependence.[3] Prescription should be limited to cases where the impairment is clinically significant and the benefits are expected to outweigh the potential harms. When starting a prescription treatment, the clinician is encouraged to discuss the temporary nature of the prescription with the patient.[28]

NONBENZODIAZEPINE RECEPTOR AGONISTS *NEUROPHARMACOLOGY*

NBBzRAs are thought to have a somewhat higher affinity for the $GABA_A$ α_1 and α_2 receptor subtypes or bind to the complex in a different way than BZDs. Therefore, NBBzRAs are considered to have a more favorable benefit-risk profile (fewer side effects, lower abuse potential) compared with BZDs.[29] The $GABA_A$ α_1 receptor subunit is associated with the most hypnotic effects. These receptors are primarily found on the lamina IV of the sensorimotor cortical regions, substantia nigra pars reticulata, olfactory bulb, ventral thalamic complex, the molecular layer of the cerebellum, pons, inferior colliculus, and globus pallidus.[30] This class of NBBzRAs, also referred to as "Z-drugs," comprise 3 compounds: (1) zopiclone and eszopiclone, (2) zolpidem, and (3) zaleplon.

Pharmacologic Properties

NBBzRAs are positive allosteric modulators at $GABA_A$ receptors but they have a chemical structure that is unrelated to other hypnotics, including BZDs. They are all rapidly absorbed after oral administration. NBBzRAs, such as BZDs, are primarily metabolized in the liver by the cytochrome P-450 (CYP) 3A4 enzyme.

Zopiclone and its active stereoisomer eszopiclone belong to the group of cyclopyrrolones. They bind to the $GABA_A$ $\alpha_{1,2,3}$ subunits. Eszopiclone has a time to maximal concentration (T_{max}) of approximately 1 to 1.5 hours, with a half-life time of approximately 6 hours. Zopiclone has a T_{max} of 1.5 to 2 hours and a half-life time of approximately 5 hours.

Zolpidem is an imidazopyridine and in therapeutic dosage binds selectively to the $GABA_A$ α subunit. T_{max} is 1 to 2 hours, with an additional 30 minutes for the extended-release formula. It has a short half-life time of approximately 2.6 hours.[31,32]

Zaleplon is a pyrazolopyrimidine. In therapeutic dosage, it binds selectively to the $GABA_A$ α_1 subunit. T_{max} is 0.7 to 1.4 hours. It has an ultrashort half-life time of 1 hour and has therapeutic effects usually within 5 to 15 minutes after ingestion.[31,32]

Clinical Effects

Clinical effects of NBBzRAs in treatment of chronic insomnia, including discontinuation effects, are comparable with BZDs.[33,34] Side effects are partial comparable with BZDs.[35] Most commonly reported side effects are amnesia, dizziness, sedation, and headache.[36] An unpleasant, altered, or metallic taste is a typical side effect of (es)zopiclone.[37,38] Somnambulism has been reported with the use of zolpidem and zaleplon.[39,40] Similar to BZDs, Z-drugs have a potentially higher risk of falls, fractures, and injuries in elderly.[41] Data on whether or not Z-drugs are associated with an increased risk of motor vehicle accidents are controversial.[42,43]

Studies evaluating objective and subjective improvements of sleep parameters of insomniacs using NBBzRAs usually report favorable outcomes. However, many of those studies have methodologic flaws, making it difficult to draw definite conclusions.[2,36]

Of the cyclopyrrolones, the clinical effects of eszopiclone are more extensively studied than those of zopiclone. However, only 6 studies fit the criteria for systematic review in the AASM clinical practice guideline. In summary, a mean reduction in SL of 14 minutes was seen, TST improved up to 57 minutes, sleep quality was better, and there was less wake after sleep onset (WASO). Studies with 2 mg eszopiclone yielded better statistical significant results than the 3 mg dose.[2]

Zolpidem, 10 mg, showed a mean reduction of SL of 5 to 12 minutes and improvement of TST by 29 minutes. In addition, improvements were seen in WASO but not in sleep efficiency or number of awakenings.[2]

For zaleplon, only 2 studies met the inclusion criteria for review, of which one only reported subjective outcomes. Objective polysomnography data showed a significant reduction of SL of approximately 10 minutes. There were no significant differences in TST or sleep quality compared with placebo.[2]

Medical Prescription

The therapeutic doses of zopiclone and eszopiclone range from 3.75 to 7.5 mg and from 1 to 3 mg, respectively. The therapeutic dose of zolpidem mainly depends on the route of administration (oral tablets, spray, sublingual) varying from 1.75 to 10 mg or 6.25 to 12.5 mg extended-release tablets.[29]

Zaleplon is dosed at 5 to 20 mg. It is advised not to be taken within 4 hours of rise-time because of the risk of residual sedation and memory impairment.[36] Because of its short half-life time, zaleplon is only suited for sleep-onset insomnia. The others are used for sleep onset and sleep maintenance insomnia. Eszopiclone is the only hypnotic sedative drug that is approved by the FDA for long-term use for the relief of insomnia.[37]

Availability and indication preferences for NBBzRAs vary worldwide. In the United States, NBBzRAs are considered as class IV drugs. As with BZDs and suvorexant, prescription of NBBzRAs should be considered only if nonpharmacologic treatments for insomnia are not available or ineffective. Similarly, prescription should be restricted to a short period and intermittent use is recommended when prescription is extended over a longer period. Similar to BDZ, caution should be taken when prescribing NBBzRAs to elderly and careful consideration in case of other drugs metabolized by CYP34 A or simultaneous use of central nervous depressants.

OREXIN RECEPTOR ANTAGONISTS

Neuropharmacology

Orexin-producing neurons are located in specific parts of the hypothalamus. These neurons project to most parts of the brain and are active during wake. Orexins stabilize wake through a strong excitatory action on wake-promoting neurons. Orexin knockout mice have many more transitions among wake, NREM, and REM states than do wild-type mice, supporting this model. Similar patterns of sleep–wake disruption are present in human narcolepsy. In addition to promoting wakefulness, orexin plays a role in goal-directed, motivated behaviors.[44,45]

Pharmacologic Properties

There are 2 types of orexin receptors (OxR1 and OxR2), which are postsynaptic G-protein-coupled receptors. They are expressed in various parts of the brain: OxRls are highly expressed in the locus coeruleus and OxR2s in the histaminergic TMN.[46,47] There are also 2 types of orexin neurotransmitters: type A and B (also known as hypocretin 1 and 2). Orexin neurotransmitter type A can bind to OxR1 and OxR2, whereas orexin neurotransmitter type B selectively binds to OxR2. The exact pathways by which dual orexin (hypocretin) receptor antagonists (DORAs) promote sleep, without causing narcoleptic features, are unknown. Presumably, antagonism of OxR2s decreases histaminergic activity in the hypothalamus, and in addition, antagonism of OxR1 decreases arousal from motivational states, therefore promoting sleep.

Suvorexant has a T_{max} of approximately 2 to 3.5 hours, depending on the ingestion of food. It binds to plasma proteins and has a half-life time of approximately 12 hours. Its kinetics are not age-dependent but gender and weight do play a role. Suvorexant is predominantly metabolized by CYP3A4 enzyme and some involvement of CYP2C19. Approximately 66% is eliminated in feces and 23% in urine.[48]

Clinical Effects

Orexin receptor antagonists are a novel drug class used to treat insomnia. So far, only suvorexant, a DORA, is registered in the United States, Japan, and Australia for the treatment of insomnia. Clinical data available for suvorexant are derived from a limited number of pivotal trials that could be subject to publication bias.[49–51]

In summary, clinical significant improvement was most noticeable in improvement of wake after sleep onset by 16 to 28 minutes, compared with placebo. This might favor suvorexant for sleep maintenance insomnia. However, the total number of awakenings was not statistically altered. TST increased by 10 minutes, compared with placebo, but this was not clinically significant. At higher doses (20 mg), it might improve sleep onset latency, with an average reduction of 22.3 minutes. Sleep efficiency at 20 mg increased on average with 10.4%. Available data were objectively controlled by polysomnography. Subjectively, TST improved but did not reach clinical significance.[49,51]

Reported side effects include somnolence, fatigue, abnormal dreams, and dry mouth but these were not significantly different from placebo.[49–52] Polysomnographic data of patients with insomnia show a reduced REM latency and an increased REM sleep duration compared with placebo. There is a limited increase of the delta power band and a limited decrease in the g and b power bands. The largest differences were seen in the first night and diminished during months 1 and 3. The clinical significance of these observations remains unclear.[53]

It should be noted that most of the presented data had an imprecision bias, mainly because of large confidence intervals. Furthermore, studies were sponsored by industry.

Medical Prescription

Suvorexant is FDA-approved for the treatment of insomnia characterized by sleep onset and/or sleep maintenance difficulties. The AASM clinical practice guideline recommends suvorexant only for the treatment of sleep maintenance insomnia.[2]

The recommended starting dose is 10 mg, taken approximately 30 minutes before bedtime, with sleep opportunity of at least 7 hours. The drug is available in 5, 10, 15, and 20 mg tablets, with 20 mg being the maximum advised daily dose. Dose reduction should be considered in obesity. When patients use moderate CYP3A4 inhibitors, the recommended starting dose is 5 mg, and the highest dose should not exceed 10 mg.[52]

The use of suvorexant is not advised in patients using strong CYP3A4 inhibitors, those with severe hepatic impairment, or with a diagnosis of narcolepsy. There are no available data on use during pregnancy or lactation, which should therefore be avoided. It is not recommended to use suvorexant simultaneously with other central nervous system depressants, including alcohol. Available data suggest that suvorexant has no major respiratory depressant effects.[54–56] However, it is unclear if this is still the case in high-risk patients (severe sleep apnea, severe chronic obstructive pulmonary disease, concomitant use of muscle relaxants). To date, there are only a few postmarketing case reports on side effects.[57,58]

MELATONIN AND MELATONIN RECEPTOR *Agonists*

Neuropharmacology

Endogenous melatonin is secreted by the pineal gland. Melatonin secretion typically starts in late afternoon, reaches a peak in the first half of the night, and disappears on awakening. As such, melatonin secretion is a hormonal signal of the central nervous system that provides different end-organs with information on the nyctohemeral phase of the circadian cycle. The physiologic function of melatonin in humans has not been fully disclosed. It is hypothesized that melatonin entrains peripheral oscillators but in vivo confirmation of this hypothesis is difficult, given the redundancy within the circadian system.[59] Neurons of the suprachiasmaticus nucleus carry melatonin receptors, indicating that melatonin can act on the central master clock itself. In in vitro studies, exogenous melatonin had 2 distinct effects on neurons of the suprachiasmaticus nucleus: an acute inhibitory effect on neuronal firing and a phase-shifting effect.[59] The acute inhibitory effect may mediate the sleep-promoting properties of melatonin, whereas the phase-shifting properties may induce a delay or advance of the sleep phase, depending on the time of administration with respect to the actual circadian phase.[60,61]

Pharmacologic properties

Natural melatonin and ramelteon are ligands with great affinity for MT1 and MT2 receptors.[61] They are present in various parts of the brain but also in other tissues, including cardiac and peripheral vessels, retina, kidneys, and other organs.[62]

The pharmacokinetics of melatonin are characterized by a low and variable bioavailability (on average, 15%). Immediate-release melatonin has T_{max} and elimination half-life close to 45 minutes.[63,64] The T_{max} of prolonged-release melatonin is affected by food intake, and ranges from 45 minutes to 3 hours in the fed state. Its elimination half-life is 3.5 to 4 hours.

The pharmacokinetics of ramelteon are characterized by rapid absorption, with T_{max} and elimination half-life, respectively, approximately 1 and 1.5 hours.[65]

Clinical effects

Experience from patients in whom pinealectomy was performed for medical reasons has shown that melatonin is not an essential factor for inducing and maintaining sleep. Many of these patients do not experience changes in subjective sleep quality or polysomnographic sleep variables following resection of the pineal gland.[66]

The natural melatonin synthesis may be reduced by drugs (eg, BZDs, nonsteroidal anti-inflammatory drugs, calcium channel blockers, and β-blockers).[67] Oral administration of melatonin or ramelteon may reduce subjective SL and increase perceived sleep quality, although effects on sleep maintenance and duration are equivocal.[68]

In a dosage up to 10 mg given at 11:30 PM, short-acting melatonin induced no significant effect on sleep architecture in healthy subjects.[69] Neither were major changes in sleep architecture observed following exogenous administration of 2 mg melatonin with prolonged-release formulation.[70] In a clinical trial, ramelteon increased the percentage of time spent in N2 by approximately 2% points, at the expense of the percentage of time spent in slow wave sleep but this is unlikely to be clinically significant.[71]

Melatonin and its agonists are considered safe drugs. Overall, side effects are not different from placebo.[2] One potential serious adverse effect with ramelteon, 8 mg, was a single case of reversible leukopenia out of 227 subjects with insomnia treated with the drug. Six-month nightly administration of prolonged-release 2 mg dose in a population of 65 to 80 year olds, and of ramelteon, 8 mg, in adults, did not produce tolerance, rebound insomnia, or withdrawal effects.[71,72] Biologic effects of melatonin outside sleep have been reviewed elsewhere.[61,73]

Medical prescription

Ramelteon is FDA-approved for the treatment of insomnia characterized by difficulty with sleep onset.[74] Prolonged-release melatonin (Circadin) is European Medicines Agency-approved for the short-term treatment of primary insomnia characterized by poor quality of sleep, in patients aged 55 years or older. In addition, short-acting melatonin is available over-the-counter in many countries. Although evidence is limited, melatonin or ramelteon may be indicated to treat sleep-onset insomnia because it slightly shortens the SL of patients with insomnia more than placebo.[2]

SEDATING ANTIDEPRESSANTS

Neuropharmacology

Sedating antidepressants promote sleep by antagonizing the effect of wake-promoting monoamines, including histamine, acetylcholine, noradrenaline, and serotonin. Evidence of the sleep-promoting effect of antagonizing histamine (H_1), muscarinic acetylcholine, noradrenaline receptors (α_1-adrenergic), and serotonin ($5HT_2$) receptors has been reviewed in a previous issue of *Sleep Medicine Clinics*.[75]

The neurons producing these monoamines are located in the ascending arousal system in the upper brainstem, its extension into the caudal hypothalamus, and in the basal forebrain. In wake (but not in REM sleep), histamine is released by neurons of the TMN and adjacent posterior hypothalamus, noradrenaline by neurons of the locus coeruleus, and serotonin by neurons of the dorsal and median raphe nuclei. Dopamine neurons located in the ventral periaqueductal gray matter are also part of this arousal system.[12]

Cholinergic neurons in the laterodorsal tegmental and pedunculopontine tegmental nuclei and the basal forebrain are active in wakefulness and REM sleep. Neurons forming the laterodorsal tegmental and pedunculopontine tegmental nuclei constitute an important modulator of the thalamic relay. In general, arousal systems project on multiple regions of the cerebrum, including the hypothalamus, thalamus, limbic system, and neocortex.[12]

Pharmacologic Properties

Doxepin and amitriptyline are sedative tricyclic antidepressants (TCAs) that also affect sleep. At doses recommended for treatment of depression, they are potent boosters of serotonergic and noradrenergic neurotransmission by blocking serotonin (5HT) and noradrenaline reuptake. They have more effect on the 5HT than on the noradrenaline reuptake, in contrast with TCAs that have stimulating effects.[76] Furthermore, doxepin and amitriptyline block histamine H receptors, which accounts for their sedative and weight gain effects. They inhibit α_1-adrenergic receptors, causing hypotension, and muscarinic M_1 receptors, causing anticholinergic side effects.[29]

At low doses, doxepin and amitriptyline exert their sedating effect through potent H_1 antagonism. At 3 to 6 mg, doxepin almost acts as a selective antagonist. Low-dose amitriptyline is less selective and exhibits stronger anti-M_1cholinergic as part of the sedating effect.[29]

Trazodone is chemically unrelated to tricyclic or other known antidepressant agents. Its antidepressant effect is probably caused by inhibition of serotonin uptake and $5HT_{2A/2C}$ antagonism. At lower (hypnotic) doses, $5HT_2$, α_1, and weak antagonism promote sleep.[29,48]

Mirtazapine has a tetracyclic chemical structure. Alpha2 antagonism results in disinhibition of 5HT and noradrenaline release. Therefore, mirtazapine is classified as a noradrenergic and specific serotonergic antidepressant. $5HT_{2A/2C}$ antagonism and potent antihistaminic action promote sleep.[48] The combined $5HT_{2C}$ and H_1 antagonism also promotes weight gain.[29] Contrarily to the TCAs, mirtazapine and trazodone have minimal to no effect on M_1 receptors.[48]

The pharmacokinetics of these drugs are diverse. T_{max} is longer for doxepin and amitriptyline (28 hours) than for trazodone and mirtazapine (1–2 hours and 1–3 hours, respectively). Doxepin, amitriptyline, and mirtazapine all have elimination half-lives close to 24 hours. Trazodone has a significantly shorter elimination half-life of approximatively 8 to 9 hours.[77] Although the pharmacokinetic profile of trazodone is more apt for use in insomnia than the other antidepressant agents, residual sedation after awakening in the morning is a frequent complaint. Because of variability in clearance, trazodone may accumulate in some individuals over time.[48]

Clinical Effects

Doxepin has been shown to increase objective TST by 26 and 32 minutes (with the 3 and 6 mg dosage, respectively) mainly because of reductions in WASO.[2] Subjective increases in TST are comparable and maintained for up to 4 weeks.[78] Reductions in objective SL are less than clinical threshold with doxepin 3 mg and 6 mg. At these dosages, adverse effects are minimal.[2] Trials in the elderly population have shown no more adverse effects than placebo during up to 4 weeks of treatment with up to 6 mg and 12 weeks with 3 mg.[78–80]

Although a positive effect of amitriptyline has been shown on the sleep of depressed patients, there are no RCTs in the treatment of insomnia without comorbidities.[81]

Placebo-controlled studies of trazodone are also scarce in insomnia. In a study of patient-reported outcomes, trazodone, 50 mg, reduced subjective SL, TST, and WASO, but less than the threshold for clinical significance.[82] A polysomnography study of trazodone, 150 mg, administered to middle-aged self-reported poor sleepers failed to show a significant improvement in objective TST versus placebo but confirms the subjective improvement in sleep quality.[83] Consistent with this observation, trazodone, 50 mg, administered to those with primary insomnia significantly improved the subjective ability to sleep. The change in polysomnographic variables was only significant for the number of nighttime awakenings (20 awakenings after 7 days of placebo vs 13 after trazodone, 50 mg) and the amount of N1 sleep. Objective sleep efficiency was unchanged.[84]

There are no studies of mirtazapine in insomnia without comorbidities. In a study of depressed patients, TST improved and WASO decreased accordingly when compared with sleep parameters before mirtazapine administration but there was no placebo control.[85] Acute administration of 30 mg mirtazapine to healthy volunteers did not improve TST versus placebo but improved other measures of sleep continuity.[86] Whether these findings are relevant for the sleep of those with insomnia is unproven.

Many antidepressants delay REM sleep and decrease its duration. This effect seems modest for low-dose doxepin because it has been shown in some, but not all studies.[79,87] A study on amitriptyline, 75 mg, showed that the REM sleep period dropped to 19 minutes, versus 83 minutes with the use of placebo.[88] No significant REM sleep duration changes were shown for mirtazapine in healthy subjects or trazodone, 50 mg, in subjects with insomnia.[84,86]

In a minority of patients, antidepressants increase restless legs syndrome symptoms and/or periodic limb movements of sleep. This effect might be higher with mirtazapine and amitriptyline than with doxepin (at dose up to 50 mg) or trazodone, 100 mg.[89]

Medical Prescription

Doxepin, amitriptyline, trazodone, and mirtazapine are approved in the United States and many other countries as antidepressants. At much lower dose than needed for their antidepressant effect, they are prescribed for the treatment of insomnia. Only low-dose doxepin (3–6 mg) is FDA approved for that indication; any other use is off label.

In the American guidelines, the use of doxepin, 3 to 6 mg, is supported for sleep maintenance but not for initiation of sleep. The use of amitriptyline, trazodone, or mirtazapine is not recommended.[2] The European guidelines report on sedating antidepressants as a group. These drugs are judged effective in the short-term treatment of insomnia, provided contraindications are carefully considered. Long-term treatment is not recommended.[3]

In older subjects, amitriptyline and doxepin greater than 6 mg are to be avoided, and mirtazapine is to be used with caution. Trazodone and doxepin up to 6 mg are not listed in the American Geriatrics Society Beers Criteria for Potentially Inappropriate Medication Use in Older Adults, and thus seem safer.[21] However, trazodone, 50 mg, slightly but significantly reduced next day memory, equilibrium, and muscle endurance versus placebo in subjects with primary insomnia younger than 65 years.[84]

ANTIPSYCHOTICS NEUROPHARMACOLOGY

Antipsychotic drugs exert their sedative effects by antagonizing the activity of wake-stimulating neurotransmitters, similarly to the antidepressants.[75]

Pharmacologic Properties

All antipsychotic medications interact with dopamine D_2 receptors (most of them are D_2 blockers), and possess numerous other pharmacologic properties, among which various degrees of H_1 histamine, M_1 cholinergic, and α_1-adrenergic receptor antagonism. This triple action can be highly sedating.[29] The second-generation antipsychotics differ from the first generation because they also possess $5HT_2$ antagonism. Therefore, they are expected to be better sleep promotors.[75]

Quetiapine is the most commonly used antipsychotic for insomnia.[90] Quetiapine is effective as an antipsychotic at doses of 300 to 800 mg. In much lower doses (25–50 mg), its hypnotic effect is preserved because of its high affinity for H_1 receptors.[29]

Clinical Effects

The effects of antipsychotic medications on sleep have mostly been investigated in psychiatric patients. These studies are not relevant to insomnia without psychiatric comorbidity, and the doses given are often much higher than the ones needed for the sedating effect. Although quetiapine is used off label in insomnia, evidence is definitely lacking.[90] A small RCT including healthy people showed improvements in subjective and polysomnographic sleep with quetiapine, 25 mg and 100 mg.[91] In insomnia without psychiatric comorbidity, only one RCT has been published so far. In this study, 7 patients took quetiapine, 25 mg daily, during 2 weeks versus 6 placebo control subjects. Compared with placebo, improvement of subjective TST and SL with quetiapine was not statistically significant.[92] Because of the small size of the study, no firm conclusion could be drawn. Although in these studies quetiapine, 25 to 75 mg, was well tolerated, a concern remains about serious adverse effects on the longer term, encompassing abuse, suicidal ideation, and metabolic adverse effects, even at low doses.[93,94] A significant increase in periodic leg movements during sleep was observed with quetiapine, 100 mg.[91]

No RCT exists on other antipsychotics prescribed for insomnia without psychiatric comorbidity.[94] Monti and colleagues[95] recently reviewed the effects of the second-generation antipsychotics in healthy subjects. The results were either nonsignificant or showed an improvement in measures of SL, WASO, and TST. Most consistent evidence of a positive effect on the sleep parameters of healthy subjects exists for olanzapine, 5 to 10 mg. Of note, the elimination half-life of olanzapine is more than 24 hours, whereas that of quetiapine is less than 8 hours.

Medical Prescription

Because of lack of evidence and potential harm even at low doses, antipsychotics are not approved or recommended for the treatment of insomnia without comorbidities.[3]

SUMMARY

Several prescription drugs are available that, at least temporarily, improve sleep duration and continuity objectively and subjectively, with acceptable side effects. Although new medication classes (eg, DORAs) are becoming available, the ideal sleeping pill still does not exist.

Will such a drug ever overthrow CBT-I as the first-line therapy for chronic insomnia? CBT-I targets many sleep mechanisms. Sleep restriction affects homeostatic sleep pressure, keeping strict bed and rise times, targets circadian timing and relaxation training reduces cognitive arousal. It is unlikely that a single drug will be able to modulate all these mechanisms simultaneously.

However, pharmacologic treatment will remain important for patients in whom CBT-I is not effective or not available. However, even then, the use of medication should always be part of a broader treatment plan in which dysfunctional sleep habits are challenged, substance use is optimized, and comorbid conditions are addressed.

In insomnia, the subjective aspects of the sleep complaint are paramount in the diagnostic criteria. Epidemiologic studies increasingly point to a link between insomnia and somatic morbidity and mortality, but until now, only in the subgroup of objectively poor sleepers.[96–99] Although pharmacologic treatment might offer some benefits to this subgroup of insomnia patients, to date, there is no evidence that hypnotics can ameliorate their health risks. It is hoped that further unraveling of the neurobiology and genetics of sleep regulation and the pathophysiology of insomnia will help the development of drugs that not only improve subjective sleep complaints but also objective health outcomes.

CLINICS CARE POINTS

- When considering the use of medications to help manage patients with insomnia, always address dysfunctional sleep habits, substance use, and comorbid conditions, if present.
- Use cognitive behavioral therapy as first-line intervention for patients presenting with chronic insomnia. Although pharmacologic therapy may be tried when cognitive behavioral therapy is not available or is ineffective, avoid chronic use of pharmacologic therapy for insomnia.

REFERENCES

1. van Straten A, van der Zweerde T, Kleiboer A, et al. Cognitive and behavioral therapies in the treatment of insomnia: a meta-analysis. Sleep Med Rev 2018; 38:3–16.
2. Sateia MJ, Buysse DJ, Krystal AD, et al. Clinical practice guideline for the pharmacologic treatment of chronic insomnia in adults: an American Academy of Sleep Medicine clinical practice guideline. J Clin Sleep Med 2017;13(2):307–49.
3. Riemann D, Baglioni C, Bassetti C, et al. European guideline for the diagnosis and treatment of insomnia. J Sleep Res 2017;26(6):675–700.
4. Morin CM, Vallieres A, Guay B, et al. Cognitive behavioral therapy, singly and combined with medi- cation, for persistent insomnia: a randomized controlled trial. JAMA 2009;301(19):2005–15.
5. Zavesicka L, Brunovsky M, Matousek M, et al. Discon tinuation of hypnotics during cognitive behavioural therapy for insomnia. BMC Psychiatry 2008;8:80.
6. Winkler A, Rief W. Effect of placebo conditions on polysomnographic parameters in primary insomnia: a meta-analysis. Sleep 2015;38(6):925–31.
7. Yeung V, Sharpe L, Glozier N, et al. A systematic review and meta-analysis of placebo versus no treatment for insomnia symptoms. Sleep Med Rev 2018;38:17–27.
8. Krystal AD. A compendium of placebo-controlled tri als of the risks/benefits of pharmacological treat ments for insomnia: the empirical basis for U.S. clinical practice. Sleep Med Rev 2009;13(4):265–74.
9. Minkel J, Krystal AD. Optimizing the pharmacologic treatment of insomnia: current status and future horizons. Sleep Med Clin 2013;8(3):333–50.
10. Wafford KA, Ebert B. Emerging anti-insomnia drugs: tackling sleeplessness and the quality of wake time. Nat Rev Drug Discov 2008;7(6):530–40.
11. Lu J, Greco MA. Sleep circuitry and the hypnotic mechanism of GABAA drugs. J Clin Sleep Med 2006;2(2):S19–26.
12. Saper CB, Scammell TE, Lu J. Hypothalamic regula tion of sleep and circadian rhythms. Nature 2005; 437(7063):1257–63.
13. Mendelson W, Laposky A. Effects of triazolam micro injections into the peri-fornicular region on sleep in rats. Sleep Hypnosis 2003;5(3):154–62.
14. Nestler EJ, Hyman S, Holtzmann DM, et al. Molecular neuropharmacology: a foundation for clinical neuroscience. 3rd edition. New York: McGraw-Hill Medical; 2015.
15. Rudolph U, Crestani F, Benke D, et al. Benzodiaze pine actions mediated by specific gamma- aminobutyric acid(A) receptor subtypes. Nature 1999; 401(6755):796–800.
16. Glass JR, Sproule BA, Herrmann N, et al. Effects of 2-week treatment with temazepam and diphenhydramine in elderly insomniacs: a randomized, placebo-controlled trial. J Clin Psychopharmacol 2008;28(2):182–8.
17. Wu R, Bao J, Zhang C, et al. Comparison of sleep condition and sleep-related psychological activity after cognitive-behavior and pharmacological therapy for chronic insomnia. Psychother Psychosom 2006;75(4):220–8.
18. Roehrs T, Bonahoom A, Pedrosi B, et al. Treatment regimen and hypnotic self-administration. Psycho Pharmacol (Berl) 2001;155(1):11–7.
19. Oswald I, French C, Adam K, et al. Benzodiazepine hypnotics remain effective for 24 weeks. Br Med J (Clin Res Ed) 1982;284(6319):860–3.

20. Janhsen K, Roser P, Hoffmann K. The problems of long-term treatment with benzodiazepines and related substances. Dtsch Arztebl Int 2015;112(1–2):1–7.
21. Campanelli C. American Geriatrics Society updated beers criteria for potentially inappropriate medication use in older adults: the American Geriatrics So- ciety 2012 beers criteria update expert panel. J Am Geriatr Soc 2012;60(4):616–31.
22. Luyster FS, Buysse DJ, Strollo PJ Jr. Comorbid insomnia and obstructive sleep apnea: challenges for clinical practice and research. J Clin Sleep Med 2010;6(2):196–204.
23. Roehrs T, Roth T. Drug-related sleep stage changes: functional significance and clinical relevance. Sleep Med Clin 2010;5(4):559–70.
24. Bastien CH, LeBlanc M, Carrier J, et al. Sleep EEG power spectra, insomnia, and chronic use of benzo diazepines. Sleep 2003;26(3):313–7.
25. Borbely AA, Mattmann P, Loepfe M, et al. Effect of benzodiazepine hypnotics on all-night sleep EEG spectra. Hum Neurobiol 1985;4(3):189–94.
26. Kilduff T, Mendelson WB. Hypnotic medications: mechanisms of action and pharmacologic effects. In: Kryger M, Roth T, editors. Principles and practice of sleep medicine. 6th edition. Philadelphia: Elsevier; 2017. p. 425–31.
27. Mazza M, Losurdo A, Testani E, et al. Polysomno graphy findings in a cohort of chronic insomnia pa tients with benzodiazepine abuse. J Clin Sleep Med 2014;10(1):35–42.
28. Royant-Parola S, Brion A, Poirot I. Prise en charge de l'insomnie: guide pratique. Issy-les-Moulineaux (France): Elsevier Masson SAS; 2017.
29. Stahl SM. Stahl's essential psychopharmacology: neuroscientific basis and practical applications. Cambridge (England): Cambridge University Press; 2013.
30. Holm KJ, Goa KL. Zolpidem: an update of its phar macology, therapeutic efficacy and tolerability in the treatment of insomnia. Drugs 2000;59(4): 865–89.
31. Wishart DS, Feunang YD, Guo AC, et al. DrugBank 5.0: a major update to the DrugBank database for 2018. Nucleic Acids Res 2018;46(D1):D1074–82.
32. Drover DR. Comparative pharmacokinetics and pharmacodynamics of short-acting hypnosedatives: zaleplon, zolpidem and zopiclone. Clin Pharmacokinet 2004;43(4):227–38.
33. Erman MK, Zammit G, Rubens R, et al. A polysomnographic placebo-controlled evaluation of the efficacy and safety of eszopiclone relative to placebo and zolpidem in the treatment of primary insomnia. J Clin Sleep Med 2008;4(3):229–34.
34. Walsh JK, Vogel GW, Scharf M, et al. A five week, polysomnographic assessment of zaleplon 10 mg for the treatment of primary insomnia. Sleep Med 2000;1(1):41–9.
35. Gunja N. In the Zzz zone: the effects of Z-drugs on human performance and driving. J Med Toxicol 2013;9(2):163–71.
36. Becker PM, Somiah M. Non-benzodiazepine receptor agonists for insomnia. Sleep Med Clin 2015; 10(1):57–76.
37. Krystal AD, Walsh JK, Laska E, et al. Sustained efficacy of eszopiclone over 6 months of nightly treatment: results of a randomized, double-blind, placebo-controlled study in adults with chronic insomnia. Sleep 2003;26(7):793–9.
38. Wadworth AN, McTavish D. Zopiclone. A review of its pharmacological properties and therapeutic efficacy as an hypnotic. Drugs Aging 1993;3(5): 441–59.
39. Toner LC, Tsambiras BM, Catalano G, et al. Central nervous system side effects associated with zolpidem treatment. Clin Neuropharmacol 2000;23(1): 54–8.
40. Chen YW, Tseng PT, Wu CK, et al. Zaleplon-induced anemsic somnambulism with eating behaviors under once dose. Acta Neurol Taiwan 2014;23(4):143–5.
41. Treves N, Perlman A, Kolenberg Geron L, et al. Z-drugs and risk for falls and fractures in older adults: a systematic review and meta-analysis. Age Ageing 2018;47(2):201–8.
42. Orriols L, Philip P, Moore N, et al. Benzodiazepine-like hypnotics and the associated risk of road traffic accidents. Clin Pharmacol Ther 2011;89(4): 595–601.
43. Chang CM, Wu EC, Chen CY, et al. Psychotropic drugs and risk of motor vehicle accidents: a population-based case-control study. Br J Clin Pharmacol 2013;75(4):1125–33.
44. Mahler SV, Moorman DE, Smith RJ, et al. Motiva tional activation: a unifying hypothesis of orexin/hypocretin function. Nat Neurosci 2014;17(10):1298–303.
45. Bonnavion P, de Lecea L. Hypocretins in the control of sleep and wakefulness. Curr Neurol Neurosci Rep 2010;10(3):174–9.
46. Sakurai T, Amemiya A, Ishii M, et al. Orexins and orexin receptors: a family of hypothalamic neuropeptides and G protein-coupled receptors that regulate feeding behavior. Cell 1998;92(4):573–85.
47. de Lecea L, Kilduff TS, Peyron C, et al. The hypocre tins: hypothalamus-specific peptides with neuroexcitatory activity. Proc Natl Acad Sci U S A 1998; 95(1):322–7.
48. Law V, Knox C, Djoumbou Y, et al. DrugBank 4.0: shedding new light on drug metabolism. Nucleic Acids Res 2014;42(Database issue):D1091–7.
49. Herring WJ, Connor KM, Ivgy-May N, et al. Suvorexant in patients with insomnia: results from two 3-month randomized controlled clinical trials. Biol Psychiatry 2016;79(2):136–48.

50. Herring WJ, Snyder E, Budd K, et al. Orexin receptor antagonism for treatment of insomnia: a randomized clinical trial of suvorexant. Neurology 2012;79(23): 2265–74.
51. Michelson D, Snyder E, Paradis E, et al. Safety and efficacy of suvorexant during 1-year treatment of insomnia with subsequent abrupt treatment discon tinuation: a phase 3 randomised, double-blind, placebo-controlled trial. Lancet Neurol 2014;13(5): 461–71.
52. Herring WJ, Connor KM, Snyder E, et al. Suvorex ant in patients with insomnia: pooled analyses of three-month data from phase-3 randomized controlled clinical trials. J Clin Sleep Med 2016;12(9):1215–25.
53. Snyder E, Ma J, Svetnik V, et al. Effects of suvorexant on sleep architecture and power spectral profile in patients with insomnia: analysis of pooled phase 3 data. Sleep Med 2016;19:93–100.
54. Sun H, Palcza J, Card D, et al. Effects of suvorexant, an orexin receptor antagonist, on respiration during sleep in patients with obstructive sleep apnea. J Clin Sleep Med 2016;12(1):9–17.
55. Sun H, Palcza J, Rosenberg R, et al. Effects of suvorexant, an orexin receptor antagonist, on breath ing during sleep in patients with chronic obstructive pulmonary disease. Respir Med 2015;109(3): 416–26.
56. Uemura N, McCrea J, Sun H, et al. Effects of the orexin receptor antagonist suvorexant on respiration during sleep in healthy subjects. J Clin Pharmacol 2015;55(10):1093–100.
57. Tabata H, Kuriyama A, Yamao F, et al. Suvorexant-induced dream enactment behavior in Parkinson disease: a case report. J Clin Sleep Med 2017; 13(5):759–60.
58. Petrous J, Furmaga K. Adverse reaction with suvorexant for insomnia: acute worsening of depression with emergence of suicidal thoughts. BMJ Case Rep 2017.
59. Pevet P. Melatonin receptors as therapeutic targets in the suprachiasmatic nucleus. Expert Opin Ther Targets 2016;20(10):1209–18.
60. Liu C, Weaver DR, Jin X, et al. Molecular dissection of two distinct actions of melatonin on the supra chiasmatic circadian clock. Neuron 1997;19(1): 91–102.
61. Liu J, Clough SJ, Hutchinson AJ, et al. MT1 and MT2 melatonin receptors: a therapeutic perspective. Annu Rev Pharmacol Toxicol 2016;56:361–83.
62. Pandi-Perumal SR, Trakht I, Srinivasan V, et al. Physiological effects of melatonin: role of melatonin receptors and signal transduction pathways. Prog Neurobiol 2008;85(3):335–53.
63. Andersen LP, Werner MU, Rosenkilde MM, et al. Pharmacokinetics of oral and intravenous melatonin in healthy volunteers. BMC Pharmacol Toxicol 2016; 17:8.
64. Harpsoe NG, Andersen LP, Gogenur I, et al. Clinical pharmacokinetics of melatonin: a systematic review. Eur J Clin Pharmacol 2015;71(8):901–9.
65. Sateia MJ, Kirby-Long P, Taylor JL. Efficacy and clin ical safety of ramelteon: an evidence-based review. Sleep Med Rev 2008;12(4):319–22.
66. Slawik H, Stoffel M, Riedl L, et al. Prospective study on salivary evening melatonin and sleep before and after pinealectomy in humans. J Biol Rhythms 2016; 31(1):82–93.
67. Auld F, Maschauer EL, Morrison I, et al. Evidence for the efficacy of melatonin in the treatment of primary adult sleep disorders. Sleep Med Rev 2017;34:10–22.
68. Ferracioli-Oda E, Qawasmi A, Bloch MH. Meta-analysis: melatonin for the treatment of primary sleep disorders. PLoS One 2013;8(5):e63773.
69. Stone BM, Turner C, Mills SL, et al. Hypnotic activity of melatonin. Sleep 2000;23(5):663–9.
70. Arbon EL, Knurowska M, Dijk DJ. Randomised clin ical trial of the effects of prolonged-release melatonin, temazepam and Zolpidem on slow-wave activity during sleep in healthy people. J Psychopharmacol 2015;29(7):764–76.
71. Mayer G, Wang-Weigand S, Roth-Schechter B, et al. Efficacy and safety of 6-month nightly ramelteon administration in adults with chronic primary insomnia. Sleep 2009;32(3):351–60.
72. Wade AG, Ford I, Crawford G, et al. Nightly treatment of primary insomnia with prolonged release mela- tonin for 6 months: a randomized placebo controlled trial on age and endogenous melatonin as predictors of efficacy and safety. BMC Med 2010;8:51.
73. Tordjman S, Chokron S, Delorme R, et al. Melatonin: pharmacology, functions and therapeutic benefits. Curr Neuropharmacol 2017;15(3):434–43.
74. Available at. https://www.fda.gov/Drugs/DrugSafety. Accessed January 22, 2018.
75. Krystal AD. Antidepressant and antipsychotic drugs. Sleep Med Clin 2010;5(4):571–89.
76. DeMartinis NA, Winokur A. Effects of psychiatric medications on sleep and sleep disorders. CNS Neurol Disord Drug Targets 2007;6(1):17–29.
77. Buysse DJ, Tyagi S. Clinical pharmacology of other drugs used as hypnotics. In: Kryger M, Roth T, editors. Principles and practice of sleep medicine. 6th edition. Philadelphia: Elsevier; 2017. p. 432–45.
78. Lankford A, Rogowski R, Essink B, et al. Efficacy and safety of doxepin 6 mg in a four-week outpatient trial of elderly adults with chronic primary insomnia. Sleep Med 2012;13(2):133–8.
79. Scharf M, Rogowski R, Hull S, et al. Efficacy and safety of doxepin 1 mg, 3 mg, and 6 mg in elderly patients with primary insomnia: a randomized, double-blind, placebo-controlled crossover study. J Clin Psychiatry 2008;69(10):1557–64.

80. Krystal AD, Durrence HH, Scharf M, et al. Efficacy and safety of doxepin 1 mg and 3 mg in a 12-week sleep laboratory and outpatient trial of elderly subjects with chronic primary insomnia. Sleep 2010;33(11):1553–61.
81. Liu Y, Xu X, Dong M, et al. Treatment of insomnia with tricyclic antidepressants: a meta-analysis of polysomnographic randomized controlled trials. Sleep Med 2017;34:126–33.
82. Walsh JK, Erman M, Erwin CW, et al. Subjective hypnotic efficacy of trazodone and zolpidem in DSMIII-R primary insomnia. Hum Psychopharmacol 1998; 13(3):191–8.
83. Montgomery I, Oswald I, Morgan K, et al. Trazodone enhances sleep in subjective quality but not in objective duration. Br J Clin Pharmacol 1983;16(2): 139–44.
84. Roth AJ, McCall WV, Liguori A. Cognitive, psychomotor and polysomnographic effects of trazodone in primary insomniacs. J Sleep Res 2011;20(4): 552–8.
85. Schmid DA, Wichniak A, Uhr M, et al. Changes of sleep architecture, spectral composition of sleep EEG, the nocturnal secretion of Cortisol, ACTH, GH, prolactin, melatonin, ghrelin, and leptin, and the DEX-CRH test in depressed patients during treat ment with mirtazapine. Neuropsychopharmacology 2006;31(4):832–44.
86. Aslan S, Isik E, Cosar B. The effects of mirtazapine on sleep: a placebo controlled, double-blind study in young healthy volunteers. Sleep 2002;25(6): 677–9.
87. Krystal AD, Lankford A, Durrence HH, et al. Efficacy and safety of doxepin 3 and 6 mg in a 35-day sleep laboratory trial in adults with chronic primary insomnia. Sleep 2011;34(10):1433–42.
88. Goerke M, Cohrs S, Rodenbeck A, et al. Differential effect of an anticholinergic antidepressant on sleep-dependent memory consolidation. Sleep 2014; 37(5):977–85.
89. Kolla BP, Mansukhani MP, Bostwick JM. The influence of antidepressants on restless legs syndrome and periodic limb movements: a systematic review. Sleep Med Rev 2018;38:131–40.
90. Walsh JK. Drugs used to treat insomnia in 2002: regulatory-based rather than evidence-based medi cine. Sleep 2004;27(8):1441–2.
91. Cohrs S, Rodenbeck A, Guan Z, et al. Sleep-promoting properties of quetiapine in healthy sub jects. Psychopharmacology (Berl) 2004;174(3):421–9.
92. Tassniyom K, Paholpak S, Tassniyom S, et al. Que tiapine for primary insomnia: a double blind, ran domized controlled trial. J Med Assoc Thai 2010;93(6):729–34.
93. Coe HV, Hong IS. Safety of low doses of quetiapine when used for insomnia. Ann Pharmacother 2012; 46(5):718–22.
94. Thompson W, Quay TAW, Rojas-Fernandez C, et al. Atypical antipsychotics for insomnia: a systematic review. Sleep Med 2016;22:13–7.
95. Monti JM, Torterolo P, Pandi Perumal SR. The effects of second generation antipsychotic drugs on sleep variables in healthy subjects and pa tients with schizophrenia. Sleep Med Rev 2017;33:51–7.
96. Vgontzas AN, Fernandez-Mendoza J, Liao D, et al. Insomnia with objective short sleep duration: the most biologically severe phenotype of the disorder. Sleep Med Rev 2013;17(4):241–54.
97. Stahl SM. Temazepam. In: Stahl SM, editor. Stahl's essential pharmacology: the prescriber's guide. 6th edition. Cambridge (UK): Cambridge University Press; 2017. p. 703–6.
98. Yasui-Furukori N, Takahata T, Kondo T, et al. Time ef fects of food intake on the pharmacokinetics and pharmacodynamics of quazepam. Br J Clin Pharmacol 2003;55(4):382–8.
99. Available at. https://www.drugs.com. Accessed February 19, 2018.

A Meta-Analysis of Mindfulness-Based Therapies for Insomnia and Sleep Disturbance Moving Toward Processes of Change

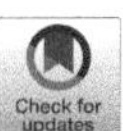

Joshua A. Rash, PhD[a], Victoria A.J. Kavanagh, BA[a], Sheila N. Garland, PhD[a,b,*]

KEYWORDS

• Insomnia • Sleep • Mindfulness • Meta-analysis • Mechanisms

KEY POINTS

- The psychological process model of sleep postulates that interventions such as mindfulness can influence sleep by altering psychological flexibility pertaining to sleep through process variables (eg, awareness, decentering, acceptance, defusion, values, readiness to change, and motivation).
- Mindfulness-based treatments are efficacious at reducing symptoms of insomnia and improving sleep quality among adults when compared with psychological placebos and waitlist control conditions.
- Mindfulness-based interventions for sleep are characterized by conceptual and methodological heterogeneity.
- Future research is needed that evaluates mediators and moderators of intervention effects in an attempt to identify the empirically supported processes of change linking mindfulness-based interventions and sleep outcomes.

INTRODUCTION

Once a term only familiar to Buddhists and experienced meditators, "mindfulness" has quickly been taken up as a goal to be attained by the mainstream and is being applied to all aspects of daily life,[1] including sleep. Some have argued that the popularity of mindfulness may also contribute to its downfall, resulting from inappropriate application and misinformation about the effectiveness of mindfulness-based therapies (MBTs) as a consequence of poor methodology and weak theoretic underpinnings.[2] Although the larger community of mindfulness researchers have sounded the alarm,[3,4] it is unknown whether this has been heard by researchers who are investigating the application of MBTs for sleep.

Mindfulness has been described as an umbrella term "used to characterize a large number of practices, processes, and characteristics, largely defined

Sleep Med Clin 14 (2019) 209-233 https://doi.org/10.1016/j.jsmc.2019.01.004 1556-407X/19/

Funding: Dr S.N. Garland is funded by a New Investigator Award from the Beatrice Hunter Cancer Research Institute.

[a] Department of Psychology, Faculty of Science, Memorial University of Newfoundland, 232 Elizabeth Avenue, St John's, Newfoundland A1B 3X9, Canada; [b] Division of Oncology, Faculty of Medicine, Memorial University of Newfoundland, 300 Prince Phillip Drive, St John's, Newfoundland A1B 3V6, Canada

* Corresponding author. Department of Psychology, Memorial University of Newfoundland, 232 Elizabeth Avenue, St John's, Newfoundland A1B 3X9, Canada.

E-mail address: sheila.garland@mun.ca

Sleep Med Clin 17 (2022) 329–353
https://doi.org/10.1016/j.jsmc.2022.06.002
1556-407X/22/

in relation to the capacities of attention, awareness, memory/retention, and acceptance/discernment."[2] The definition of mindfulness most often cited comes from the seminal work by Jon Kabat-Zinn who characterized mindfulness as paying attention, on purpose, in the present moment without judgment.[5] Although this definition may be the most commonly cited, there remains little consensus on what mindfulness is, the specific mechanisms of effect, and how to measure the construct.[6] This creates several problems for researchers who are interested in applying and/or modifying and testing an intervention in a particular population such as those with insomnia and/or poor sleep.

Herein, the authors present a unifying model that can be used to understand how mindful practices, processes, and characteristics might be relevant to the normal sleep process and how acceptance-based and mindfulness-based interventions may be used to target the mechanisms that perpetuate insomnia. Further, they undertook a review of the literature and performed a meta-analysis of randomized controlled trials (RCTs) evaluating the effect of MBTs on sleep among adults with insomnia or sleep problems with the following objectives:

1. To describe the methodological quality of the available research. The authors were particularly interested in assessing the frequency that research reported modifications to the intervention to make it specific to sleep and whether investigators assessed whether the mindfulness training was associated with, in part or in whole, sleep outcomes.
2. To assess the immediate (ie, postintervention) and sustained (ie, at follow-up) effects of MBTs for insomnia and sleep disturbance compared with waitlist or attention/education controls. Given the limited number and the variability in the nature of active comparison interventions, the authors thought it is premature to compare MBTs with active controls at this time.
3. To propose a series of recommendations to guide future research in this area.

The Relationship Between Mindfulness and Sleep: Toward a Psychological Process Model of Sleep

From a theoretic perspective, there are several plausible mechanisms through which MBTs might operate to improve insomnia and associated daytime impairment. An understanding of normal sleep and the development of chronic insomnia is important to elucidating these mechanisms.

Sleep is a naturally unfolding process that is governed by homeostatic and circadian regulation.[7] Under normal circumstances, sleep-related reduction in arousal occurs automatically and passively (ie, without attention, intention, or effort).[8] The sleep system can be thought of as a self-calibrating system that maintains a degree of flexibility and returns to a homeostatic set-point following acute perturbations (eg, acute stressors that increase physiologic and cognitive/emotional arousal).

There have been 9 models proposed to explain the development of chronic insomnia.[9] Insomnia is theorized to be a disorder characterized by somatic, cognitive, and cortical hyperarousal.[8,10,11] Evidence from autonomic, neuroendocrine, immunology, and neuroimaging studies have generally supported the notion that insomnia is characterized by a failure to de-arouse before sleep.[11,12] According to the 3P,[13] 4P,[14] and neurocognitive models,[10] predisposing factors (eg, hyperreactivity, proclivity to ruminate) serve as a diathesis toward the development of chronic insomnia that interact with precipitating factors and trigger acute disturbance in sleep continuity (eg, life stressors, psychiatric illness). Chronic insomnia is believed to develop within the context of perpetuating factors that interfere with the plasticity and automaticity of sleep and prevent the process of nighttime de-arousal at the behavioral (eg, maladaptive habits and safety behaviors, such as spending excessive time in bed), cognitive (eg, dysfunctional beliefs about sleep and its consequences), and emotional levels (eg, paired associations between the bed and worry or frustration).[15–18]

Factors that perpetuate insomnia can be categorized as sleep-interfering, sleep-interpreting, and metacognitive processes.[17,19] Sleep-interfering processes include arousal-producing processes that interfere with sleep. Sleep-interpreting processes include dysfunctional beliefs, expectations and attributions concerning sleep, and the causes and consequences of poor sleep.[17] Metacognitive processes refer to the way that people relate to their thoughts about sleep, including rigidity in sleep-related behaviors and beliefs, attachment to sleep-related needs and expectations, and absorption in solving the sleep problem.[19] In reality, these processes feed into one another and result in a vicious cycle. For example, compared with good sleepers, people with insomnia endorse unhelpful beliefs about (1) the negative consequences of insomnia; (2) fear of losing control over sleep; and (3) helplessness about the unpredictability of sleep.[16,20,21] They describe their thoughts as intrusive, uncontrollable, and negative.[22,23] Individuals who suffer from insomnia report devoting greater effort toward sleep,[24] rigidity in beliefs about sleep, and attachment toward sleep-related needs and expectations.[19,25] Perhaps unsurprisingly, relative to controls, individuals with insomnia report the use of a higher number of sleep-interfering processes, including worry, thought suppression, and rumination.[26–30]

MBTs may improve sleep by facilitating psychological flexibility, improving metacognitive processes that contribute to insomnia, and promoting sleep-related de-arousal. Psychological flexibility refers to (1) conscious and open contact with thoughts and feelings, (2) an awareness of the available responses in any situation, and (3) changing or persisting in behavior when doing so serves one's goals and values.[31,32] Psychological flexibility contains a set of 6 interrelated subprocesses, including (1) acceptance—the ability to open up to unwanted experiences without struggle or avoidance, (2) cognitive defusion—the ability to notice thoughts as thoughts rather than becoming wrapped up in their meaning, (3) being present—open, nonjudgmental contact with the present, (4) self-as-observer—seeing oneself as more than a collection of thoughts and feelings, (5) values—understanding chosen qualities of purposive action, and (6) committed action—development of larger patterns of effective actions linked to chosen values.[31,32] A cross-sectional assessment of 159 adults with chronic pain (79% with clinical insomnia) reported associations between components of psychological flexibility and symptoms of insomnia in the expected directions (ie, an inverse association between psychological flexibility and symptoms of insomnia).[33] Adopting psychological flexibility as an underlying model, MBTs can be used to explicitly target sleep-interfering, sleep-interpreting, and metacognitive processes that maintain insomnia, including: (1) fostering a willingness to accept unpleasant experiences, thoughts, and beliefs pertaining to sleep and the possibility that safety behaviors (eg, excess time spent in bed) may contribute to the sleep problem rather than the sleep solution; (2) facilitating psychological distance from entrenched beliefs about sleep (ie, cognitive defusion, decentering, or disengagement) by promoting present focused, nonjudgmental awareness of thoughts, physical sensations, and feelings. This state of equanimity can serve to reduce the struggle with feelings, entanglement with arousing thoughts, and reliance on ineffective metacognitive processes, such as thought suppression; and (3) promoting committed action to values to reduce the focus on perceived daytime impairment.[19,25,34]

The adoption of an overarching psychological process model of sleep (PPMS; **Fig. 1**) to the treatment of insomnia is only useful to the extent that the model generates testable hypotheses that enrich our understanding of the disorder and its treatment. When viewed from this perspective, MBTs are viewed as targeting the process variables (ie, awareness, decentering, acceptance, defusion, values, readiness to change, motivation) that affect psychological flexibility[35] and have indirect effects on insomnia through reduction of sleep-related arousal. As such, it is important to perform a critical evaluation of the processes of change between MBTs and outcomes following the treatment of insomnia in order to advance our understanding of precision treatments for insomnia. This approach aligns with transdiagnostic treatments.[36] Treatments that target transdiagnostic processes (eg, cognitive rigidity and regulation of emotion) that underpin a broad range of diagnostic presentations, including insomnia and psychopathology, may be particularly effective among individuals with insomnia and medical/psychiatric comorbidity because they address a broader range of symptomatology.[37,38] One notable observational single-cohort study evaluated the processes of change in sleep problems following the delivery of group acceptance and commitment therapy (ACT) for 252 patients with chronic pain and concomitant sleep problems, many of whom experienced comorbid depression. Treatment occurred on 4 days per week over 4 weeks and included a prominent mindfulness component along with 2 hours of content on sleep that focused on sleep-related cognitions.[39] Significant improvement was observed for insomnia severity (*d* = 0.45), sleep interference (*d* = 0.61), sleep efficiency (d = 0.32), pain (d = 0.72), and symptoms of depression (d = 1.03), most of which were maintained at 9-

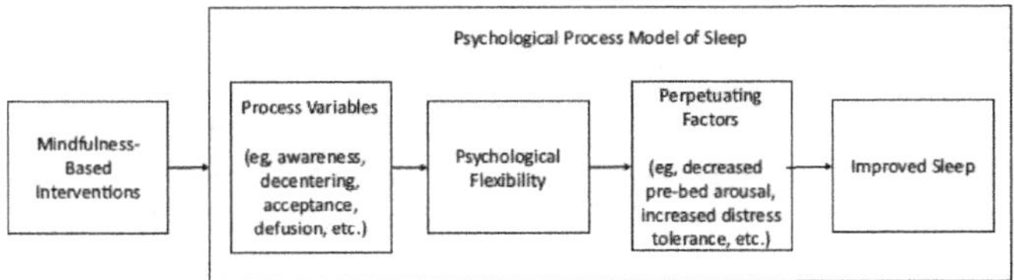

Fig. 1. How MBTs interact with the psychological process model of sleep.

month follow-up. Importantly, change was observed on measures of psychological flexibility (including acceptance and cognitive defusion), which were associated with sleep-related improvement.

The proposed PPMS can be used to move past simply assessing whether MBTs can improve sleep and begin guiding future research questions on how MBTs exert their effect. It is also possible that applying such a mechanistic model will improve overall treatment efficacy but this remains to be tested. While looking to the future, it is important to characterize the current literature pertaining to MBTs for insomnia and sleep disturbance to serve as a heuristic to inform the design of future trials. Two previous reviews and meta-analyses of the efficacy of MBTs specifically for sleep have been conducted but these were characterized by limitations, including (1) the inclusion of study designs other than RCTs, (2) small or insufficient sample sizes, and (3) a failure to exclude studies where sleep was not the primary intervention target.[40,41] These limitations negatively affect the ability to draw firm conclusions. To appreciate the current state of the research applying MBTs to insomnia and sleep disturbance, the authors conducted a systematic review and meta-analysis of the literature with a focus on RCTs with sleep as the primary intervention target.

METHODS

Search Strategy

A thorough literature search was performed using 3 electronic databases—PubMed, Medline, and PsycInfo. Given the authors' interest in recent literature, search dates were restricted to January 01, 2010 to August 31, 2018. Searches were enhanced by scanning bibliographies of identified articles.

Search terms were constructed to include the combination of keywords and controlled vocabulary for 3 search themes, including mindfulness (eg, mindfulness or acceptance), sleep disturbance (eg, insomnia, sleep quality, and sleep disturbance), and RCTs. Terms within each theme were combined using the Boolean operator "OR." Themes were combined using the Boolean operator "AND."

Trial Selection

Articles were included if they met inclusion criteria for (1) trial design: reporting on an RCT; (2) trial population: adults older than 18 years with sleep disturbance, with clinically relevant levels of insomnia (as defined by the Diagnostic and Statistical Manual for Mental Disorders,[42] International Classification of Sleep Disorders,[43] or the insomnia severity index [ISI])[21] or sleep disturbance (as defined by the Medical Outcomes Study Sleep Scale [MOS-SS],[44] Pittsburgh Sleep Quality Index [PSQI],[45] or sleep diary) at baseline; (3) delivery of an intervention where mindfulness/acceptance was a prominent component, including mindfulness-based stress reduction (MBSR), mindfulness-based cognitive therapy (MBCT), and ACT; and (4) outcome: measures of sleep (eg, sleep diary) or insomnia symptoms (eg, ISI) as a primary or secondary outcome. Only research published in English language journals were included.

Data Extraction

Details of each trial were extracted using a standardized extraction form. This form included the following information: author and year of published report, methods (eg, design of RCT, number of treatment arms, trial duration and follow-up, blinding, allocation concealment, method of randomization and attrition), participant characteristics (eg, sample size, age, sex distribution), control details, and outcomes. A separate table was used to record raw outcome data on symptoms of insomnia and sleep quality.

Quality Ratings

All trials were rated using a scale originally developed to assess the quality of psychological treatments for chronic pain.[46] The measure contains 2 subscales. The subscale measuring treatment quality evaluates stated rationale for treatment, manualization, therapist training, and patient engagement (scores range from 0 to 9 with higher scores reflecting greater rigor). The subscale measuring trial design and methods includes 8 items and evaluates inclusion/exclusion criteria, attrition, sample description, minimization of bias (randomization method, allocation bias, blinding of assessment, and equality of treatment expectations), selection of outcomes, length of follow-up, analyses, and choice of control (scores range from 0 to 26 with higher scores reflecting greater rigor). Scores on both subscales are summed to measure overall trial quality (scores range from 0 to 35). All trials were independently rated and consensus reached after initial comparison ratings.

Quantitative Data Synthesis

Procedures and formula for conducting a meta-analysis were based on recommendations by Lipsey and Wilson.[47] True effects estimates were computed as adjusted standardized mean differences (Hedge's g) using random effects models.

Three steps were taken to calculate Hedge's g. First, the mean within-group difference was calculated as change from pretest to posttest within each trial. Second, prepost within-group standard deviations were pooled to calculate the standard deviation of change scores according to recommendations.[48] Finally, Hedge's *g* between the MBT and control groups was computed from the between-group change scores and associated standard deviation.

Pooling of effects and meta-analytic comparison was performed on trials that compared MBTs with inactive control conditions and psychological placebos (ie, attention/education controls). Meta-analysis was not performed on trials comparing an MBT with an active comparator because of the variability in active comparators. Separate meta-analyses were performed for effects at postintervention and follow-up. Fail-safe Ns were calculated to assess for publication bias using Orwin's formula.[49] The recommended criterion effect size of 0.20 was used.

Statistical analysis was performed using the random effects model performed with RevMan5.3 software (Review Manager (RevMan) [Computer program]. Version 5.3. Copenhagen: The Nordic Cochrane Centre, The Cochrane Collaboration, 2014). Heterogeneity was assessed using the I^2 index, chi-square, and tau^2 tests.[50] According to recommendations, substantial heterogeneity was assumed if I^2 exceeded 50%.[50]

Qualitative Analysis of Mindfulness and Sleep Components

The included articles were also evaluated based on the recommendations of Van Dam and colleagues[2] to improve reporting of mindfulness-based interventions. Extracted information included instructor details, experience and qualifications, mindfulness techniques used, home practice recommendations and tracking, use of supportive materials, monitoring of adverse events, and whether or not the participants had previous meditation experience. An additional column was added to specify whether the intervention was adapted or modified to include sleep-specific interventions or recommendations.

RESULTS

Summary of Included Trials

The search of the literature yielded 16 publications reporting on 13 trials conducted since 2010 that reported on 864 adults (542 women and 304 men). **Table 1** depicts the characteristics of included trials. Nine trials assessed the effect of MBTs on insomnia, with the remaining 4 investigating sleep disturbance more generally. Eight trials used an active control condition,[51–59] 3 an inactive control,[60–62] and 2 included both active and inactive control conditions.[63–66] Seven trials were conducted with adults with insomnia,[55,59,61,64,65] 2 of which were limited to older adults.[51,62] The remaining trials tested the intervention in cancer survivors,[53,57] veterans,[56,58] postmenopausal women,[52] and women with fibromyalgia.[60]

There was a great deal of heterogeneity between interventions tested. Three trials tested traditional MBSR interventions,[54,55,62] one trial used a modified MBSR protocol,[51] 3 trials tested combinations of MBTs with behavioral sleep approaches,[59,64,65] one combined mindfulness with relaxation training,[52] 2 used ACT practices tailored for sleep,[60,61] and 3 trials by the same group trained participants in focusing their awareness/attention without any formal meditation training.[56–58] The duration of the interventions ranged from a minimum of 2 weekly 1.5 hour sessions[58] to the maximally intensive 2.5 hour weekly classes for 8 weeks with daily assigned homework and a 6 hour silent retreat.[55,64] The overwhelming majority of the inventions tested were delivered in group format with only one delivered to individuals,[65] and one trial did not specify.[58]

Nine trials[51–53,56–59,61,65] included a measure of mindfulness but only 3 examined whether the measure of mindfulness was related to the sleep outcomes.[51,54,63] Three trials assessed whether self-reported minutes of meditation practice was associated with sleep outcomes.[55,59,64]

Trial Quality

Ratings of trial quality are presented in **Table 2**. Ratings for the reporting of treatment quality ranged from a low of 3 to a high of 9 (out of a possible 9). The areas of lowest quality were whether the treatment was manualized and whether formal checks on adherence to the manual by the therapists (ie, treatment fidelity) was conducted via direct observations, tape recording, or supervisory processes. The other most common area where trials were lacking was the inclusion of formal assessment of patient engagement, described as formal checks on homework or skills practice.

Reporting of trial design and methods was also quite variable with a low of 13 to a high of 24 (out of a possible 26). Areas that trials were largely lacking were related to improper randomization and blinding procedures (the use of an independent person to create the allocation sequence or the use of sequentially numbered opaque sealed

Table 1
Study details

First Author, Date	Sample/Sex Population	Intervention Details Follow-up Period	Control/Comparison Details	Sleep Outcome Mindfulness Outcome	Results	Relation Between Sleep and Mindfulness
RCTs that assessed effect of mindfulness on insomnia symptoms with active control						
Garcia et al,[52] 2018	30 Postmenopausal women w/ insomnia (19 MRTI; 11 control)	Group 8 wk (30 min/wk in class; up to 40 min/d at home) MRTI follow-up: none	Group 8 wk Attention control general discussion in class (30 min) and crossword puzzles (up to 40 min)	Sleep: PSQI, ISI, polysomnography Mindfulness: MAAS	Relative to control, MRTI improved symptoms of insomnia and sleep quality. No differences between groups were observed for PSG variables. MAAS scores increased in the MRTI group only	Not reported
Garland et al,[53] 2014, Garland et al,[54] 2015	111 (80 F; 31 M) patients with cancer w/insomnia (64 MBSR; 47 CBT-I)	Group 8 wk (90 min/wk) + 6 h silent retreat. MBSR follow-up: 3 mo	Group 8 wk (90 min/wk) CBT-I	Sleep: actigraphy, DBAS, ISI, PSQI, sleep diary Mindfulness: FFMQ	MBSR was inferior to CBT-I immediately after treatment but not at 3 mo follow-up. As a single-group, MBSR resulted in improvement in symptoms of insomnia, sleep quality, and dysfunctional beliefs about sleep at 3 mo follow-up	Both groups increased "acting with awareness" and "nonjudging." Increases in mindfulness were associated with decreases in DBAS scores. Nonjudging was associated with decreased insomnia severity
Gross et al,[55] 2011	27 (22 F; 8 M) adults w/insomnia (18 MBSR; 9 pharmacotherapy)	Group 8 wk (2.5 h/wk) + 6 h silent retreat MBSR. Information on sleep hygiene follow-up: 3 mo	3 mg of eszopiclone (nightly for 8 wk) pharmacotherapy information on sleep hygiene	Sleep: sleep diary, actigraphy, ISI, PSQI, DBAS, SSES mindfulness: none	MBSR used in conjunction with readings on sleep showed similar results to that of pharmacotherapy	Significant correlation between reduction in dysfunctional sleep beliefs and meditation practice during intervention period

Ong et al,[66] 2014; Ong et al,[64] 2018	54 (40 F; 14 M) adults w/insomnia (13 MBSR; 15 MBTI; 16SM)	Group 8 wk (2.5 h/wk) + 6 h silent retreat. MBSR or MBTI follow-up: 3 mo, 6 mo	Individual 16 wk (8 wk SM, 8 wk BT) delayed control	Sleep: GSES, BAS, HAS, FSS, ESS mindfulness: none	MBSR and MBTI were superior to SM on all subjective and objective sleep measures but no significant differences found between MBSR and MBTI. MBTI was noninferior to BT for reducing sleep effort, dysfunctional sleep beliefs, and hyperarousal	Significant correlation between more minutes of meditation and reduced dysfunctional sleep beliefs in MBTI group only
Wong et al,[65] 2016 Lee et al,[63] 2018	64(36 F; 21 M) adults w/insomnia (12 immediate MBT; 17 immediate CT; 14 delayed MBT; 14 delayed CT)	4 wk individual CBT-I followed by immediate MBT or CT follow-up: 3 mo	4 wk individual CBT-I followed by 4 wk waiting then assignment to MBT or CT	Sleep: ISI, PSQI, APSQ, SAMI, DBAS, SRBQ, sleep diary, actigraphy mindfulness: KIMS, NRI	After initial treatment with CBT-I, further treatment with MBT or CT produced further impairment, relative to WLC. No differences were observed between MBT and CT. MBT improved mindfulness skills (KIMS) and DBAS	Baseline insomnia severity and sleep beliefs, but not mindfulness, predicted posttreatment insomnia severity

(*continued on next page*)

Table 1
(continued)

First Author, Date	Sample/Sex Population	Intervention Details Follow-up Period	Control/Comparison Details	Sleep Outcome Mindfulness Outcome	Results	Relation Between Sleep and Mindfulness
Wong et al,[59] 2017	216 (169 F; 47 M) adults w/insomnia (111 MBCT-I; 105 PEEC)	Group 8 wk (2.5 h/wk) MBCT-I follow-up: 5 mo, 8 mo	Group 8 wk (2.5 h/wk) PEEC	Sleep: ISI, sleep diary mindfulness: FFMQ	The MBCT-I group was significantly better than the PEEC group posttreatment but not at 3 and 6 mo follow-ups. The MBCT-I group had greater reductions in WASO posttreatment and 3 mo. No other significant differences between PEEC and MBCT-I were observed. No change demonstrated on the FFMQ	No differences in insomnia was seen in those who practiced their mediations 3×/week and those who did not
RCTs that assessed effect of mindfulness on sleep disturbance with active control						
Black et al,[51] 2015	49 (33 F; 16 M) older adults w/sleep disturbance (24 MAPs; 25 SHE)	Group 6 wk (2 h/wk) MAPS follow-up: none	Group 6 wk (2 h/wk) SHE	Sleep: FSI, PSQI, AIS mindfulness: FFMQ	Relative to SHE, MAPS improved sleep quality, insomnia symptoms, depressed mood, and fatigue	Mindfulness increased in MAPS but not SHE group. In the MAPS group, increased nonreactivity was associated with reductions in sleep disturbance and insomnia symptoms

Nakamura et al,[58] 2011	58 (3 F; 55 M) US Veterans with sleep disturbance (33 MBB; 25 SHE)	2 wk (1.5 h/wk) MBB follow-up: none	2 wk (1 h/wk) SED and monitoring using sleep diary	Sleep: MOS-SS mindfulness: FFMQ	Larger reductions in sleep disturbance and greater increases in mindfulness were reported in the MBB group compared with the SED group at follow-up	Not reported
Nakamura et al,[57] 2013	57 (43 F; 14M) cancer survivors with sleep disturbance (19 MBB; 20 MM; 18 SHE)	Group 3 wk (2 h/wk) MBB or MM follow-up: none	Group 3 wk (2 h/wk) SED	Sleep: MOS-SS mindfulness: FFMQ	Sleep disturbance improved in both the MBB and MM groups compared with SED, and mindfulness increased in MBB but not the MM group relative to SHE.	Not reported
Nakamura et al,[56] 2017	60 (6 F; 54 M) Gulf war veterans with sleep disturbance (33 MBB; 27 SHE)	Group 3 wk (2 h/wk) MBB follow-up: 3 mo	Group 3 wk (2 h/wk) SED	Sleep: MOS-SS, MFI mindfulness: FFMQ	No overall differences in sleep disturbance between MBB and SED immediately after treatment but MBB reported greater improvement than SED at follow-up. No reliable change in mindfulness	Not reported
RCTs that assessed effect of mindfulness on insomnia symptoms with inactive control						
Amutio et al,[60] 2018	39 female adults w/ fibromyalgia w/ insomnia (20 FM; 19 control)	Group 7 wk (2 h/wk) FM follow-up: 3 mo	WLC	Sleep: AIS, PSQI, ESS, SII Mindfulness: none	The FM group improved sleep quality, sleepiness, sleep impairment, and subjective insomnia from pretest to posttest. These improvements continued during follow-up	Not reported

(*continued on next page*)

Table 1
(*continued*)

First Author, Date	Sample/Sex Population	Intervention Details Follow-up Period	Control/Comparison Details	Sleep Outcome Mindfulness Outcome	Results	Relation Between Sleep and Mindfulness
deok Baik,[61] 2015	25 (16 F; 9 M) adults w/insomnia (14ACT; 11 control)	Group 2 wk (3–4 h/wk) ACT follow-up: none	WLC, monitored sleep	Sleep: ISI, PSAS, sleep diary mindfulness: AAQ-II, EQ	There was no effect of group on insomnia symptoms, presleep arousal, or sleep diary variables. Time effects were seen for both groups on measures of acceptance and mindfulness	Not reported
Zhang, 2015	60 (25 F; 35 M) older adults w/insomnia (30 MBSR; 30 control)	Group 8 wk (2 h/wk) + 2 h silent retreat MBSR follow-up: none	WLC	Sleep: PSQI mindfulness: none	Relative to WLC, MBSR improved PSQI total score and daytime dysfunction, but no other PSQI subscales	Not reported

Abbreviations: AAQ-II, acceptance and action questionnaire II; ACT, acceptance and commitment therapy; AIS, Athens Insomnia Scale; APSQ, Anxiety And Preoccupation With Sleep Questionnaire; BAS, beliefs and attitudes about sleep scale; BT, behavioral therapy; CBT-I, cognitive behavior therapy for insomnia; CT, cognitive therapy; DBAS, dysfunctional beliefs and attitudes about sleep scale; EQ, experiences questionnaire; ESS, Epworth sleepiness scale; F, female; FF-MQ, Five Facet Mindfulness Questionnaire; FM, flow meditation; FSI, fatigue symptom inventory; FSS, fatigue severity scale; GSES, Glasgow sleep effort scale; HAS, hyper arousal scale; ISI, insomnia severity index; ISQ, Insomnia Symptom Questionnaire; KIMS, Kentucky inventory of mindfulness skills; M, male; MAAS, mindfulness awareness attention scale; MAPS, mindfulness awareness practices intervention; MBB, mind body bridging; MBCT, mindfulness based cognitive therapy; MBCT-I, mindfulness-based cognitive therapy for insomnia; MBSR, mindfulness-based stress reduction; MBTI, mindfulness based therapy for insomnia; MFI, multidimensional fatigue inventory; MOS-SS, Medical Outcomes Study Sleep Scale; MM, mindfulness meditation; MRTI, mindfulness and relaxation training for insomnia; NRI, nonreactivity to inner-experience; PEEC, psycho education with exercise control; PSAS, presleep arousal scale; PSD, Pittsburgh sleep diary; PSG, polysomnography; PSQI, Pittsburgh Sleep Quality Index; SAMI, sleep associative monitoring index; SED, sleep education; SHE, sleep hygiene education; SII, sleep impairment index; SM, self-monitoring; SRBQ, sleep-related behavior questionnaire; SSES, sleep self-efficacy scale; TCQIR, thought control.

Table 2
Study quality rating scale

Quality Rating	Amutio et al,[60] 2018	deok Baik,[61] 2015	Black, 2015	Garcia et al,[52] 2018	Garland et al,[53] 2014	Gross et al.[55] 2011	Nakamura et al,[58] 2011	Nakamura et al,[57] 2013	Nakamura et al,[56] 2017
Treatment Quality									
Treatment content 0,2	1	2	2	1	2	2	1	2	2
Treatment duration 0,1	1	1	1	1	1	1	1	1	1
Manualization 0,2	0	2	2	2	2	2	0	0	0
Manual adherence 0,1	0	1	0	0	0	0	0	0	0
Therapist training 0,2	1	2	2	0	2	2	1	1	1
Patient engagement 0,1	1	1	0	1	0	1	0	0	0
Overall treatment quality	4	9	7	5	7	8	3	4	4
Quality of Design and Methods									
Sample criteria 0,1	1	1	1	1	1	1	1	1	1
Evidence criteria met 0,1	1	1	1	1	1	1	1	1	1
Attrition 0,2	0	0		1	2	1	1	2	2
Rates of attrition 0,1	1	0	1	1	1	1	1	1	1
Sample characteristics 0,1	1	1	1	1	1	1	0	1	1
Group equivalence 0,1	1	1	1	1	1	0	1	0	1
Randomization 0,2	0	1		0	1	2	1	1	1
Allocation bias 0,1	1	0	1	0	1	1	0	0	0
Measurement bias 0,1	0	0	1	0	0	0	0	0	0
Treatment expectations 0,1	0	0	0	0	0	0	0	0	1
Justification of outcomes 0,2	2	2	2	2	2	2	2	2	2
Validity of outcomes 0,2	2	2	2	2	2	2	2	2	2
Reliability 0,2	2	2	2	2	2	2	2	2	2
Follow-up 0,1	0	0	0	0	0	0	0	0	0
Power calculation 0,1	0	0	1	0	1	0	0	0	1
Sample size 0,1	0	0	1	1	1	0	0	0	0

(*continued on next page*)

Table 2
(continued)

Quality Rating	Amutio et al,[60] 2018	deok Baik,[61] 2015	Black, 2015	Garcia et al,[52] 2018	Garland et al,[53] 2014	Gross et al.[55] 2011	Nakamura et al,[58] 2011	Nakamura et al,[57] 2013	Nakamura et al,[56] 2017
Data analysis 0,1	0	1	1	1	1	1	1	1	1
Statistics reporting 0,1	1	1	1	1	1	1	1	1	1
Intent to treat analysis 0,1	1	0	1	1	1	0	1	1	1
Control group 0,2	0	0	2	1	2	1	0	2	1
Overall design quality	14	13	24	17	22	17	15	18	20
Quality score	18	22	31	22	29	25	18	22	24

Quality Rating	Ong et al,[64] 2018	Wong et al,[65] 2016	Wong et al,[59] 2017	Zhang et al,[62] 2015
Treatment Quality				
Treatment content 0,2	2	2	2	1
Treatment duration 0,1	1	1	1	1
Manualization 0,2	1	2	1	2
Manual adherence 0,1	1	0	1	0
Therapist training 0,2	2	2	2	1
Patient engagement 0,1	1	0	1	0
Overall treatment quality	8	7	8	5
Quality of Design and Methods				
Sample criteria 0,1	1	1	1	1
Evidence criteria met 0,1	1	0	1	1
Attrition 0,2	2	1	2	1
Rates of attrition 0,1	1	1	1	1
Sample characteristics 0,1	1	0	1	1
Group equivalence 0,1	1	0	1	1
Randomization 0,2	2	1	2	1
Allocation bias 0,1	1	0	1	0
Measurement bias 0,1	0	0	1	0

Treatment expectations 0,1		1			0	0	0
Justification of outcomes 0,2		2			2	2	2
Validity of outcomes 0,2		2			2	2	2
Reliability 0,2	2	2	2	2			
Follow-up 0,1	1	0	1	0			
Power calculation 0,1	1	0	1	1			
Sample size 0,1	0	0	1	1			
Data analysis 0,1	1	0	1	1			
Statistics reporting 0,1	1	1	1	1			
Intent to treat analysis 0,1	1	1	1	1			
Control group 0,2	2	2	2	0			
Overall design quality	24	14	25	18			
Quality score	32	21	33	23			

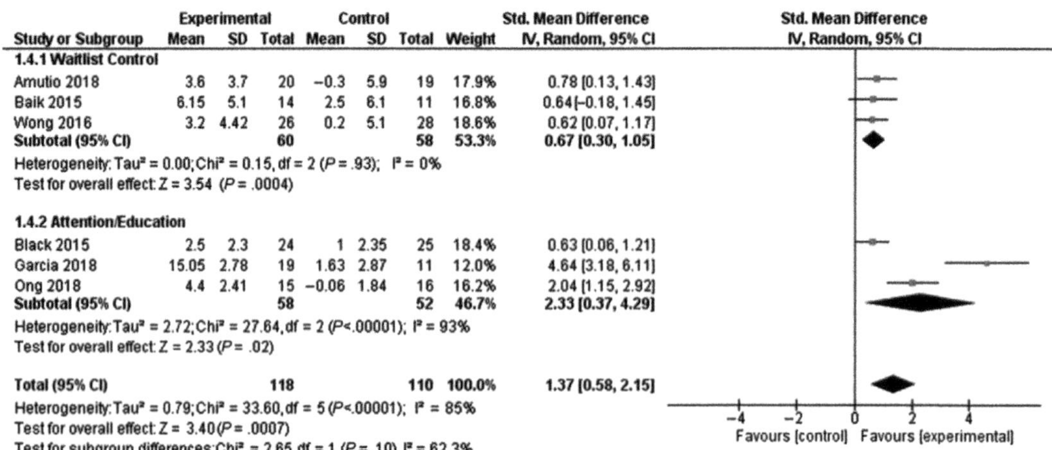

Fig. 2. Forest plot depicting the effect of MBTs on sleep disturbances relative to waitlist and attention/education controls at post-intervention, with heterogeneity across trials (I^2= 81%, $c^2(4) = 21.48$, $P < .01$; see **Fig. 4**). A sensitivity test removing the article by Garcia and colleagues[52] diminished variability to 3% but did not change the overall effect.

envelopes and using a third party who is blind to the patient's trial group for the collection of trial data), lack of a priori power calculations, and insufficient duration of follow-up (<6 months). Only 2 of the trials[56,64] included a measurement of participant treatment expectations, which is arguably a critical component of evaluations of behavioral trials.

The overall rating of trial quality was 24.62 across the 13 trials included. The original scale[46] did not include published cut-offs for overall quality; however, average scores for excellent, average, and poor trials across the validation sample were 22.70, 18.71, and 12.10, respectively. Thus, included trials would be considered excellent in trial quality when compared with RCTs of psychological interventions for adults with chronic pain. Combined, only 4 trials[51,53,59,64] had a total quality rating score in the top quarter (>26/35).

Meta-Analysis Symptoms of Insomnia

Six trials (n = 228; 76% women) reported on symptoms of insomnia, 5 using the ISI and 1 using the Athens Insomnia Scale, and provided sufficient data for the computation of unbiased effect sizes[51,52,60,61,64,65] (**Fig. 2**). Meta-analysis of 3 trials with waitlist controls[60,61,65] indicated a main effect (g = 0.67, 95% confidence interval [CI] = 0.30–1.05, $Z = 3.54$, $P < .01$) of MBTs for insomnia (n = 60) relative to waitlist controls (n = 58) at postintervention, with no heterogeneity across trials ($I^2 = 0\%$, $c^2(2) = 0.15$, $P = .93$). Meta-analysis of 3 trials with attention/education controls[51,52,64] indicated a main effect (g = 2.33,

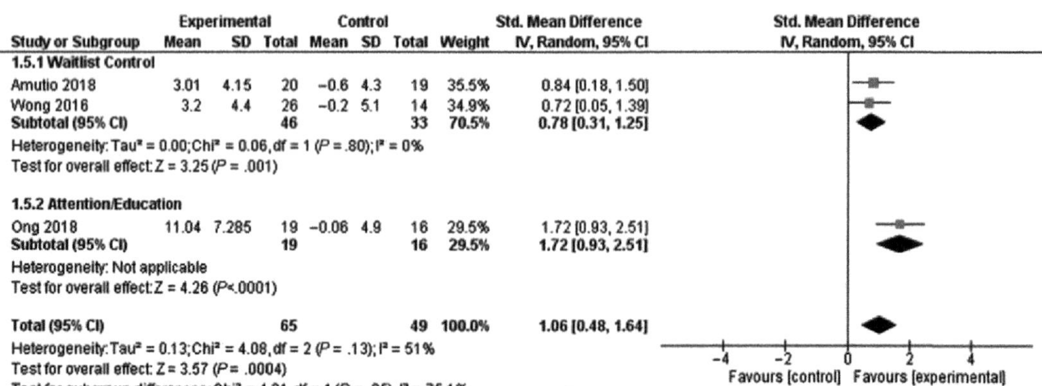

Fig. 3. Forest plot depicting the effect of MBTs on change in symptoms of insomnia from pretest to 3-month follow-up. Separate forest plots are presented for waitlist and attention/education control conditions.

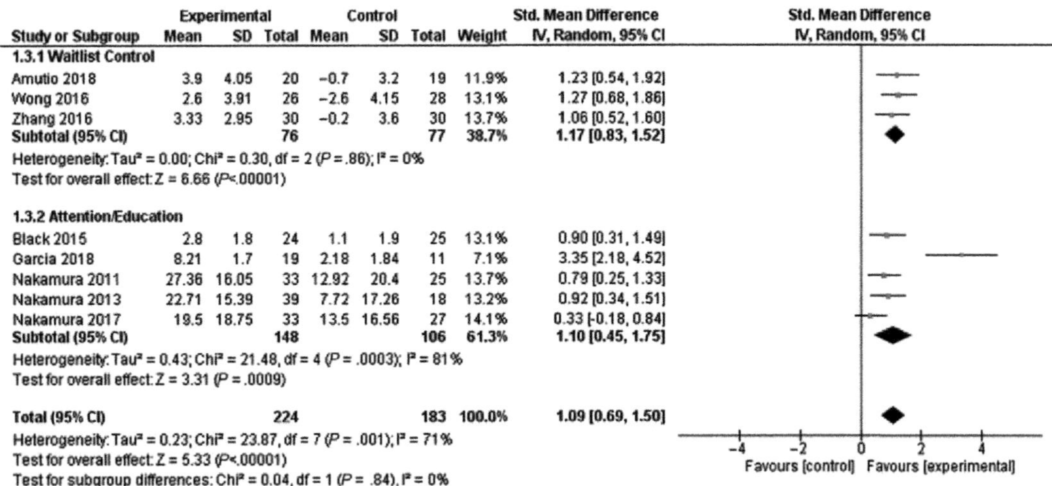

Fig. 4. Forest plot depicting the effect of MBTs on change in sleep quality from pretest to posttest. Separate forest plots are presented for waitlist and attention/education control conditions.

95% CI = 0.37–4.29, z = 2.33, *P* = .02) of MBTs on insomnia (n = 58) relative to attention/education controls (n = 52) at postintervention, with significant heterogeneity across effects (I^2 = 93%, $c^2(2) = 27.64$, $P < .01$).

Three trials reported on the effect of MBTs on symptoms of insomnia at 3-month follow-up[60,65,66] (**Fig. 3**). The effects of MBTs (n = 65) on symptoms of insomnia endured at 3-month follow-up (g = 1.06, 95% CI = 0.48–1.64) when compared with control (n = 49). It should be noted that this comparison is somewhat biased given that 2 trials[65,66] did not assess the control group at 3-month follow-up (ie, change in symptoms of insomnia due to MBT from baseline to 3-month follow-up was compared with change in control group from baseline to postintervention).

Sleep Quality

Eight trials (n = 407; 52% women) reported on sleep quality, 5 using the PSQI and 3 using the MOS-SS SPI-II, and provided sufficient data for the computation of unbiased effect sizes.[51,52,56–58,60,62,65] Meta-analysis of 3 trials[60,62,65] indicated a main effect (g = 1.17, 95% CI = 0.83–1.52, Z = 6.66, *P* < .01) of MBTs on sleep quality (n = 76) relative to waitlist control (n = 77) at postintervention, with no heterogeneity across trials (I^2 = 0%, $c^2(2) = 0.30$, *P* = .86; **Fig. 4**). Meta-analysis of 5 trials[51,52,56–58] indicated a main effect (g = 1.10, 95% CI = 0.45–1.75, z = 3.31, *P* < .01) of MBTs on sleep quality of insomnia from pretest to posttest. Separate forest plots are presented for waitlist and attention/education control conditions.

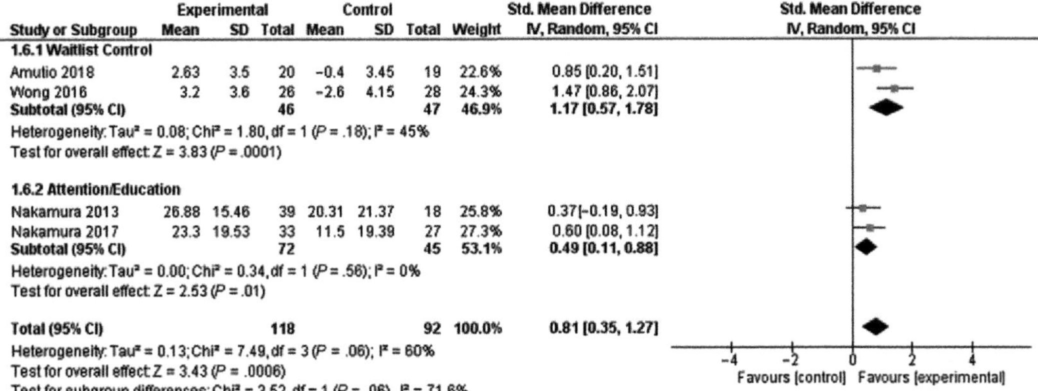

Fig. 5. Forest plot depicting the effect of MBTs on change in sleep quality from pretest to 3-month follow-up. Separate forest plots are presented for waitlist and attention/education control conditions.

Table 3
Mindfulness intervention design features

First Author, Year		Instructor Information				Intervention Details			Participant Information
	Instruction Experience	Mindfulness Training	Clinical Qualifications	Mindfulness Details	Specific Sleep Instructions	Meditation Practice/Log	Types of Materials	Monitoring of Adverse Events	Prior Experience with Meditation
Amutio et al,[60] 2018	Referred to as extensive	Referred to as extensive	Not reported	Formal meditation: body scan, breath awareness ACT exercises and Zen meditation metaphors	Not reported	Home practice: 10 min/d of body scan, 30 min/d of full-body awareness breathing Log: daily record of level of engagement with at-home practices	Not reported	Not reported	Excluded if currently undergoing any mindfulness training
deok Baik,[61] 2015	Two previous training sessions	Not reported	Psychology graduate students	Formal meditation: sitting, Metta, and Tonglen meditation Awareness of body sensations, breathing, labeling thoughts, acceptance, commitment, and cognitive defusion	Tailoring of ACT exercises and metaphor for sleep	Home practice: 10–20 min/d rs Log: diary of sessions and total minutes	Not reported	Not reported	Not reported
Black et al,[51] 2015	Not reported	Certified[a] mindfulness teacher with 20 y mindfulness practice	Not reported	Formal meditation: sitting, mindful eating, walking meditation, and mindful movement	Not reported	Home practice: started with 5 min/d and increased to 20 min/d by wk 6. Log: diary of number of independent sessions and total minutes	Mindfulness book, audio recordings for guided meditation	Not reported	Not reported

Garcia et al,[52] 2018	Referred to as experienced	Not reported	Not reported	Formal meditation: seated relaxation, body scan, and breathing, breath awareness	Practice at night lying in bed just before sleeping	Home practice: varied by wk from 8-40 min, 1–3 times/d Log: when and for how long meditated	Audio recordings for guided meditation	Not reported	Not reported
Garland et al,[53] 2014; Garland et al,[54] 2015	10 + years of experience delivering MBSR	Certified[a] MBSR instructor from CFM	Nurse	Formal meditation: body scan, sitting, walking, movement, and Hatha yoga	No specific instructions were provided for sleep	Home practice: 45 min/d Log: not reported	Workbook, readings, audio recordings for guided meditation	Not reported	Excluded if they had prior experience with MBSR or CBT-I
Gross et al,[55] 2011	Not reported	Certified[a] MBSR instructor from CFM	Not reported	Formal meditation: body scan, standing, sitting, walking, and gentle yoga	Emphasized sleep and sleep stress readings from Full Catastrophe Living by Jon Kabat Zinn, which recommends breath focus in bed to reduce sleep effort	Home practice: 45 min/d at least 6 d/wk for 8 wk followed by 20 min/d for 3 mo Log: duration was tracked with electronic logger (HOBO® data logger Onset Computer Corporation, Bourne, MA, USA)	Workbook, readings, audio recordings for guided meditation	Adverse events tracked and none were reported	Not reported
Nakamura et al,[58] 2011	**Not reported**	**Certified[6] MBB instructor**	**Licensed clinical social worker**	**Focused** awareness/ attention exercises (no	**Encouraged to** practice exercises before bed	**Home practice: as** much as possible Log: not reported	**Mind-Body map**	**Not reported**	**Not reported**

(*continued on next page*)

Table 3
(continued)

First Author, Year	Instructor Information					Intervention Details			Participant Information
	Instruction Experience	Mindfulness Training	Clinical Qualifications	Mindfulness Details	Specific Sleep Instructions	Meditation Practice/Log	Types of Materials	Monitoring of Adverse Events	Prior Experience with Meditation
				formal meditation practice)					
Nakamura et al,[57] 2013	MBB: not reported MM: referred to as experienced	Certified[b] MBB instructor "years" of meditation experience	Licensed clinical social worker	Focused awareness/ attention exercises (no formal meditation practice) formal meditation: sitting, walking, body scan, and awareness training	Not reported	Home practice: as much as possible log: not reported	Mind-body map, reference to a textbook used copy of book "full catastrophe living," audio recordings for guided meditation, handouts	Not reported	Excluded if had Prior exposure to MBB, MM, MBSR, or MBCT
Nakamura et al,[56] 2017	Not reported	Certified[b] MBB instructors	Licensed clinical social workers	Focused awareness/ attention exercises (no formal meditation practice)	Encouraged to practice exercises before bed and/or during the middle of night	Home practice: encouraged to practice as much as possible Log: not reported	Reference to following procedures of previous studies	Not reported	Not reported
Ong et al,[66] 2014; Ong et al,[64] 2018	MBSR: first instructor—2 y teaching experience; second instructor—15 y teaching	MBSR: One instructor-200 h of MBSR training MBTI: 100 h of mindfulness	MBSR: first instructor—PhD; second instructor—MD MBTI: PhD	Both groups formal meditation: breathing, body scan, walking, and gentle yoga	None Provided additional sleep restriction and stimulus control instructions	Both groups Home practice: 30–35 min/d 6 d/wk Log: duration of meditation	Both groups A copy of book "Full Catastrophe Living," audio recordings for guided	A DSMB reviewed adverse events	Not reported

	experience MBTI: taught previous MBTI groups						meditation, handouts		
Wong et al,[65] 2016; Lee et al,[63] 2018	Not reported	Referred to training but did not provide details	Registered psychologist	Formal meditation: sitting, body scan, focused attention, 3-min breathing space	Practice before going to bed, after they awoke in the morning (out of the bed) and/or any other times during the day	Home practice: 3-min breathing space 3 times/d, listen to mindfulness audio 6 d/wk Log: not reported	Audio recordings for guided meditation	Not reported	Not reported
Wong et al,[59] 2017	2 y of experience teaching MBCT	Referred to qualified but did not provide details	Clinical psychologists	Formal meditation: eating, body scan, sitting, breathing, and walking, 3 min breathing space (80% of content was meditation)	Psychoeducation, sleep restriction and stimulus control instructions (20% of content was CBT-I)	Home practice: daily mediation practice Log: duration of meditation	Audio recordings for guided meditation	Adverse events tracked and none were reported	Not reported
Zhang, 2015	Not reported	Certified[a] MBSR instructor from CFM	Not reported	Formal meditation: sitting, standing, walking, and body scan	Not reported	Home practice: 45 min/d Log: not reported	Audio recordings for guided meditation	Not reported	Excluded if had previous contemplative, meditation, or Zen training

Abbreviations: ACT, acceptance and commitment therapy; CBT-I, cognitive behavioral therapy for insomnia; CFM, center for mindfulness; MBB, mind-body bridging; MBCT, mindfulness-based cognitive therapy; MBSR, mindfulness-based stress reduction; MBTI, mindfulness based therapy for insomnia; MD, Doctor of Medicine; MM, mindfulness meditation; PhD, Doctor of Philosophy.

[a] **This can range extensively from intensive programs offered at (or based on) the CFM in Medicine, Health Care, and Society at UMass Medical School to certificates provided by an online course necessitating** more specific information about credentials.

[b] Certification requires the completion of a Mind-Body Bridging training course, which consists of approximately 40 h of training.

Three trials reported on the effect of MBTs on sleep quality at 3-month follow-up,[56,60,65] and one trial at 2-month follow-up.[57] The effect of MBTs on sleep quality endured at follow-up (g = 0.81, 95% CI = 0.35–1.27, z = 3.43, $P < .01$) when pooled across inactive controls and psychological placebos (**Fig. 5**). It is important to note that one trial did not assess the control group at 3-month follow-up.[65]

Mindfulness Intervention Details and Sleep-Specific Components

Table 3 depicts the mindfulness intervention design features. The reporting of information related to instructor experience, mindfulness training, and clinical qualifications was highly variable and sometimes vague. Only 6 trials[52,55,56,58,61,65] reported specific instructions to practice mindfulness skills in bed or during the middle of the night if awake. When stated, home practice recommendations ranged from 10 to 45 minutes per day. A little more than half of the trials (n = 7)[51,52,55,59-61,64] reported using logs to track meditation practice, whereas only 3 trials tracked adverse events.[51,59,66] Only 4 trials reported whether previous/current meditation experience was an inclusion criteria.[53,57,60,62]

DISCUSSION

A systematic review of the literature for studies that reported on an MBT for the treatment of insomnia or sleep disturbance in adults yielded 13 trials published since 2010. Trials reported on diverse populations (eg, veterans, cancer survivors, individuals with fibromyalgia, and postmenopausal women) and used diverse MBTs (eg, MBSR, mindful bridging, MBCT, MBTI, ACT). Average trial quality was excellent, although substantial heterogeneity was observed between trials. Although the authors were unable to assess the effect of MBTs compared with other active treatments (such as cognitive behavior therapy for insomnia), the results of their meta-analysis indicated that MBTs are significantly more effective for reducing insomnia severity compared with attention/education and waitlist controls. The strength of this conclusion is limited by the significant heterogeneity among included trials. It can be concluded with stronger evidence that MBTs are significantly better than waitlist control groups and that the effects seem to be durable at 3 months postintervention. A similar pattern of results was observed for overall sleep quality.

This article represents an effort to present a unifying and testable theory for how mindfulness can be applied to the treatment of insomnia and sleep problems. MBTs are complimentary to behavioral and cognitive-behavioral approaches to treatment and can be used to augment existing treatments.[66,67] If MBTs operate at the level of psychological flexibility then they may exert their greatest effects on insomnia by facilitating patient adherence with challenging behavioral sleep interventions (eg, sleep restriction and stimulus control) while promoting mindful and nonjudgmental awareness of experience.[68] With this in mind, it will be important to progress from evaluating whether MBTs are effective for the treatment of insomnia and other sleep complaints to more refined questions as follows:

1. Are MBTs more effective when they are specifically tailored to sleep? Data pertaining to this question will inform whether mindfulness operates at the level of global psychological flexibility or psychological flexibility pertaining to solving the problem of perceived poor sleep.

Are MBTs an effective stand-alone treatment of insomnia? If so, does the addition of behavioral treatments for sleep significantly improve outcomes when added to MBTs?

What are the putative mechanisms (ie, processes of change) through which MBTs operate to improve sleep among individuals with insomnia or sleep disturbance?

For which individuals are MBTs most likely to be effective? For example, research evaluating MBTs for insomnia has focused on women (65% of the overall sample reviewed), and it is still unclear whether the effectiveness of MBTs for insomnia vary by patient sex.

Recommendation #1: Thoroughly Describe the Theory Justifying Why the MBT Being Tested Is Appropriate for the Treatment of Insomnia or Sleep Disturbance.

It behooves researchers to provide more detailed justification for why the MBT is being proposed as a treatment of insomnia and/or poor sleep in their population of choice. The PPMS presents several testable hypotheses related to the theorized processes of change that can guide future research in this area.

Recommendation #2: Describe Whether the MBT Has Been Modified to Specifically Target the Proposed Mechanisms of Change and Solidify These in Manuals that Can Be Adopted by Others.

Manualization is an important precursor to knowledge dissemination because it allows others to recreate the intervention and test its applicability with other clinical groups in research and real-world settings. The results of this review suggest that important information about how MBTs are being applied to the treatment of insomnia and sleep disturbance is not consistently reported.

This includes such information as whether people were being instructed to practice mindfulness before bed, while trying to sleep, or if they awaken during the night. This is not a small detail to overlook. Mindfulness as a practice is not specifically designed to assist with sleep onset in the same way as sleeping medication, and instruction to use it in this manner may be counterproductive. Further, mindfulness is not always conducive to the de-arousal that is required to facilitate sleep, especially in the skill development stage when people may get frustrated that the processes of letting go, nonattachment, and nonreactivity do not occur as naturally or quickly as they had hoped.[34] In this way, mindfulness close to, or while in bed, may actually make the process of sleep more difficult. It is also important to note that engaging in mindfulness practice is in contrast to instruction provided by stimulus control therapy, a standard treatment recommended by the American Academy of Sleep Medicine,[69] which recommends that the bed not be paired with anything other than sleep or sex. Perhaps there are people or situations for which one method might be preferred to the other. This is yet to be determined and will continue to be so until there is a better reporting of how mindfulness is being tailored to sleep and whether it is being advocated as a bona fide first-line treatment or adjuvant to traditionally used behavioral therapies.

Recommendation #3: Identify and Measure the Specific Sleep Targets that MBT Are Being Used to Address.

Future research is needed that moves beyond omnibus effects of MBTs for insomnia and toward the identification of mediators and moderators of treatment effects in order to better understand the process of change. The measurement of mindfulness has been criticized for being semantically ambiguous[2] yet most of the trials reviewed herein included general mindfulness measures. Mindfulness questionnaires do not consistently relate to the extent of mindfulness practice, have different response patterns in nonmeditators and those people with previous meditation experience, and may be especially influenced by social desirability.[2] Moreover, measures of mindfulness do not capture the range of putative mechanisms such as duration, frequency and setting of mindfulness practice, acceptance, and cognitive defusion that may underly the effects of MBTs for insomnia. Given the identified problems with measuring mindfulness, a shift toward measuring empirically supported processes of change such as those hypothesized in the PPMS is recommended. Identification of these targets, along with transparent reporting of parameters of mindfulness practice, would represent a movement toward precision medicine and facilitate further testing and refinement of interventions by allowing for (1) the development of comparison interventions that are matched for nonspecific factors and (2) determining the optimal dose and setting for mindfulness practice. A similar proposal has been made in the field of health behavior change.[70] Further, defining the mechanisms may inform future work to identify potential biological processes of change.

Recommendation #4: Pay Attention to the Issue of Clinician Training and Measure Treatment Fidelity.

Unlike with pharmacologic trials, nonpharmacologic treatments present difficulties due to complexity and variability of the intervention and interventionists. A meta-analysis of 46 studies with 1281 therapists and more than 14,000 patients reported that therapists account for 5% of variability in treatment outcomes.[71] Moreover, interventionist allegiance to therapies has been observed to account for 12% of variance in outcomes[72] and as much as a standardized mean difference in effect of 0.30.[73] Given the importance of therapist effects, assessing fidelity to the intervention protocol is essential to evaluate the feasibility and reproducibility of the intervention in clinical practice, as well as the true unbiased effect size. This issue is so important that it has become a recommended reporting standard for nonpharmacologic interventions.[74] This includes reporting on the credentials and training of the interventionist, as well as measuring fidelity to the principles of the intervention. More pragmatically, MBT instructors are often required to maintain their own meditation practice, which poses limits to the pool of available MBT providers and represents a potential barrier to the scalability of MBTs for insomnia.

Recommendation #5: Include Measures of Participant Expectancy and Participant Preference for Treatment.

Patient expectancy and preference are at the center of pluralistic field of psychological, behavioral, and complementary therapies; however, expectancy and preference have often been overlooked as important factors influencing outcomes in randomized trials, including those in the area of sleep medicine. Matching patients with their preferred treatment has been associated with increased retention[75,76] and improved outcomes in the treatment of psychological disorders.[77,78] Patient preference is particularly important for psychological or behavioral interventions such as MBTs, which require engagement and active participation.[79] When compared with cognitive behavioral therapy for insomnia, MBSR was not inferior at the 3-month follow-up point but only for those patients who were seeking or willing to try and persist in their assigned treatment approach.[53] This suggests that patient preferences have the potential to significantly affect treatment engagement and outcomes. Further, a recent meta-analysis demonstrated a strong expectancy/placebo effect for insomnia treatments.[80] As such, there is a need for studies that examine the role of patient preferences and expectancy in order to optimize treatment and answer important questions about how to best deliver these evidence-based interventions within the context of patient-centered care.

Recommendation #6: Avoid Assuming that MBT Are Devoid from the Potential for Harm and Specifically Ask About Adverse Events.

Only recently have sleep researchers investigating nonpharmacologic interventions for insomnia turned their attention to possible adverse effects of treatment. Specifically, a key component of CBT-I, sleep restriction, has been associated with acute reductions in objective total sleep time, increased daytime sleepiness, and objective performance impairment in some,[81,82] but not all,[83] trials. There is a similar concern of unintended harm being raised in the area of mindfulness research. Several potential harms, including depersonalization and reexperiencing of trauma, as a result of participating in MBTs have been reported, leading the NIH to caution that "meditation could cause or worsen certain psychiatric problems."[84] It is noted in a review that only 3 trials assessed adverse events. This is an area in need of immediate attention.

SUMMARY

MBTs are increasingly being investigated as a viable treatment of insomnia or sleep disturbance. To date, 13 trials have been published since 2010, and they suggest that MBTs are efficacious for improving symptoms of insomnia and sleep quality relative to psychological placebos and inactive control conditions with medium to large effects. Limited evidence suggests that these effects are sustained at 3-month follow-up. Despite this, limited data have been collected evaluating the empirically supported mechanisms or processes of change. As such, it is unclear whether MBTs have general effects that carry over to sleep or whether they target psychological processes that specifically facilitate sleep. The collection of such information is essential to move toward personalized medicine. With this in mind, the authors propose a testable model in the PPMS that they hope will advance the next generation of research into MBTs for insomnia. In order to accomplish this goal, it is incumbent on researchers to (1) adequately detail the rationale for the MBT being offered, (2) measure the putative mechanisms or processes of change, (3) ensure that the MBT is manualized and delivered in a standardized manner, (4) report interventionist qualifications and assess potential interventionist effects, and (5) evaluate the effect of patient preference or expectation.

CLINICS CARE POINTS

- Mindfulness-based therapies may be used to improve sleep and insomnia in some individuals, particularly those with a preference for these therapies or an expection of benefit.
- The quality of the program and it's inclusion of sleep specific components may affect the observed results.
- It is unclear whether mindfulness-based therapies directly improve sleep or improve other comorbid symptoms with the secondary benefit of sleep improvement.

DISCLOSURE

The authors do not have any commercial or financial conflicts of interest.

REFERENCES

1. Farb NAS. From retreat center to clinic to board room? Perils and promises of the modern mindful ness movement. Religions 2014;5(4):1062–86.
2. Van Dam NT, van Vugt MK, Vago DR, et al. Mind the hype: a critical evaluation and prescriptive agenda for research on mindfulness and meditation. PerSpect Psychol Sci 2018;13(1):36–61.
3. Davidson RJ, Kaszniak AW. Conceptual and methodological issues in research on mindfulness and meditation. Am Psychol 2015;70(7):581–92.
4. Dimidjian S, Linehan MM. Defining an agenda for future research on the clinical application of mindful ness practice. Clin Psychol Sci Pract 2003;10(2): 166–71.
5. Kabat-Zinn J. Full catastrophe living (revised version): using the wisdom of your body and mind to face stress, pain, and illness. New York: Bantam Books; 2013.
6. Lutz A, Jha AP, Dunne JD, et al. Investigating the phenomenological matrix of mindfulness-related

practices from a neurocognitive perspective. Am Psychol 2015;70(7):632–58.

7. Borbely AA, Daan S, Wirz-Justice A, et al. The two-process model of sleep regulation: a reappraisal. J Sleep Res 2016;25(2):131–43.
8. Espie CA. Insomnia: conceptual issues in the devel opment, persistence, and treatment of sleep disor der in adults. Annu Rev Psychol 2002;53:215–43.
9. Perlis ML, Ellis JG, Kloss JD, et al. Etiology and pathophysiology of insomnia. In: Kryger M, Roth T, Dement WC, editors. Principles and practice of sleep medicine. 6th edition. Philadelphia: Elsevier; 2017. p. 769–84.
10. Perlis ML, Giles DE, Mendelson WB, et al. Psycho physiological insomnia: the behavioural model and a neurocognitive perspective. J Sleep Res 1997; 6(3):179–88.
11. Riemann D, Spiegelhalder K, Feige B, et al. The hy perarousal model of insomnia: a review of the concept and its evidence. Sleep Med Rev 2010; 14(1):19–31.
12. Bonnet MH, Arand DL. Hyperarousal and insomnia: state of the science. Sleep Med Rev 2010;14(1): 9–15.
13. Spielman AJ, Caruso LS, Glovinsky PB. A behavioral perspective on insomnia treatment. Psychiatr Clin North Am 1987;10(4):541–53.
14. Spielman AJ, Yang C, Glovinsky PB. Assessment techniques for insomnia. In: Kryger M, Roth T, Dement WC, editors. Principles and practice of sleep medicine. 5th edition. Philadelphia: Elsevier; 2011. p. 1632–45.
15. Buysse DJ, Germain A, Hall M, et al. A neurobiological model of insomnia. Drug Discov Today Dis Models 2011;8(4):129–37.
16. Harvey AG. A cognitive model of insomnia. Behav Res Ther 2002;40(8):869–93.
17. Lundh LG, Broman JE. Insomnia as an interaction between sleep-interfering and sleep-interpreting processes. J Psychosom Res 2000;49(5):299–310.
18. Morin CM, Espie CA. Insomnia: a clinical guide to assessment and treatment. New York: Kluwer Academic; 2004.
19. Ong JC, Ulmer CS, Manber R. Improving sleep with mindfulness and acceptance: a metacognitive model of insomnia. Behav Res Ther 2012;50(11): 651–60.
20. Carney CE, Edinger JD, Morin CM, et al. Examining maladaptive beliefs about sleep across insomnia patient groups. J Psychosom Res 2010;68(1):57–65.
21. Morin CM, Stone J, Trinkle D, et al. Dysfunctional be liefs and attitudes about sleep among older adults with and without insomnia complaints. Psychol Ag Ing 1993;8(3):463–7.
22. Harvey AG. Pre-sleep cognitive activity: a comparison of sleep-onset insomniacs and good sleepers. Br J Clin Psychol 2000;39(Pt 3):275–86.
23. Kuisk LA, Bertelson AD, Walsh JK. Presleep cogni tive hyperarousal and affect as factors in objective and subjective insomnia. Percept Mot Skills 1989; 69(3 Pt 2):1219–25.
24. Broomfield NM, Espie CA. Towards a valid, reliable measure of sleep effort. J Sleep Res 2005;14(4): 401–7.
25. Lundh LG. The role of acceptance and mindfulness in the treatment of insomnia. J Cogn Psychother 2005;19(1):29–39.
26. Harvey AG. I can't sleep, mymins is racing! an investigation of strategies of thought control in insomnia. Behav Cogn Psychother 2001;29(1):3–11.
27. Nicassio PM, Mendlowitz DR, Fussell JJ, et al. The phenomenology of the pre-sleep state: the development of the pre-sleep arousal scale. Behav Res Ther 1985;23(3):263–71.
28. Taylor DJ, Lichstein KL, Durrence HH, et al. Epide miology of insomnia, depression, and anxiety. Sleep 2005;28(11):1457–64.
29. Thomsen DK, Mehlsen MY, Christensen S, et al. Rumination—relationship with negative mood and sleep quality. Personal Individual Dif 2003;34(7): 1293–301.
30. Carney CE, Edinger JD, Meyer B, et al. Symptom-focused rumination and sleep disturbance. Behav Sleep Med 2006;4(4):228–41.
31. Hayes SC, Luoma JB, Bond FW, et al. Acceptance and commitment therapy: model, processes and outcomes. Behav Res Ther 2006;44(1):1–25.
32. Hayes SC, Villatte M, Levin M, et al. Open, aware, and active: contextual approaches as an emerging trend in the behavioral and cognitive therapies. Annu Rev Clin Psychol 2011;7:141–68.
33. McCracken LM, Williams JL, Tang NKY. Psychological flexibility may reduce insomnia in persons with chronic pain: a preliminary retrospective study. Pain Med 2011;12(6):904–12.
34. Lundh LG. Insomnia. In: McCracken LM, editor. Mindfulness and acceptacne in behavioral medicine: current theory and practice. Oakland (CA): New Harbinger; 2011. p. 131–58.
35. McCracken LM, Vowles KE. Acceptance and commitment therapy and mindfulness for chronic pain: model, process, and progress. Am Psychol 2014;69(2):178–87.
36. Harvey AG, Buysse DJ. Treating sleep problems: a transdiagnostic approach. New York: Guilford Publications; 2017.
37. Riemann D. Insomnia and comorbid psychiatric dis orders. Sleep Med 2007;8(Suppl 4):S15–20.
38. Taylor DJ, Mallory LJ, Lichstein KL, et al. Comorbid ity of chronic insomnia with medical problems. Sleep 2007;30(2):213–8.
39. Daly-Eichenhardt A, Scott W, Howard-Jones M, et al. Changes in sleep problems and psychological flex ibility following interdisciplinary acceptance and

commitment therapy for chronic pain: an observa tional cohort study. Front Psychol 2016;7:1326.
40. Gong H, Ni CX, Liu YZ, et al. Mindfulness meditation for insomnia: a meta-analysis of randomized controlled trials. J Psychosom Res 2016;89:1–6.
41. Haller H, Winkler MM, Klose P, et al. Mindfulness-based interventions for women with breast cancer: an updated systematic review and meta-analysis. Acta Oncol 2017;56(12):1665–76.
42. American Psychiatry Association A. Diagnostic and statistical manual of mental disorders: DSM-IV. Washington, DC: American Psychiatry Association; 1994.
43. Association ASD. The international classification of sleep disorders: diagnostic and coding manual. 2nd edition. New York: American Sleep Disorders Association; 2005.
44. Hays RD, Martin SA, Sesti AM, et al. Psychometric properties of the medical outcomes study sleep measure. Sleep Med 2005;6(1). 41—4.
45. Buysse DJ, Reynolds CF 3rd, Monk TH, et al. The Pittsburgh sleep quality index: a new instrument for psychiatric practice and research. Psychiatry Res 1989;28(2):193–213.
46. Yates SL, Morley S, Eccleston C, et al. A scale for rating the quality of psychological trials for pain. Pain 2005;117(3):314–25.
47. Lipsey MW, Wilson DB. Practical meta-analysis. Thousand Oaks (CA): Sage Publications, Inc; 2001.
48. Higgins JP, Green S. Cochrane handbook for sys te-matic reviews of interventions. Wiley Online Li- brary: Cochrane Collaboration; 2008.
49. Orwin RG. A fail-safe N for effect size in meta-analysis. J Educ Stat 1983;8(2):157–9.
50. Higgins JP, Thompson SG. Quantifying heterogene ity in a meta-analysis. Stat Med 2002;21(11): 1539–58.
51. Black DS, O'Reilly GA, Olmstead R, et al. Mindfulness meditation and improvement in sleep quality and daytime impairment among older adults with sleep disturbances: a randomized clinical trial. JAMA Intern Med 2015;175(4):494–501.
52. Garcia MC, Kozasa EH, Tufik S, et al. The effects of mindfulness and relaxation training for insomnia (MRTI) on postmenopausal women: a pilot study. Menopause 2018;25(9):992–1003.
53. Garland SN, Carlson LE, Stephens AJ, et al. Mindfulness-based stress reduction compared with cogni tive behavioral therapy for the treatment of insomnia comorbid with cancer: a randomized, partially blinded, noninferiority trial. J Clin Oncol 2014; 32(5):449–57.
54. Garland SN, Rouleau CR, Campbell T, et al. The comparative impact of mindfulness-based cancer recovery (MBCR) and cognitive behavior therapy for insomnia (CBT-I) on sleep and mindfulness in cancer patients. Explore (NY) 2015;11(6):445–54.
55. Gross CR, Kreitzer MJ, Reilly-Spong M, et al. Mindfulness-based stress reduction versus pharmacotherapy for chronic primary insomnia: a randomized controlled clinical trial. Explore (NY) 2011;7(2): 76–87.
56. Nakamura Y, Lipschitz DL, Donaldson GW, et al. Investigating clinical benefits of a novel sleep-focused mind-body program on gulf war illness symptoms: a randomized controlled trial. PsychoSom Med 2017;79(6):706–18.
57. Nakamura Y, Lipschitz DL, Kuhn R, et al. Investigating efficacy of two brief mind-body intervention programs for managing sleep disturbance in cancer survivors: a pilot randomized controlled trial. J Cancer Surviv 2013;7(2):165–82.
58. Nakamura Y, Lipschitz DL, Landward R, et al. Two sessions of sleep-focused mind-body bridging improve self-reported symptoms of sleep and PTSD in veterans: a pilot randomized controlled trial. J Psychosom Res 2011;70(4):335–45.
59. Wong SY, Zhang DX, Li CC, et al. Comparing the effects of mindfulness-based cognitive therapy and sleep psycho-education with exercise on chronic insomnia: a randomised controlled trial. Psychother Psychosom 2017;86(4):241–53.
60. Amutio A, Franco C, Sanchez-Sanchez LC, et al. Ef fects of mindfulness training on sleep problems in patients with fibromyalgia. Front Psychol 2018;9: 1365.
61. deok Baik K. Evaluating acceptance and commitment therapy for insomnia: a randomized controlled trial. Bowling Green (OH): Bowling Green State University; 2015.
62. Zhang JX, Liu XH, Xie XH, et al. Mindfulness-based stress reduction for chronic insomnia in adults older than 75 years: a randomized, controlled, single-blind clinical trial. Explore (NY) 2015;11(3):180–5.
63. Lee CW, Ree MJ, Wong MY. Effective insomnia treatments: investigation of processes in mindfulness and cognitive therapy. Behav Change 2018;35(2): 1–20.
64. Ong JC, Xia Y, Smith-Mason CE, et al. A randomized controlled trial of mindfulness meditation for chronic insomnia: effects on daytime symptoms and cognitive-emotional arousal. Mindfulness 2018;9(6): 1 11.
65. Wong MY, Ree MJ, Lee CW. Enhancing CBT for chronic insomnia: a randomised clinical trial of addi tive components of mindfulness or cognitive ther apy. Clin Psychol Psychother 2016;23(5): 377–85.
66. Ong JC, Manber R, Segal Z, et al. A randomized controlled trial of mindfulness meditation for chronic insomnia. Sleep 2014;37(9):1553–63.

67. Ong JC. Mindfulness-based therapy for insomnia. Washington, DC: American Psychological Association; 2017.
68. Dalrymple KL, Fiorentino L, Politi MC, et al. Incorporating principles from acceptance and commitment therapy into cognitive-behavioral therapy for insomnia: a case example. J Contemp Psychother 2010;40(4):209–17.
69. Morgenthaler T, Kramer M, Alessi C, et al. Practice parameters for the psychological and behavioral treatment of insomnia: an update. An American Academy of Sleep Medicine Report. Sleep 2006; 29(11):1415–9.
70. Sheeran P, Klein WM, Rothman AJ. Health behavior change: moving from observation to intervention. Annu Rev Psychol 2017;68:573–600.
71. Baldwin SA, Imel ZE. Therapist effects: findings and methods. 5th edition. Hoboken (NJ): Wiley; 2013.
72. Munder T, Fluckiger C, Gerger H, et al. Is the allegiance effect an epiphenomenon of true efficacy differences between treatments? A meta-analysis. J Couns Psychol 2012;59(4):631–7.
73. Falkenstrom F, Markowitz JC, Jonker H, et al. Can psychotherapists function as their own controls? Meta-analysis of the crossed therapist design in comparative psychotherapy trials. J Clin Psychiatry 2013;74(5):482–91.
74. Boutron I, Moher D, Altman DG, et al. Extending the CONSORT statement to randomized trials of nonpharmacologic treatment: explanation and elabora tion. Ann Intern Med 2008;148(4):295–309.
75. Sidani S, Bootzin RR, Epstein DR, et al. Attrition in randomized and preference trials of behavioural treatments for insomnia. Can J Nurs Res 2015; 47(1):17–34.
76. Steidtmann D, Manber R, Arnow BA, et al. Patient treatment preference as a predictor of response and attrition in treatment for chronic depression. Depress Anxiety 2012;29(10):896–905.
77. McHugh RK, Whitton SW, Peckham AD, et al. Patient preference for psychological vs pharmacologic treatment of psychiatric disorders: a meta-analytic review. J Clin Psychiatry 2013;74(6):595–602.
78. Williams R, Farquharson L, Palmer L, et al. Patient preference in psychological treatment and associations with self-reported outcome: national cross-sectional survey in England and Wales. BMC Psy chiatry 2016;16:4.
79. Kowalski CJ, Mrdjenovich AJ. Patient preference clinical trials: why and when they will sometimes be preferred. Perspect Biol Med 2013;56(1):18–35.
80. Yeung V, Sharpe L, Glozier N, et al. A systematic re view and meta-analysis of placebo versus no treat ment for insomnia symptoms. Sleep Med Rev 2018;38:17–27.
81. Kyle SD, Miller CB, Rogers Z, et al. Sleep restric- tion therapy for insomnia is associated with reduced objective total sleep time, increased daytime somnolence, and objectively impaired vigilance: implications for the clinical manage- ment of insomnia disorder. Sleep 2014;37(2):229–37.
82. Kyle SD, Morgan K, Spiegelhalder K, et al. No pain, no gain: an exploratory within-subjects mixed-methods evaluation of the patient experience of sleep restriction therapy (SRT) for insomnia. Sleep Med 2011;12(8):735–47.
83. Whittall H, Pillion M, Gradisar M. Daytime sleepiness, driving performance, reaction time and inhibitory control during sleep restriction therapy for Chronic Insomnia Disorder. Sleep Med 2018;45: 44–8. *A A Q.*
84. Health NCfCaI. Meditatin: in depth. 2017. NCCIH Pub No.: D308. Available at: https://nccih.nih.gov/health/meditation/overview.htm#hed5. Accessed October 10, 2018.

Cognitive Behavioral Therapy for Insomnia in School-Aged Children and Adolescents

Julia Dewald-Kaufmann, PhD[a,b,*], Ed de Bruin, PhD[c], Gradisar Michael, PhD[d]

KEYWORDS

• Insomnia • Children • Adolescents • Sleep problems
• Cognitive behavioral therapy for insomnia (CBT-i)

KEY POINTS

- Insomnia is a common sleep disorder in school-aged children and adolescents with severe consequences on daytime functioning.
- Diagnostic tools should include clinical interviews, questionnaires, and sleep diaries. Objective sleep assessments (actigraphy, polysomnography) can additionally be used, especially when other sleep disorders (eg, sleep apnea) may be suspected.
- Cognitive behavioral therapy for insomnia (CBT-i) seems to be effective in school-aged children and adolescents; however, only a limited number of randomized controlled trials exist.
- More replication research, especially in clinical settings, is needed to systematically evaluate the effects of CBT-i in children and adolescents.

INTRODUCTION

One of the most prevalent sleep disorders in children and adolescents is "insomnia," which can be briefly described as problems with initiating and/or maintaining sleep with associated daytime consequences. These are typical insomnia symptoms, and when experienced for long enough and when they interfere with an important area of the young person's life (eg, schooling), then a diagnosis of an insomnia disorder may be warranted. The prevalence rates of insomnia symptoms are high and range up to 30% in children[1–3] and from ~ 40%[4] to 66%[5] in adolescents, whereas prevalence rates for the full insomnia disorder diagnosis vary between ~ 9% and 23%.[4,6–8] Differences in prevalence rates may be explained by differences in assessment methods and definitions of "sleep problems" and "insomnia" (eg, assessment of symptoms or sleep disorders, using different diagnostic classifications).[6,9] If not treated, insomnia symptoms during childhood and adolescence are often persistent and constitute a risk factor for negative daytime consequences, including cognitive deficits, behavioral problems, school problems, somatic problems, and emotional problems.[10–15] Although an insomnia disorder includes both problems with initiating and/or maintaining sleep, school-aged children and adolescents mostly suffer from

Sleep Med Clin 14 (2019) 155–165 https://doi.org/10.1016/j.jsmc.2019.02.002 1556-407X/19/© 2019 Elsevier Inc.

[a] Department of Psychiatry and Psychotherapy, University Hospital, LMU Munich, Nussbaumstr. 7, Munich 80336, Germany; [b] Hochschule Fresenius, University of Applied Sciences, Infanteriestr. 11a, Munich 80797, Germany; [c] Research Institute of Child Development and Education, University of Amsterdam, Nieuwe Achtergracht 127, Amsterdam 1018 WS, the Netherlands; [d] School of Psychology, Flinders University, GPO Box 2100, Adelaide 5001, South Australia

* Corresponding author. Department of Psychiatry and Psychotherapy, University Hospital, LMU Munich, Nussbaumstr. 7, Munich 80336, Germany.

E-mail address: Julia.dewald-kaufmann@hs-fresenius.de

Sleep Med Clin 17 (2022) 355–365
https://doi.org/10.1016/j.jsmc.2022.06.003
1556-407X/22/© 2022 Elsevier Inc.

problems with initiating sleep. In addition, children often have behavioral difficulties including bedtime resistance and reluctance/refusal to sleep alone.[1,16]

In the second edition of the International Classification of Sleep Disorders-2 (ICSD-2),[17] the diagnosis of Behavioral Insomnia of Childhood (with limit-setting and sleep-onset association type) captured sleep problems of school-aged children and young adolescents quite well. Indeed, many types of insomnia disorders were provided in the ICSD-2. However, with the introduction of the third edition (ICSD-3), most insomnia disorders were removed in favor of a more simplified approach. This meant specific insomnia disorder subtypes and a special pediatric category no longer exist in the ICSD-3, in which simply a distinction is now made between short-term insomnia and chronic insomnia.[18] These two diagnoses solely differ on the criteria of frequency (chronic insomnia requires sleeping problems at least three times per week) and the time frame criterion of problems lasting for at least 3 months for chronic insomnia. Most children and adolescents who seek treatment experience sleep problems over a longer time period and therefore fulfill the criteria of a chronic insomnia diagnosis. For example, Paine and Gradisar[16] found that school-aged children with insomnia were experiencing their sleep problem for 5.7 years, indicating an average age of onset at 3.7 years. Although different etiologic adult models[19] and attempts for models in young children exist,[20] no specific model for school-aged children and adolescents has been developed so far, but an interplay of multiple intrinsic and extrinsic factors is assumed to be crucial.

The recommended first-line treatment of insomnia in adults is cognitive behavioral therapy for insomnia (CBT-i),[21,22] which is a non-pharmacologic treatment that aims to change behavioral (eg, sleep hygiene, bedtime routine) and cognitive (eg, modification of thoughts) patterns to improve the individual's sleep. Adult studies show that CBT-i has beneficial and clinically meaningful effects on sleep[22–25] and even on cognitive performance.[26] Furthermore, the effects of CBT-i do not have the drawbacks of pharmacotherapy, such as habituation and dependence.[22,27] However, the number of studies systematically evaluating the effects of CBT-i in children and adolescents is relatively small, and so far no consensus statement has been published for these age groups, which may be because there are so few studies with these populations, however, this may change. Meltzer and Mindell[28] published a systematic review and meta-analysis on sleep treatments in children and adolescents, which showed that 12 of the 16 included studies focused on infants and young children (birth to 5 years), whereas only 4 studies addressed school-aged children. No randomized controlled trial (RCT) with adolescents could be included in their study at that time. Furthermore, out of the four studies on school-aged children, only one study applied CBT-i explicitly[16] and one study used a brief sleep intervention, which included aspects of CBT-i.[29] A more recent systematic review on CBT-i in adolescents included nine studies investigating the effects of CBT-i in adolescents,[30] with only one RCT that applied CBT-i in adolescents with insomnia without a comorbid disorder.[31]

Before considering CBT-i as a treatment option, children and adolescents should be screened, optimally by parent reports and self-reports, and if necessary treated for physical conditions (eg, allergies, breathing problems, chronic illnesses) that can cause sleeping problems. Because it has been shown that improving sleep has beneficial effects on emotional problems (eg, mood, anxiety),[16,32,33] it is recommended to treat insomnia problems even if it co-occurs with other mental disorders. Still, clinicians should keep comorbidity and situational influences in mind and adapt treatment individually, when needed. In children and adolescents with complaints indicating a delayed sleep-wake phase disorder, dim light melatonin onset (DLMO) should also be assessed, because patients may need exogenous melatonin to fall asleep.[34,35] If a circadian rhythm delay is suspected, the authors recommend clinicians to treat this factor before undertaking CBT-i with the following paper contained within this journal.[36] The diagnostic process of insomnia optimally includes screening questionnaires (self-reports and parent reports), a clinical interview, and sleep diaries (**Table 1**).

In this article, the authors first review the evidence for cognitive and behavioral trials for school-aged children and adolescents and then discuss the practical application of these techniques in each of these populations.

COGNITIVE BEHAVIORAL THERAPY FOR INSOMNIA IN SCHOOL-AGED CHILDREN

Empirical Evidence

The age range of school-aged children recruited into clinical trials evaluating CBT-i has ranged between 5 and 13 years of age.[16,45] It is suggested that fewer school-aged children will be able to grasp the concepts and skills needed for complex cognitive therapy skills, yet this is likely to increase from age 7 years.[16] It is also recognized that the

Table 1
Diagnostic tools used in the diagnostic process of insomnia in school-aged children and adolescents

Assessment Tool	
Sleep disorders and sleep disturbances questionnaires[3]	*Specification of Assessment*
	Sleep Disturbance Scale for Children[37]*:* 6.5–15.3 y, parent report *Children's Sleep Habit Questionnaire*[38]*:* 4–12 y, parent report *Behavioral Evaluation of Disorders of Sleep Scale*[39]*:* 5–12 y, parent report
Sleepiness questionnaires[a]	*Cleveland Adolescent Sleepiness Questionnaire*[40]*:* 11–17 y, self-report *Pediatric Daytime Sleepiness Scale*[41]*:* 11–15 y, self-report
Sleep hygiene	*Adolescent Sleep Hygiene Scale*[42]*:* 12–18 y, self-report
Clinical interview	Sleep schedule (bedtime, wake time, naps), evening activities (eg, exercise, social media use, TV), bedtime routine, sleeping environment (eg, lighting, temperature, adequate sleep opportunity), nature of sleep problem (eg, initiating and/or maintaining sleep), night time fears, bedtime refusal and/or need for parental presence, sleepiness and daytime impairments that target diagnostic criteria (eg, emotional problems, school performance), safety behaviors (eg, caffeine, alcohol, medication use), family and social functioning (eg, stress, life events). Information on what measures have already been taken to improve sleep; prior sleep therapies. Information from parents and teachers on daytime functioning can also be helpful. The clinical interview should also be used to screen for other sleep disorders (eg, apnea, narcolepsy) that should be treated differently.
Sleep diaries[b]	Bedtime, sleep onset latency, number and duration of night time awakenings, wake time, sleep duration, naps. Separate assessment for weekdays and weekends are needed, especially for adolescents.
Actigraphy	Objective assessment of bedtime, sleep onset latency, number and duration of night time awakenings, wake time, sleep duration, and naps can provide additional information. Separate assessment for weekdays and weekends are needed. Actigraphy always requires information from sleep diaries.
Polysomnography	Gives information about sleep architecture, sleep quality, and other sleep-related characteristics (eg, breathing). Can be considered if other sleep disorders (eg, sleep apnea) are suspected.
Other technologies (eg, apps, Fitbit)	Aim to measure sleep and wake times; however, their reliability and validity for sleep have not been established. These technologies are therefore not advised for sleep assessment.

[a] Further information and a systematically evaluated list of sleep questionnaires can be found in Spruyt and Gozal, 2011.[43]
[b] See, for example, Carney et al, 2012.[44]

upper end of this age range overlaps with early adolescence (denoted by the onset of puberty). For older school-aged children, the evidence is reviewed here based on the facts that (1) these children do not possess a delayed circadian rhythm contributing to their sleep problem and (2) these children's worries are more centered on issues common in younger school-aged children (eg, fears of harm to self or family members, fears of separation from parents).

Besides the relatively high prevalence rates and the effectiveness of CBT-i in adults, only two RCTs have been conducted to investigate the effectiveness of CBT-i in school-aged children.[28] In the first study, Paine and Gradisar[16] had 42 children between 7 and 13 years randomly assigned to receive either six sessions of CBT-i or a waiting list control group. Their results indicate positive effects in the CBT-i group for sleep (sleep latency, wake after sleep onset, sleep efficiency) and anxiety. These improvements were maintained at the 1-month and 6-month follow-ups. However, no changes occurred in total sleep time. In one other RCT, school-aged children with insomnia were treated with CBT-i: Schlarb and colleagues[45] implemented CBT-i, consisting of three sessions for children and three for parents in 112 children (age range 5–11.5 years). Interventions in this study included sleep restriction, stimulus control therapy, sleep hygiene, relaxation, and cognitive therapy. Results from this study show improvements in sleep problems, sleep onset latency, sleep efficiency, and nocturnal awakenings, but, similar to the study by Paine and Gradisar[16] no changes in total sleep time were found. Improvements persisted also at the 3-, 6-, and 12-month follow-up assessments. In summary, the limited empirical evidence for CBT-i in school-aged children points toward beneficial effects when treating insomnia; however, more controlled intervention studies are needed to further support these findings. Although other studies have applied sleep interventions for school-aged children (for a review, see Ref[28]), these studies (1) did not necessarily focus on children diagnosed with (only) insomnia and/or (2) did not use a combination of behavioral and cognitive techniques. Nevertheless, they frequently used the same techniques as those in the reviewed RCTs and likewise found positive effects on sleep.

Practical Application of Cognitive Behavioral Therapy for Insomnia in School-Aged Children

Concerning school-aged children's sleep, parents' behavior plays an essential role.[46] Often parents are not aware of their dysfunctional parenting behavior and develop or maintain a child's sleep problem (eg, child refuses to sleep in the absence of the parent). Furthermore, parents can forget to positively reinforce healthy sleep behaviors (eg, child goes to bed independently, child sleeps through the night). Thus, children with sleeping problems may experience an imbalance of little positive reinforcement of desirable sleep behaviors and yet too much positive reinforcement of undesirable behaviors, which may perpetuate the sleeping problems. Therefore, CBT-i for school-age children includes both interventions that relate to the parents and interventions that relate to the child.

Children with insomnia often have problems with initiating sleep, which may take the form of long sleep latencies when trying to sleep independently of a parent. This problem can be addressed by faded bedtimes, an intervention in which bedtimes are scheduled at a later time so the child becomes more sleepy when attempting sleep.[47,48] This technique aims to increase children's sleep pressure and consequently decrease sleep onset latencies and is similar to sleep restriction therapy for adolescents and adults.[49] After sleep latencies decrease, bedtimes can gradually be shifted to an earlier time point, where there is a balance between an appropriate amount of time to fall asleep (eg, <20 min) and no daytime consequences. The implementation of a positive routine before the child's bedtime is also considered to have positive effects on children's sleep, because children enter their bed more relaxed. Consequently, a positive association with the sleeping process (here lying in bed) may occur. Furthermore, moving rewarding components (positive activity with the parent) to a daytime activity helps to extinguish its association with sleep.[47] This intervention is similar to stimulus control therapy for adolescents and adults.[50,51] Positive reinforcement also plays a role when it comes to graduated extinction, during which children are gradually exposed to sleeping alone in their bed, whereas negative reinforcement (reduced anxiety due to parental attendance) is removed and replaced by positive reinforcement (eg, rewards for successful achievements and practices).[16] **Table 2** provides the step-by-step instructions for both faded bedtimes and graduated extinction.

Because many children suffer from unpleasant, sleep incompatible feelings and thoughts (eg, "If *I do not fall asleep I will fail at school"),* one important cognitive technique is thought challenging. In the first step, the dysfunctional thought is identified and then in the second step challenged by looking for evidence and against these thoughts and/or even replacing it with a more functional/helpful thought. **Box 1** presents a clinical example of thought challenging for a 10-year-old patient with insomnia. As mentioned previously, school-aged children are more likely to engage with cognitive therapy techniques as they become older. As a general rule of thumb, these techniques can be used with children aged 7 years and older,[16] but there are also capable 6-year-olds who can elicit and challenge thoughts and likewise 9-year-olds (and even adults) who have difficulty with such techniques.

Table 2
Stepwise procedure: faded bedtimes and graduated extinction

Faded Bedtimes	Graduated Extinction
1. Delay the child's bedtime by 15 min and keep this new bedtime consistent for 1 wk. 2. Ensure the child's wake up time is consistent across the 7 d of the wk. 3. Avoid the child napping 4. After 1 wk, if the child's sleep latency is >20 min, repeat Step 1 above 5. If the child's sleep latency becomes <20 min, keep to this new bedtime. 6. If daytime consequences occur (eg, sleepiness at school), then advance bedtimes by 15 min for 1 wk 7. Continue Step 6 if daytime consequences still occur 8. The goal is to strike the balance between the length of the child's sleep latency and the severity and/or frequency of their daytime consequences	1. If a child is in the parent's bed, move them to a mattress on the floor next to the parent. After practicing this step to a point where the child is experiencing less fear/anxiety, move the mattress near the bedroom door (either inside or outside the bedroom). After this is practiced enough, move the mattress further toward the child's bedroom (eg, a room near the parents' bedroom). When practiced enough, keep gradually moving the mattress closer to the child's bedroom, until they are in their own bed. *Note*: often a family might decide to go from parents' bed to a room next to the parents' bed, and then straight to the child's bedroom, as it is more convenient. 2. If a child is in their own bedroom, but needs the parent close by, then the following steps can be taken: a. Parent may be lying down under the covers with the child. b. Parent lies down on top of the covers with the child. c. Parent sits up on top of the covers with the child. d. Parent sits next to the bed, but lays their hand on the child. e. Parent sits next to the bed, but no contact with the child. f. Parent sits near the end of the child's bed or near the bedroom door. g. Parent is outside the bedroom door (eg, sitting on a chair). h. Parent gets to reclaim their night and do what they want for themselves.

(*continued on next page*)

In addition to these behavioral and cognitive interventions, CBT-i includes psychoeducation, especially on sleep hygiene, which refers to information about sleeping behaviors and the bedtime routine, because it has been shown that children and adolescents with insomnia often suffer from poor sleep hygiene.[52,53] The general sleep hygiene rules, which should be adapted for each age group, are shown in **Box 2**. In addition, it is important to inform children and their parents about various aspects of sleep, including individual differences in sleep need, sleep homeostatic pressure (as a treatment rationale for faded bedtime), and sleep architecture (ie, cycling from light-to-deep-to-light stages of sleep). Psychoeducation, and especially sleep hygiene rules, should be provided and discussed in detail before the other CBT-i interventions, as understanding the underlying mechanisms may increase motivation and compliance.

Box 1
Thought challenging of a child

Therapist: What worries you about not being able to fall asleep quickly at night?

Child: That I won't get enough sleep and fail my Maths test.

Therapist: So, every night you have a bad sleep, you're likely to fail a test?

Child: Maybe.

Therapist: OK, so what we can do is see how true that thought is by looking at what's happened in the past. How many times have you failed your test?

Child: Once.

Therapist: OK. So earlier, your mum said that you've had a sleep problem for the last 2 years.

How many tests have you had in the past 2 years?

Child: Ummm... probably, about 10.

Therapist: So, you have five tests each year?

Child: I guess not. Maybe it is like 12 or 13.

Maybe 14?

Therapist: OK. But even so. Although you have had a sleep problem over the past 2 years, you have failed 1 test out of about 14.

Child: Yeah.

Therapist: So even though you have slept not so great, you passed 13 tests out of 14.

Child: Yeah, I guess I have.

Therapist: So what are the chances of passing a test, even if you have not slept so great?

Child: I guess they are not so bad.

Box 2
Sleep hygiene rules

- A continuous place to sleep (eg, children and adolescents should have their own bed)
- Regular bedtimes: Bedtimes should be roughly the same each day (also on weekends)
- Avoidance of lying in bed for too long (eg, >30 min), waiting to fall asleep
- Sleep supporting environment (eg, cool air temperature, very dim to no light, minimal noise/sound)
- Avoidance of drinks with caffeine
- Reduction of light before bedtimes (including TV, smartphone, computer usage)
- Reduction of stimulating activities before bedtimes
- Adequate physical activity during the day
- No napping throughout the day

COGNITIVE BEHAVIORAL THERAPY FOR INSOMNIA IN ADOLESCENTS

Empirical Evidence

Similar to the research on CBT-i in children, the scientific literature on the effectiveness of CBT-i in adolescents is rare. Given the positive results from the adult literature and the high prevalence rates of insomnia in adolescents, this constitutes a rather surprising finding. In a recent meta-analysis, Blake and colleagues[30] found nine studies that used adolescent cognitive behavioral sleep interventions, which included only four RCTs, and only one of these RCTs included adolescents with an isolated insomnia diagnosis.[31] The other studies that included adolescents with "insomnia symptoms"/"sleep problems" (with or without comorbid conditions),[50,54–57] adolescents with insomnia and a comorbid psychiatric diagnosis,[58] adolescents with delayed sleep phase disorder[59] were pilot studies[54,57,58,60] and/or uncontrolled studies.[50,54,56,57,61] Still, the results from this meta-analysis showed preliminary positive effects for CBT-i in adolescents, which can be seen in increased sleep durations, decreased sleep onset latencies, decreased wake times after sleep onset, and thus improved sleep efficiency. Furthermore, positive effects were found for sleep quality and daytime functioning, including daytime sleepiness and depressive and anxiety symptoms.[62]

Focusing on the only RCT to date that included adolescents with an insomnia diagnosis, de Bruin and colleagues[31] compared CBT-i (provided as online therapy or group therapy) with a waiting list control group in a sample of 116 adolescents (age range: 12–19 years). The intervention lasted for six treatment sessions over 6 weeks, as well as a booster session 2 months after the last treatment session. The program included the following components: psychoeducation/sleep hygiene advice, exercise for worry, thought challenging (ie, cognitive therapy), mindfulness-based relaxation, restriction of time in bed, stimulus control, and finally relapse prevention. Compared with the waiting list control group, both treatment groups improved significantly on sleep efficiency, sleep onset latency, wake after sleep onset, and total sleep time.[31] These improvements were maintained up to a 1-year follow-up, and improvements were also found in symptoms of psychopathology.[33] Using Internet-based CBT-i was shown to be more cost-effective than group therapy,[63]

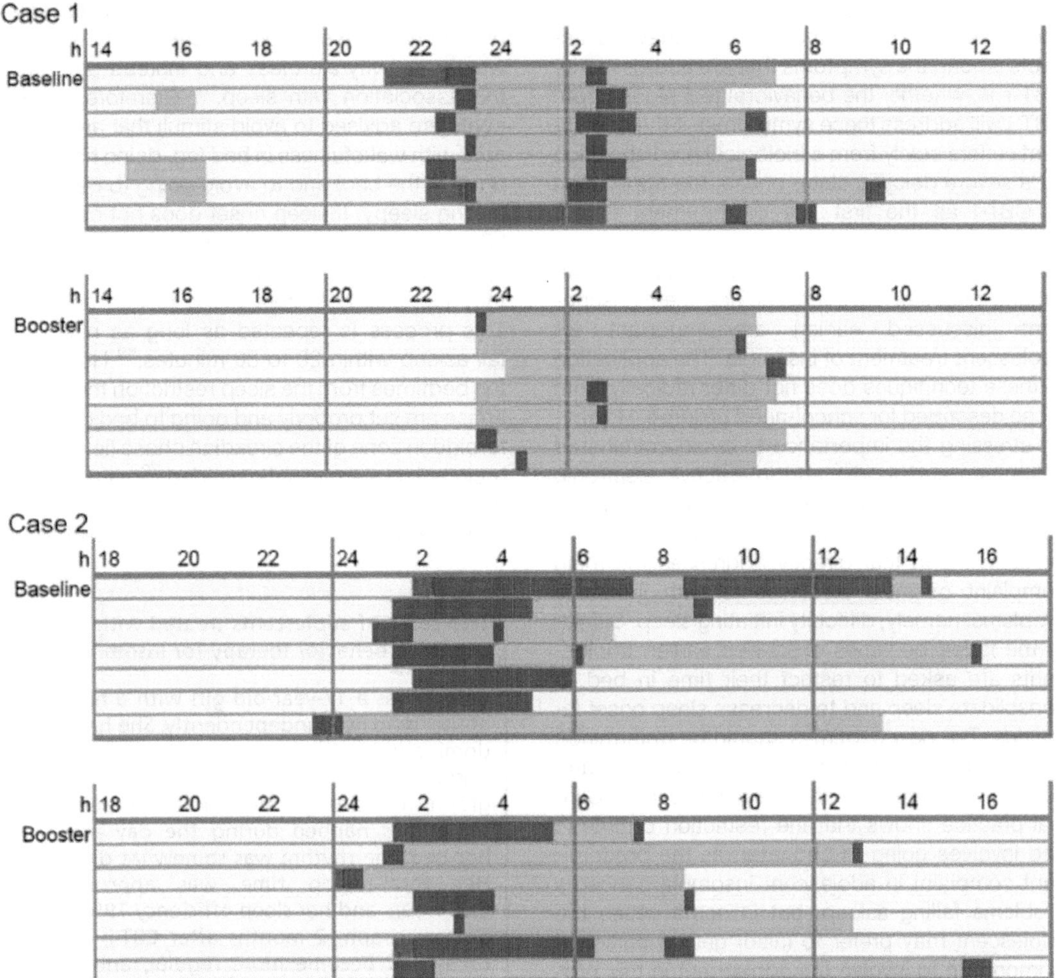

Fig. 1. Sleep diaries of two cases (described in **Box 3**) of adolescents with insomnia before and after CBT-i.

has the advantage to increase availability and access to treatment, and may also be characterized by high acceptability in adolescent populations. One should be aware that using Internet-based CBT-i requires adolescents to use their computer or mobile phone, possibly close to bedtime, which may contradict sleep hygiene advice; however, the effects of electronic media use on sleep are still not fully understood.[64,65]

Practical Application of Cognitive Behavioral Therapy for Insomnia in Adolescents

Before undertaking CBT-i for adolescents, the authors recommend that clinicians first assess for, and treat, any significant delay in their sleep timing (>2 hour difference between weekday vs. weekend bedtimes) that may be due to a delayed circadian rhythm. The rationale behind this is that although cognitive and behavioral techniques are likely to reduce the sleep latency of an adolescent with a delayed circadian rhythm, they are unlikely to advance the timing of their sleep onset time (which may be well past midnight). This delayed sleep onset will perpetuate the restricted sleep of the school-attending adolescent and may prove to become a barrier to treatment. By undertaking chronobiological treatments for the delayed sleep timing,[36] this may provide not only an improvement in an adolescent's sleep phase and duration but also some benefits to any secondary insomnia symptoms.[66]

There exists a gray area between more mild symptoms of delayed sleep phase and insomnia, especially in adolescents. The distinction between the two—even with a DLMO assessment—is not always easy to make and both can be a predisposing or perpetuating factor for the other.[66] Therefore, the predominant complaint should serve as an important factor to decide which to address first, insomnia or delayed sleep phase, or to address both simultaneously. As a principle rule of thumb for the application of CBT-i, clinicians should decide whether there exists behavioral aspects among the symptoms that are addressed by CBT-i (ie, whether the behavioral techniques from CBT-i will address these symptoms). If the adolescent suffers solely from a biological predisposition for a severe delayed sleep phase, the application of CBT-I as the first line of treatment is not recommended.

Similar to CBT-i for children, thought challenging and sleep hygiene advice (see descriptions discussed earlier) are important for adolescent treatment of insomnia. The application of these techniques does not differ radically from those described for school-aged children. However, stressing the importance to avoid caffeinated beverages and food[67] and interactive electronic media usage[68] is more relevant in this age group. Furthermore, sleep restriction therapy refers to an intervention that directly addresses the main complaint of most adolescents with insomnia problems, namely, difficulty initiating sleep. Similar to the faded bedtimes described earlier, adolescents are asked to restrict their time in bed to consolidate sleep and to decrease sleep onset latencies. The new bedtimes should be determined based on sleep diaries or actigraphy data and have to be discussed with the adolescent.[57] Clinical practice shows that the restriction of time in bed involves going to bed later, as the predominant complaint in adolescent insomnia concerns problems falling asleep, but in some cases the adolescent may prefer to (also) get up earlier. It is important to involve the adolescent in this process, because their agreement to the protocol is needed to ensure compliance. This is essential because clinical practice shows that adolescents often experience sleep restriction as a challenging therapeutic technique. Furthermore, it is important to tailor bedtimes to daytime requirements (eg, school) and change the sleeping habits the adolescent has adopted (eg, long naps or a behaviorally shifted circadian rhythm). It is generally advised to restrict sleep until a sleep efficiency (time in bed/total sleep time*100) of 85% to 90% is reached (depended on other personal and lifestyle factors such as age, school start times, and leisure activities) and then extending bedtimes gradually (eg, by approximately 15 minutes earlier each week).[57,69,70] Sleep restriction should be repeated immediately when sleep efficiency decreases to 80%. **Fig. 1** shows sleep restriction for two clinical cases, highlighting the need to (1) adapt the protocol to the individual, (2) define treatment success differently, and (3) take other comorbidities for further treatment into account (**Box 3**).

Stimulus control therapy aims to disassociate dysfunctional associations between the bed and waking activity/alertness and instead strengthen the association with sleep.[51] Therefore, adolescents are advised to avoid stimuli that are associated with wakefulness in bed (eg, doing homework on or in the bed) and to avoid going to bed before feeling sleepy. If sleep onset does not occur after 20 to 30 minutes, adolescents are asked to get up for about 15 to 20 minutes and stay awake until they feel sleepy, before going to bed again.[69,71] This process is repeated as long as needed to fall asleep within 20 to 30 minutes.[69] However, if the bedtimes from the sleep restriction therapy exercise are set properly and going to bed during the forbidden zone of the circadian phase (ie, peak 24-h circadian alertness) is avoided,[72] stimulus control therapy is rarely needed. In addition, it has been shown that behavioral relaxation techniques

Box 3
Two cases of adolescents treated with cognitive behavior therapy for insomnia

Case 1 was a 17-year-old girl with a history of abuse, who lived independently. She had a predominant complaint of waking after sleep onset and short total sleep time. In the top graph, it is clearly visible that at baseline she sometimes napped during the day and that her bedtime rhythm was somewhat disrupted. Her total sleep time was approximately 6:00 hours and her sleep efficiency 79%. In the bottom graph, 2 months after CBT-i, her bed times had become more regular, and she refrained from napping during the day. Total sleep time had increased to 6:50 hours and sleep efficiency to 95%.

Case 2 was a 14-year-old boy with anxiety problems, who lived alone with his mother. The top graph shows a severe disruption of regular bedtime routines, with long sleep onset latencies and some nights with no sleep at all. The predominant problem seemed to be the absence of daytime routines, which was compounded by the exemption from school for most days because of complex family problems and the infrequent (bedtimes-) support from his mother because of her work hours. At baseline total sleep time was approximately 5:10 hours and sleep efficiency 46%. At 2 months after CBT-i, these increased to 7:20 hours and 72%, respectively.

Although both cases showed significant improvements, they also show that after CBT-i there could be residual sleep problems and that sleep problems of adolescents are often strongly influenced by the context, such as parents, family, and school.

(eg, body scan) can reduce sleep onset latencies, whereas the cognitive technique of constructive worry (writing down worries and solutions instead of worrying in bed) does not, because relaxation decreases psychophysiologic arousal when being applied before bedtime.[73]

SUMMARY

Insomnia is one of the most prevalent sleep disorders in school-aged children and adolescents. Although CBT-i is the first-line treatment for adults and existing studies show promising effects also for children and adolescents, the number of RCTs in these younger age groups is rather small. CBT-i techniques for school-aged children and adolescents include bedtime shifts (including sleep restriction), stimulus control, thought challenging, psychoeducation about sleep, sleep hygiene, and relaxation techniques. The inclusion of parents, especially in school-aged children with insomnia, is highly recommended. The authors strongly urge the scientific community to conduct further controlled trials, including dismantling trials that evaluate the relative effectiveness of individual CBT-i components (eg, thought challenging, sleep restriction therapy)[74]; so clinicians can be more confident in using these techniques to better the sleep health of young people. Furthermore, more research is needed to investigate specific characteristics and models of child and adolescent insomnia.

CLINICS CARE POINTS

- Use questionnaires, including self-reports and parent reports, as well as clinical interviews and sleep diaries to help diagnose insomnia in school-aged children and adolescents. Screen for physical conditions, such as allergies, breathing problems, chronic illnesses, that can cause sleep disturbances.
- Adapt treatments to the individual's comorbidities and situational influences. Treat insomnia problems even if it co-occurs with other mental disorders.

DISCLOSURE

G. Michael has a book contract with the Little Brown Book Company on this topic and has received consultancies from the Australian Psychological Society; there are no other conflicts of interest to declare.

REFERENCES

1. Blader JC, Koplewicz HS, Abikoff H, et al. Sleep problems of elementary school children. A commu nity survey. Arch Pediatr Adolesc Med 1997;151:473–80.
2. Liu X, Liu L, Owens JA, et al. Sleep patterns and sleep problems among schoolchildren in the United States and China. Pediatrics 2005;115:241–9.
3. Spruyt K, O'Brien LM, Cluydts R, et al. Odds, prevalence and predictors of sleep problems in school-age normal children. J Sleep Res 2005;14:163–76.
4. Chung KF, Kan KKK, Yeung WF. Insomnia in adolescents: prevalence, help-seeking behaviors, and types of interventions. Child Adolesc Ment Health 2014;19: 57–63.
5. Short MA, Gradisar M, Gill J, et al. Identifying adolescent sleep problems. PLoS One 2013;8: e75301.
6. Hysing M, Pallesen S, Stormark KM, et al. Sleep patterns and insomnia among adolescents: a population-based study. J Sleep Res 2013;22:549–56.
7. Johnson EO, Roth T, Schultz L, et al. Epidemiology of DSM-IV insomnia in adolescence: lifetime prevalence, chronicity, and an emergent gender difference. Pediatrics 2006;117:e247–56.
8. Ohayon MM, Roberts RE. Comparability of sleep disorders diagnoses using DSM-IV and ICSD classi fications with adolescents. Sleep 2001;24:920–5.
9. Dohnt H, Gradisar M, Short MA. Insomnia and its symptoms in adolescents: comparing DSM-IV and ICSD-II diagnostic criteria. J Clin Sleep Med 2012;8:295–9.
10. Gregory AM, Sadeh A. Sleep, emotional and behavioral difficulties in children and adolescents. Sleep Med Rev 2012;16:129–36.
11. Beebe DW. Cognitive, behavioral, and functional consequences of inadequate sleep in children and adolescents. Pediatr Clin North Am 2011;58:649–65.
12. Roberts RE, Roberts CR, Chen IG. Impact of insomnia on future functioning of adolescents. J Psychosom Res 2002;53:561–9.
13. Dewald JF, Meijer AM, Oort FJ, et al. The influence of sleep quality, sleep duration and sleepiness on school performance in children and adolescents: a meta-analytic review. Sleep Med Rev 2010;14. -i 7Q on 1/9-89.
14. ShochatT, Cohen-Zion M, Tzischinsky O. Functional consequences of inadequate sleep in adolescents: a systematic review. Sleep Med Rev 2014;18:75–87.
15. Simola P, Liukkonen K, Pitkaranta A, et al. Psychosocial and somatic outcomes of sleep problems in children: a 4-year follow-up study. Child Care Health Dev 2014;40:60–7.
16. Paine S, Gradisar M. A randomised controlled trial of cognitive-behaviour therapy for behavioural insomnia of childhood in school-aged children. BeHav Res Ther 2011;49:379–88.
17. American Academy of Sleep Medicine. The inter- national classification of sleep disorders, 2nd edition:

diagnostic and coding manual. Westches- ter (IL): American Academy of Sleep Medicine; 2005.
18. American Academy of Sleep Medicine. The international classification of sleep disorders, 3nd edition: Diagnostic and coding manual. Westchester (IL): American Academy of Sleep Medicine; 2014.
19. Perlis M, Shaw PJ, Cano G, et al. Models of insomnia. Principles Pract Sleep Med 2011;5:850–65.
20. Sadeh R, Anders TF. Infant sleep problems: origins, assessment, Infant Mental Health. Journal 1993;14: 17–34.
21. Morgenthaler T, Kramer M, Alessi C, et al. Practice parameters for the psychological and behavioral treatment of insomnia: an update. An american academy of sleep medicine report. Sleep 2006;29:1415–9.
22. Mitchell MD, Gehrman P, Perlis M, et al. Compara- tive effectiveness of cognitive behavioral therapy for insomnia: a systematic review. BMC Fam Pract 2012; 13:40.
23. Koffel EA, Koffel JB, Gehrman PR. A meta-analysis of group cognitive behavioral therapy for insomnia. Sleep Med Rev 2015;19:6–16.
24. Okajima I, Inoue Y. Efficacy of cognitive behavioral therapy for comorbid insomnia: a meta-analysis. Sleep Biol Rhythms 2018;16(1):21–35.
25. Trauer JM, Qian MY, Doyle JS, et al. Cognitive behavioral therapy for chronic insomnia: a systematic review and meta-analysis. Ann Intern Med 2015;163:191–204.
26. Herbert V, Kyle SD, Pratt D. Does cognitive behav ioural therapy for insomnia improve cognitive perfor mance? A systematic review and narrative synthesis. Sleep Med Rev 2018;39:37–51.
27. Riemann D, Perlis ML. The treatments of chronic insomnia: a review of benzodiazepine receptor ago- nists and psychological and behavioral therapies. Sleep Med Rev 2009;13:205–14.
28. Meltzer LJ, Mindell JA. Systematic review and meta-analysis of behavioral interventions for pediatric insomnia. J Pediatr Psychol 2014;39:932–48.
29. Quach J, Hiscock H, Ukoumunne OC, et al. A brief sleep intervention improves outcomes in the school entry year: a randomized controlled trial. Pediatrics 2011;128:692–701.
30. Blake MJ, Sheeber LB, Youssef GJ, et al. Systematic review and meta-analysis of adolescent cognitive-behavioral sleep interventions. Clin Child Fam Psy Chol Rev 2017;20:227–49.
31. de Bruin EJ, Bogels SM, Oort FJ, et al. Efficacy of cognitive behavioral therapy for insomnia in adolescents: a randomized controlled trial with internet therapy, group therapy and a waiting list condition. Sleep 2015;38:1913–26.
32. Blake MJ, Snoep L, Raniti M, et al. A cognitive-behavioral and mindfulness-based group sleep intervention improves behavior problems in at-risk adolescents by improving perceived sleep quality. Behav Res Ther 2017;99:147–56.
33. de Bruin EJ, Bogels SM, Oort FJ, et al. Improvements of adolescent psychopathology after insomnia treatment: results from a randomized controlled trial over 1 year. J Child Psychol Psychia-Try 2018;59:509–22.
34. Smits MG, van Stel HF, van der Heijden K, et al. Melatonin improves health status and sleep in children with idiopathic chronic sleep-onset insomnia: a randomized placebo-controlled trial. J Am Acad Child Adolesc Psychiatry 2003;42:1286–93.
35. van Maanen A, Meijer AM, Smits MG, et al. Effects of melatonin and bright light treatment in childhood chronic sleep onset insomnia with late melatonin onset: a randomized controlled study. Sleep 2017; 40. https://doi.org/10.1093/sleep/zsw038.
36. Gradisar M, Smits M, Bjorvatn B. Assessment and treatment of delayed sleep phase disorder in adolescents: recent innovations and cautions. Sleep Med Clin 2014;9:199–210.
37. Bruni O, Ottaviano S, Guidetti V, et al. The sleep disturbance scale for children (sdsc). Construction and validation of an instrument to evaluate sleep dis- turbances in childhood and adolescence. J Sleep Res 1996;5:251–61.
38. Owens JA, Spirito A, McGuinn M. The children's sleep habits questionnaire (cshq): psychometric properties of a survey instrument for school-aged children. Sleep 2000;23:1043–51.
39. Schreck KA, Mulick JA, Rojahn J. Development of the behavioral evaluation of disorders of sleep scale. J Child Fam Stud 2003;12:349–59.
40. Spilsbury JC, Drotar D, Rosen CL, et al. The cleveland adolescent sleepiness questionnaire: a new measure to assess excessive daytime sleepiness in adolescents. J Clin Sleep Med 2007;3:603–12.
41. Drake C, Nickel C, Burduvali E, et al. The pediatric daytime sleepiness scale (pdss): sleep habits and school outcomes in middle-school children. Sleep 2003;26:455–8.
42. LeBourgeois MK, Giannotti F, Cortesi F, et al. The relationship between reported sleep quality and sleep hygiene in Italian and american adolescents. Pediatrics 2005;115:257–65.
43. Spruyt K, Gozal D. Pediatric sleep questionnaires as diagnostic or epidemiological tools: a review of currently available instruments. Sleep Med Rev 2011;15:19–32.
44. Carney CE, Buysse DJ, Ancoli-Israel S, et al. The consensus sleep diary: standardizing prospective sleep self-monitoring. Sleep 2012;35:287–302.
45. Schlarb AA, Bihlmaier I, Velten-Schurian K, et al. Short- and long-term effects of cbt-i in groups for school-age children suffering from chronic insomnia: the kiss-program. Behav Sleep Med 2018;16:380–97.

46. Moore M. Behavioral sleep problems in children and adolescents. J Clin Psychol Med Settings 2012;19:77–83.
47. Kuhn BR, Elliott AJ. Treatment efficacy in behavioral pediatric sleep medicine. J Psychosom Res 2003; 54:587–97.
48. Sadeh A. Cognitive-behavioral treatment for child- hood sleep disorders. Clin Psychol Rev 2005;25:612–28.
49. Miller CB, Espie CA, Epstein DR, et al. The evidence base of sleep restriction therapy for treating insomnia disorder. Sleep Med Rev 2014;18:415–24.
50. Bootzin RR, Stevens SJ. Adolescents, substance abuse, and the treatment of insomnia and daytime sleepiness. Clin Psychol Rev 2005;25:629–44.
51. Bootzin RR, Perlis ML. Stimulus control therapy. In: Perlis M, Aloia M, Kuhn B, editors. Stimulus control therapy. Behavioral treatments for sleep disorders. New York: Academic Press; 2011. p. 21–30.
52. de Bruin EJ, van Kampen RK, van Kooten T, et al. Psychometric properties and clinical relevance of the adolescent sleep hygiene scale in Dutch adolescents. Sleep Med 2014;15:789–97.
53. Mindell JA, Meltzer LJ, Carskadon MA, et al. Devel opmental aspects of sleep hygiene: findings from the 2004 national sleep foundation sleep in America poll. Sleep Med 2009;10:771–9.
54. Bei B, Byrne ML, Ivens C, et al. Pilot study of a mindfulness-based, multi-component, in-school group sleep intervention in adolescent girls. Early Interv Psychiatry 2013;7:213–20.
55. Blake M, Waloszek JM, Schwartz O, et al. The sense study: post intervention effects of a randomized controlled trial of a cognitive-behavioral and mindfulness-based group sleep improvement intervention among at-risk adolescents. J Consult Clin Psychol 2016;84:1039–51.
56. Britton WB, Bootzin RR, Cousins JC, et al. The contribution of mindfulness practice to a multicom- ponent behavioral sleep intervention following sub- stance abuse treatment in adolescents: a treatment-development study. Subst Abus 2010;31:86–97.
57. de Bruin EJ, Oort FJ, Bogels SM, et al. Efficacy of internet and group-administered cognitive behavioral therapy for insomnia in adolescents: a pi lot study. Behav Sleep Med 2014;12:235–54.
58. Clarke G, McGlinchey EL, Hein K, et al. Cognitive-behavioral treatment of insomnia and depression in adolescents: a pilot randomized trial. Behav Res Ther 2015;69:111–8.
59. Gradisar M, Dohnt H, Gardner G, et al. A randomized controlled trial of cognitive-behavior therapy plus bright light therapy for adolescent delayed sleep phase disorder. Sleep 2011;34:1671–80.
60. Schlarb AA, Liddle CC, Hautzinger M. Just - a multimodal program for treatment of insomnia in adolescents: a pilot study. Nat Sci Sleep 2011;3:13–20.
61. Roeser K, Schwerdtle B, Kubler A, et al. Further ev idence for the just program as treatment for insomnia in adolescents: results from a 1-year follow-up study. J Clin Sleep Med 2016;12:257–62.
62. Blake MJ, Blake LM, Schwartz O, et al. Who benefits from adolescent sleep interventions? Moderators of treatment efficacy in a randomized controlled trial of a cognitive-behavioral and mindfulness-based group sleep intervention for at-risk adolescents. J Child Psychol Psychiatry 2018;59:637–49.
63. De Bruin EJ, van Steensel FJ, Meijer AM. Cost-effectiveness of group and internet cognitive behavioral therapy for insomnia in adolescents: results from a randomized controlled trial. Sleep 2016;39:1571–81.
64. Bartel K, Scheeren R, Gradisar M. Altering adoles cents' pre-bedtime phone use to achieve better sleep health. Health Commun 2019;34(4):456–62.
65. Harris A, Gundersen H, Mork-Andreassen P, et al. Restricted use of electronic media, sleep, performance, and mood in high school athletes-a random ized trial. Sleep Health 2015;1:314–21.
66. Richardson C, Micic G, Cain N, et al. Cognitive "insomnia" processes in delayed sleep-wake phase disorder: do they exist and are they responsive to chronobiological treatment? J Consult Clin Psychol 2018. https://doi.org/10.1037/ccp0000357.
67. Bonnar D, Gradisar M. Caffeine and sleep in adoles cents: a systematic review. J Caffeine Res 2015;5: 105–14.
68. Hale L, Kirschen GW, LeBourgeois MK, et al. Youth screen media habits and sleep: sleep-friendly screen behavior recommendations for clinicians, ed ucators, and parents. Child Adolesc Psychiatr Clin N Am 2018;27:229–45.
69. Palermo TM, Bromberg MH, Beals-Erickson S, et al. Development and initial feasibility testing of brief cognitive-behavioral therapy for insomnia in adolescents with comorbid conditions. Clin Pract Pediatr Psychol 2016;4:214–26.
70. Schutte-Rodin S, Broch L, Buysse D, et al. Clinical guideline for the evaluation and management of chronic insomnia in adults. J Clin Sleep Med 2008;4:487–504.
71. De Bruin EJ, Watermann D, Meijer AM. Slimslapen: cognitieve gedragstherapie voor insomnia (cgt-i) bij adolescenten. In: Breat C, Bogels S, editors. Slimslapen: cognitieve gedragstherapie voor insomnia (cgt-i) bij adolescenten. Protocollaire behandeling voor kinderen en adolescenten met psychische klachten, deel 2. Amsterdam (the Netherlands): Boom; 2013. p. 277–312.
72. Lack LC, Lushington K. The rhythms of human sleep propensity and core body temperature. J Sleep Res 1996;5:1–11.
73. Bartel K, Huang C, Maddock B, et al. Brief school-based interventions to assist adolescents' sleep- onset latency: comparing mindfulness and constructive worry versus controls. J Sleep Res 2018;27:e12668.
74. Gradisar M, Richardson C. Cbt-i cannot rest until the sleepy teen can. Sleep 2015;38:1841–2.

Drugs Used in Parasomnia

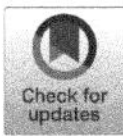

Paola Proserpio, MD[a,*], Michele Terzaghi, MD[b], Raffaele Manni, MD[b], Lino Nobili, MD, PhD[a,c]

KEYWORDS

• Disorders of arousal • REM behavior disorder • Sleep-related eating disorder • Sleep enuresis • Benzodiazepines • Clonazepam • Melatonin • Antidepressant drugs

KEY POINTS

- Nonrapid eye movement (NREM) parasomnias, especially during childhood, are often benign conditions, and pharmacologic therapy is usually unnecessary.
- There are no properly powered randomized controlled studies evaluating the efficacy of pharmacologic therapy for NREM parasomnias.
- The most commonly used drugs for NREM parasomnias are intermediate-acting and long-acting benzodiazepines and antidepressants. Anecdotal cases reported the efficacy of melatonergic agents and hydroxytryptophan.
- The pharmacologic treatment of rapid eye movement sleep behavior disorder is symptomatic, and the most commonly used drugs are clonazepam and melatonin.

INTRODUCTION

Parasomnias are defined as "undesirable physical events or experiences that occur during entry into sleep, within sleep, or during arousal from sleep."[1] Depending on the sleep stage of occurrence, they are classified as nonrapid eye movement (NREM)-related parasomnias (confusional arousals, sleepwalking, sleep terrors, and sleep-related eating disorder [SRED]), rapid eye movement (REM)-related parasomnias (REM sleep behavior disorder [RBD], recurrent isolated sleep paralysis, and nightmare disorder), and other parasomnias (exploding head syndrome [EHS], sleep-related hallucinations, and sleep enuresis [SE]).[1]

Parasomnias are not generally associated with a primary complaint of insomnia or excessive sleepiness, although this last one may be present in some of them. However, parasomnias can be associated with possible resulting injuries, adverse health, and negative psychosocial effects. Moreover, the clinical consequences of parasomnias can affect the patient, parents, or both.

Parasomnias, especially disorders of arousal (DOA) during childhood, are often relatively benign and transitory and do not usually require a pharmacologic therapy. A relevant aspect in both NREM and REM parasomnia treatment is to prevent sleep-related injuries by maintaining a safe environment. Physicians should always evaluate the possible presence of favoring and precipitating factors (sleep disorders and drugs). A pharmacologic treatment may be indicated in case of frequent, troublesome, or particularly dangerous events. The aim of this article is to review current available evidence on pharmacologic treatment of different forms of parasomnia.

Sleep Med Clin 13 (2018) 191-202 https://doi.org/10.1016/j.jsmc.2018.02.003 1556-407X/18/© 2018 Elsevier Inc.

[a] Sleep Medicine Center, Department of Neuroscience, Niguarda Hospital, Piazza Ospedale Maggiore 3, 20162 Milano, Italy; [b] Sleep Medicine and Epilepsy, IRCCS Mondino Foundation, Via Mondino 2, 27100 Pavia, Italy; [c] Department of Neuroscience (DINOGMI), University of Genoa, Child Neuropsychiatry Unit, IRCCS Istituto G. Gaslini, Genoa 5-16147, Italy
* Corresponding author. Child Neuropsychiatry Unit, IRCCS Istituto G. GASLINI, DINOGMI, University of Genoa, Genoa, Italy
E-mail address: paola.proserpio@ospedaleniguarda.it

Sleep Med Clin 17 (2022) 367–378
https://doi.org/10.1016/j.jsmc.2022.06.004
1556-407X/22/© 2022 Elsevier Inc.

NONRAPID EYE MOVEMENT PARASOMNIAS

Disorder of Arousal from Nonrapid Eye Movement Sleep

DOA are the subgroup of parasomnias arising from NREM sleep, encompassing confusional arousals, sleep terrors, and sleep walking.[1] They are most prevalent during childhood and normally cease by adolescence but onset or persistence during adulthood is well recognized.[2] More than one type may coexist within the same patient.[3] Many clinical features are common to these manifestations.[4,5] First, they generally occur during deep NREM sleep (N3) and, thus, most often take place in the first third of the night. During the episode, patients are usually unresponsive to the environment and completely or partially amnestic after the event. A positive family history is frequently found in DOA. Finally, any factor that deepens (sleep deprivation, stress, febrile illness, medications, alcohol) or fragments sleep (external or internal stimuli, sleep disorders, mental activity) may increase the occurrence of DOA.

DOA are generally considered benign phenomena. However, especially in adults, they can be characterized by complex behavior with potentially violent or injurious features[6] or be associated with significant functional impairment, such as daytime sleepiness, fatigue, and distress.[7] Therefore, evaluation and treatment are recommended in these cases, especially when violent manifestations are frequent or very disturbing for the patient or other family members.

The management of DOA is not well codified. No drug has yet been approved, and there are no properly powered randomized controlled studies evaluating the efficacy of behavioral or pharmacologic interventions for DOA.[8] Current treatment recommendations are based on scarce evidence derived from expert opinions, case reports, and only few case series. To date, the largest retrospective case series, analyzing treatment options and efficacy in DOA, refers to a population of 103 adults.[9]

Only recently, a self-administered scale has been developed with the aim of providing a valid and reliable tool able to assess the diagnosis and severity of NREM parasomnia as well as to monitor the efficacy of treatment.[10] Considering that evidence is lacking for off-label use of pharmacologic agents, clinicians may wish to ensure that patients are fully informed about all therapeutic options.[8]

Nonpharmacologic treatment

As previously discussed, if the episodes are rare, or not associated with harm potential, treatment is often unnecessary. Management includes reassuring patients about the usual benign nature of the episodes. Parents or bed partners should be instructed to keep calm and not to insist in trying to awaken the patient because this may aggravate or lengthen the episodes.[11] Precautions should be taken to ensure a safe sleep environment. Simple safety measures can include the removal of obstructions in the bedroom, securing windows, sleeping on the ground floor, and installing locks or alarms on windows, doors, and stairways.[4,11]

Every priming or triggering factor should be investigated and avoided. For instance, every effort should be made to ensure regular and adequate sleep routines, to prevent sleep loss or disruption of the sleep–wake cycle. Sleep disorders (sleep apnea or periodic leg movements) must be recognized and treated.[12] Moreover, patients should avoid the intake of drugs or substances that could favor the occurrence of episodes (alcohol, hypnotics, antipsychotics, antidepressants, antihistamines).

Some investigators proposed "scheduled awakenings" in the case of DOA occurring nightly and consistently at or around the same time each night.[13] In adults, a psychological approach may be considered (hypnosis, relaxation therapy, or cognitive behavioral therapy), although studies evaluating its efficacy have provided contrasting results.[14,15]

Pharmacologic treatment

The main indications for a pharmacologic treatment in patients with DOA encompass the following: (1) persistence of frequent episodes despite resolution and removal of all potential predisposing and precipitating factors, (2) high risk of injury for the patient or the family, (3) significant functional impairment (such as insomnia, daytime sleepiness, weight gain from nocturnal eating), and (4) potential legal consequences related to sexual or violent behavior.

As illustrated above, if drug therapy is planned, patients or their parents should be advised that drugs for DOA are considered "off label" and, if the decision is to prescribe, a patient's written consent is recommended.

Benzodiazepines (BZD): Intermediate and long-acting agents in the BZD class of sedative hypnotics are the most frequently used treatment of DOA,[4,11,16] although they have never been approved for this indication. They act by increasing the chloride conductance through GABA A receptors,[17] thus inducing a hypnotic-sedative effect. It is worth reminding that BDZ may have muscle-relaxing properties and should be used with caution if comorbid sleep-disordered breathing is suspected. The use of

BZD in the treatment of DOA is apparently paradoxic, considering that other sedative-hypnotics such as non-BZD receptor agonists can induce amnestic nocturnal behavior.[18] The exact mechanism by which BZD suppress DOA is unknown. Probably, their effectiveness may be related to sedative effects or to decreases in slow-wave sleep.[19] Alternatively, they may work through the suppression of cortical arousals.[16]

Among the BZD class, clonazepam at 0.5 to 2 mg is the most common medication used in the treatment of DOA. However, studies (mainly conducted in adults) in the last 2 decades showed conflicting results. To date, only small case series, analyzing the efficacy of BDZ in children,[20] have been published. In 1989, Schenck and colleagues[21] studied 100 consecutive adults referred to their sleep disorders center for repeated nocturnal injury. All patients underwent full polysomnography recordings. Fifty-four of these patients were diagnosed with either sleep terrors or sleepwalking. Clonazepam was prescribed for 28 of these patients and a rapid and sustained response was observed in 83.6% of them. A few years later, the same group published the results of a study designed to look for safety and abuse of BZDs taken for sleep disorders.[22] They analyzed 170 adults with sleep-related injuries of whom 69 had either sleepwalking or sleep terrors and were treated with BDZ, essentially clonazepam (n = 58) but also alprazolam. Most patients (86%) reported good control after an average follow-up of 3.5 years. The mean dose for clonazepam at the end of the study was 1.10 ± 0.96 mg. Interestingly, the risk of dosage escalation was low. In a more recent case series, Attarian and Zhu[9] analyzed the response to various therapeutic modalities in 103 adults with DOA. They found that clonazepam (0.5–2 mg) was used in 55% of the patients with a high response to treatment (73.7%).

Conversely, in another report, 5 patients with sleepwalking treated with clonazepam reported persistence of nocturnal episodes after 1 year of follow-up.[15]

Clonazepam has also been used successfully in somnambulism induced by neuroleptics[23] and in DOA with behaviors such as driving and sleep violence.[22,24]

Anecdotal data have shown that patients with DOA respond to diazepam (2–5 mg).[25] However, in a small double-blind placebo-controlled crossover study of diazepam in sleepwalking, results failed to show significant difference between placebo and diazepam,[26] although investigators stated that in some participants, there was an alleviation of self-reported symptoms. Other BZDs that have been shown to be effective include triazolam (0.25 mg) at bedtime[27] and flurazepam.[28]

Antidepressant drugs: Antidepressant drugs are occasionally effective in the treatment of DOA.[4,29] In the already mentioned recent largest case series study,[9] 4 patients responded to sertraline and 2 responded to clomipramine.

Anecdotal data reported efficacy of tricyclic antidepressant (imipramine or clomipramine) and trazodone. For instance, 2 patients with a history of sleep terrors and sleepwalking, in both of whom diazepam therapy failed, responded well to imipramine.[30] Conversely, trazodone provided a remarkable relief of symptoms in a 7-year-old girl who suffered from a severe sleep terror disorder, previously treated unsuccessfully with imipramine.[31]

Serotoninergic antidepressants, especially paroxetine, have been reported to be particularly effective in the treatment of sleep terrors. Indeed, a small case series showed a significant reduction of sleep terror events in 6 patients.[32] The investigators suggested that selective serotonin reuptake inhibitors (SSRIs) may improve sleep terrors by virtue of serotonergic effects on the mesencephalic periaqueductal gray matter. Considering sleepwalking, a single case report showed the efficacy of paroxetine,[33,34] whereas other evidence reported a paroxetine-inducing somnambulism.[35]

The mechanism by which antidepressant medications would influence DOA remains unclear, especially in light of these contradictory results. Indeed, the different efficacy of serotonin in sleepwalking and sleep terrors could suggest possible distinct pathophysiologic mechanisms at the basis of these manifestations.[4]

Other drugs: Single case reports have shown the efficacy of other pharmacologic treatments, such as melatonin, hydroxytryptophan, and ramelteon.

Melatonin (W-acetyl-5-methoxytryptamine) is an endogenous hormone produced by the pineal gland and released exclusively at night. Exogenous melatonin supplementation is well tolerated and has no significant adverse effects and a low potential for dependence. Melatonin has been shown to synchronize the circadian rhythms and improve the onset, duration, and quality of sleep. Thus, melatonin seems to represent an alternative treatment of sleep disorders with significantly less side effects.[36] Moreover, melatonin has been shown to be particularly useful for the treatment of sleep disorders in children with neurodevelopmental disabilities.[37] To date, only 2 case reports showed its efficacy in the treatment of DOA. In particular, Jan and colleagues[38] described a 12-year-old patient affected by Asperger syndrome and a chronic sleep-phase onset delay in whom melatonin was effective in the treatment of sleepwalking and sleep terror episodes. However, its efficacy could be related mainly to the correction of the circadian disorder and the consequent improvement of the underlying sleep deprivation. More recently, Ozcan and Donmez[39] reported the efficacy of treatment with melatonin for 2 weeks in a 36-month-old patient with sleep terror.

An open pharmacologic trial conducted in 45 children with sleep terror demonstrated the efficacy of L-5-hydroxytryptophan, a precursor of serotonin, in 83.9% of patients after 6 months of therapy.[40] The investigators hypothesized that this drug could induce a long-term improvement of sleep terrors through a stabilization of the sleep microstructure and a modulation of the arousal level in children.

Finally, Sasayama and colleagues[41] recently reported a boy with attention-deficit/hyperactivity disorder whose night terrors and sleepwalking were effectively treated with ramelteon, a melatonin receptor agonist, probably improving sleep deprivation.

Sleep-related Eating Disorder

SRED is an NREM sleep parasomnia characterized by frequent episodes of dysfunctional and involuntary eating and drinking that occur after an arousal during NREM sleep associated with diminished levels of consciousness and subsequent recall, with problematic health consequences.[1] This sleep disorder generally starts in young adults, with a female predominance.[42] SRED is sometimes associated with the use of psychotropic drugs (triazolam, zolpidem, amitriptyline, olanzapine, and risperidone) and other sleep disorders, including parasomnias, narcolepsy, restless legs syndrome, and periodic leg movements.[43] Thus, the first goal of treatment is to eliminate any precipitating factors and to recognize and treat any comorbid sleep disorders. Indeed, the removal of any offending drug together with the treatment of sleep disturbances has been shown to resolve many cases of SRED.[43,44] Moreover, the nonpharmacologic treatment plan should also include education regarding proper sleep hygiene, the maintenance of a safe sleep environment, and the limitation of other precipitating factors, such as cigarette smoking or alcohol intake.[45–47]

The preferred drugs used for the treatment of SRED are represented by dopamine agonists, BZDs, topiramate, and SSRI.[47,48(p2)]

A randomized, double-blind, placebo-controlled crossover study of pramipexole (0.180.36 mg/d) on 11 SRED subjects demonstrated improvement in sleep quality and actigraphic measures.[49] Nevertheless, the number and duration of waking episodes related to eating behaviors were unchanged, and no weight loss was observed. A more recent study confirmed the efficacy of dopamine agonist in 3 patients with SRED.[50] Interestingly, other dopaminergic agents, such as carbidopa/L-dopa and bromocriptine as monotherapy, were effective in 25% of the patients with SRED associated with sleepwalking, and in combination with BZDs (mainly clonazepam), opiates, or both in approximately 87% of subjects.[51]

SSRI (fluoxetine, paroxetine, and fluvoxamine) were reportedly effective in 2 different studies.[51,52]

Substantial reduction of sleep-related eating episodes and significant weight loss have been achieved in subjects treated with topiramate, an antiepileptic drug that induces weight loss.[50,53–55] In particular, Winkelman[55] reported that 68% of patients responded to topiramate, with a mean dose of 135 mg/d but the discontinuation rate was high because of side effects, including dullness, paresthesia, and daytime sleepiness. In a more recent study, 20 patients with SRED were treated with topiramate, 17 of whom showed cessation or a clear reduction in night eating episodes, whereas 6 (30%) had to discontinue medication because of adverse effects (eg, dizziness, visual problems, and worsening of preexisting depressive symptoms).[50] Physicians should follow up patients regularly with SRED treated with topiramate in order to promptly recognize and treat side effects.[47] It is unclear how topiramate works to decrease SRED manifestations. It was hypothesized that the drug may work by suppressing arousals produced by underlying sleep disorders or by acting as an anorexigenic agent, through either glutamatergic antagonism or serotonergic agonism.[54] Moreover, topiramate has been reported to stimulate insulin release and increase insulin sensitivity, both of which may contribute to appetite regulation and weight loss.[56]

Zapp and colleagues[57] recently described a case of a patient with SRED associated with the use of various antidepressants and sleep apnea that completely vanished after treatment with ago-melatine or melatonin extended release.

RAPID EYE MOVEMENT PARASOMNIAS

Rapid Eye Movement Sleep Behavior Disorder

RBD treatment is currently based on a symptomatic approach because interventions to prevent or slow the conversion toward neurodegenerative diseases in susceptible subjects are not available at the moment.

Sleep-related injuries are frequent and reported in up to 65% of RBD cases,[58–60] so that RBD subjects should be offered a treatment immediately following the diagnosis. Symptomatic treatment is aimed at preventing injuries to the patient and/or to the bed partner by reducing the frequency and severity of dream-enacted behaviors. Effects on dream content and sleep quality should also be considered when optimizing RBD pharmacologic interventions.

In the management of RBD subjects, clinicians should also be aware of the possibility that ongoing pharmacologic treatment with antidepressants, particularly SSRIs, can have an impact on RBD, worsening its manifestations.[61]

Despite the importance of establishing treatment, research found a limited number of drugs effective in RBD, and current knowledge about efficacy and tolerability profile of drugs used in RBD subjects is still based on low-level evidence data based on case reports and case series.[62] Thus, adequately powered controlled trials addressing drug effects in this category are needed.

Clonazepam

The effectiveness of clonazepam on RBD was reported in the seminal article from Schenck and colleagues,[63] and since then, it has been widely used for RBD treatment as first-choice therapy. Its efficacy is reflected in a complete remission of symptoms in 55% to 90% of RBD subjects.[60] In a recent open-label study of the effect of clonazepam up to 3 mg, the figure of RBD subjects defined as responders (ie, absence of injuries and potential injurious behaviors to self and/or to bed partner) was reported to be 66.7%.[64] Clonazepam doses are between 0.25 and 4.0 mg at bedtime, with 0.5 mg appearing to be a suitable dosage for most of the subjects.[65]

Although RBD symptoms occur after discontinuation of clonazepam,[62] they usually are easily controlled by the resumption of therapy. Tolerance and withdrawal symptoms only rarely occur, even if complaints of insomnia and unsatisfactory sleep quality can be reported.[62] Main side effects, such as early morning sedation, incoordination, falls, confusion, memory impairment, sexual dysfunctions, and worsening of sleep-disordered breathing, can occur.[62] Clonazepam does not influence the occurrence of dreams with emotional or sorrowful content but results in a reduction of the frequency of nightmares and dreams with violent and frightening content, paralleled by the reduction in potential injurious behaviors.[64] In consideration of the side-effect profile of the drug, caution is needed in elderly subjects for the possibility to impair both postural instability and cognitive performances, up to the occurrence of confusional states in subjects with cognitive decline.[66]

Furthermore, clonazepam should be prescribed at the lowest effective dose in patients with sleep apnea, and respiratory pattern should be assessed during the treatment.

Melatonin

Exogenous melatonin has been shown as being approximately equally effective at reducing RBD severity in respect to clonazepam.[62,65,67] In a comparative study to clonazepam, melatonin resulted in better tolerability, with subjects taking clonazepam reporting more frequently drowsiness, instability, and neuropsychological impairment.[65] Differently from clonazepam, melatonin has univocal evidence of restoring REM sleep muscle atonia.[68] Melatonin dosages are 2 to 12 mg at bedtime. Melatonin at a median dosage of 6 mg proved to be as effective in reducing RBD behavior as clonazepam (0.5 mg).[65] These doses are usually well tolerated, despite dose-dependent side effects, such as morning headache, sleepiness, delusions, and hallucinations.[69] Because of its profile of effectiveness and tolerability, melatonin is a valid option in RBD subjects and can be preferred to clonazepam in the case of background disease features, consisting of sleep-disordered breathing, disorders of gait and unsteadiness, or cognitive impairment.

Melatonergic agents

Because of the effectiveness and tolerability profile of exogenous melatonin, melatoninergic agents are expected to benefit RBD subjects. Effects of ramelteon at doses of 8 mg/d (in improving RBD control in subjects affected by extrapyramidal disorders[70]) were not confirmed on objective polysomnographic assessment of RBD behavior and REM sleep without atonia (RSWA), despite a subjective reduction in dream enactment frequency and severity.[71,72] In the same way, agomelatine (25 mg) proved to improve RBD symptoms in idiopathic RBD but did not change RBD motor events frequency and RSWA on polysomnographic assessment.[73]

Dopamine agonists

Controversial results were carried out by efforts in treating RBD with pramipexole. Pramipexole was reported to reduce RBD symptoms[74–76] and seems to be effective mainly in the form of RBD with limited loss of atonia.[75] However, no changes were found in RBD subjects with extrapyramidal disorders on clinical or polysomnographic grounds.[77] All in all, pramipexole should be considered when other treatments have failed to control RBD. Because its efficacy in restless legs syndrome, pramipexole can be considered for the initial treatment of subjects with comorbid restless legs syndrome but deserves a short-interval follow-up visit to assess RBD evolution.

Acetylcholinesterase inhibitors

Use of acetylcholinesterase inhibitors for RBD treatment is based on the notion that cholinergic mechanisms are central for the initiation and coordination of REM sleep.[78] Furthermore, in dementia with Lewy bodies, in which cholinergic transmission is impaired, administration of acetylcholinesterase inhibitor was reported to potentially restore correct sleep patterns and resolve nocturnal confusional events.[79,80]

However, conflicting data are reported in the literature about the efficacy of acetylcholinesterase inhibitor in RBD.

Acetylcholinesterase inhibitors donepezil and rivastigmine were reported to reduce RBD behavior.[62,81–84] However, no changes in RBD in subjects with comorbid neurodegenerative diseases could be found,[69] and even the occurrence of de novo RBD was reported in a patient with Alzheimer disease.[85] Altogether, considering the limited and conflicting data about the efficacy of acetylcholinesterase inhibitors in RBD, these drugs should be used as a third-line treatment analogously to pramipexole, in cases of clonazepam or melatonin failure. Because the possibility that RBD occurs in the context of cognitive impairment, acetylcholinesterase inhibitors can be used in symptomatic RBD patients requiring concurrent treatment of cognitive impairment or hallucinations (ie, dementia with Lewy bodies and Parkinson disease dementia).

Cannabidiol

There has been evidence that suggests that cannabis may have therapeutic potential in several neurologic disorders, and sleep in particular.[86] Data on the effect of cannabinoids on RBD are limited but the efficacy of cannabidiol, the nonintoxicating constituent of cannabis, in ameliorating RBD in subjects with Parkinson disease was reported, together with a good tolerability profile.[87]

Miscellaneous

For BZDs other than clonazepam, temazepam as monotherapy or in association to zopiclone,[88,89] triazolam,[60] and alprazolam[22] were used in RBD, suggesting that they may have a class-specific effect. Zopiclone seems to be effective and well tolerated in reducing RBD symptoms.[88] Herbal derivatives, as Yi-Gan San[90] or Yokukansan, which contain exactly measured mixtures of dried herbs, can be effective in improving RBD symptoms. Sodium oxybate can be an effective add-on option for the treatment of idiopathic RBD, refractory to conventional therapies, despite a lack of improvement in polysomnographic parameters.[91,92]

Nightmare Disorder

The therapeutic approach to nightmares encompasses nonpharmacologic as well as pharmacologic options. Although psychotherapy and cognitive behavior interventions have traditionally been the treatment of choice, drugs alone or in combination therapy can be used as an alternative to psychological interventions.

In the evaluation of nightmares, it should be kept in mind that numerous drugs can trigger nightmares and vivid dreams, among which are catecholaminergic agents, β-blockers, barbiturates, dopaminergic agents, and alcohol and even some antidepressants. Several drugs classes, including SSRIs, tricyclic antidepressants, antipsychotics, and adrenergic agonists, were studied in nightmare disorder.[93–95] Some lines of evidence show that risperidone, trazodone, clonidine, quetiapine, fluvoxamine, mirtazapine, and terazosin can be helpful.[95] However, data are limited, and the quality of evidence is poor.[62]

Prazosin

Prazosin is a centrally acting selective α_1-adrenergic antagonist and has been considered efficacious as pharmacologic treatment of nightmares, especially in cases of posttraumatic nightmares, with a good profile of tolerability.[96–98] The relapse of nightmares following discontinuation of prazosin was reported, showing the need for long-term use.[99] However, recent data put into discussion the results from previous studies,[100] and data showing no effect of prazosin on nightmare frequency were reported.[95]

Cannabinoids

The use of tetrahydrocannabinol in the treatment of nightmares associated with posttraumatic stress disorder was reported to result in the reduction of nightmare recurrence and intensity.[101–104] A good profile of tolerability accompanied the drug,[104] with dry mouth, headache, and dizziness being the more frequently reported symptoms.

Recurrent Isolated Sleep Paralysis

It should be carefully considered whether to pharmacologically treat sleep paralysis episodes or not. Most of the patients with sleep paralysis do not experience clinically significant distress, and basic treatment is avoidance of sleep deprivation and other precipitants. In the case of recurrent sleep paralysis and significant clinical distress, the cost/benefit balance of drug therapy should be considered. A substantial lack of systematic data in this field leads personal experience to have a central role in the choice of the drug.

Pharmacologic intervention is based on the possibility of suppressing REM sleep, and tricyclic antidepressants (clomipramine, imipramine, desmethylimipramine)[105–107] and SSRIs (fluoxetine, femoxetine, and viloxazine)[107–109] can be considered. Sodium oxybate is a possible therapy for sleep paralysis in narcolepsy.[110]

OTHER PARASOMNIAS

Exploding Head Syndrome

EHS is characterized by a "sudden, loud imagined noise or sense of a violent explosion in the head occurring as the patient is falling asleep or waking during the night."[1]

To date, no open or controlled clinical trials for EHS treatment are available but several case studies of effective treatment have been conducted.[111,112] In many cases, reassurance about the benign nature of EHS could lead to a remission of EHS episodes. Tricyclic antidepressants (clomipramine, amitriptyline) are reported to decrease the frequency and intensity of attacks in some patients.[111,113] Moreover, calcium channel blockers (flunarizine and slow-release nifedipine) may also be useful.[114,115] Finally, anticonvulsants have been prescribed in some cases. Topiramate reduced the intensity of auditory sounds from loud bangs to much softer buzzing sounds but without a complete remission.[116] Carbamazepine was described to be effective in 3 cases.[112]

Sleep-Related Hallucinations

Sleep-related hallucinations are "hallucinatory experiences that occur at sleep onset (hypnagogic) or on awakening from sleep (hypnopompic)."[1] They can be associated with narcolepsy but a high prevalence in the normal population is also described. Complex nocturnal visual hallucinations are often associated with different disorders, especially in elderly, such as visual loss (Charles Bonnet syndrome), Lewy body disorders, and pathologic abnormality of the mesencephalon and diencephalon (peduncular hallucinosis).

Little objective information is available regarding the management of sleep-related hallucinations. Reassurance is frequently sufficient. Tricyclic antidepressants have been suggested for hypnagogic and hypnopompic hallucinations.

Sleep Enuresis

SE is characterized by "recurrent involuntary voiding that occurs during sleep. In primary SE, recurrent involuntary voiding occurs at least twice a week during sleep after 5 years of age in a subject who has never been consistently dry during sleep for 6 consecutive months. SE is considered secondary in a child or adult who had previously been dry for 6 consecutive months and then began wetting at least twice a week. Both primary and secondary enuresis must be present for a period of at least 3 months."[1] Moreover, SE is defined as *monosymptomatic* when the subject has no associated daytime symptoms of bladder dysfunction (such as wetting, increased voiding frequency, urgency, jiggling, squatting, and holding maneuvers). However, usually, when a meticulous history is obtained, most children have at least some mild daytime void symptoms, and their SE is classifiable as nonmonosymptomatic.[117]

The management of SE starts from some simple strategies, such as lifting or wakening, rewarding dry nights, bladder training (including retention control training), and fluid restriction.[117–119] However, it has been suggested that children should be encouraged to maintain an adequate fluid intake because fluid restriction can worsen bladder function.[120] Alarm systems that alert and awaken the child if any moisture is detected are considered a first-line treatment, and its effect seems to be more gradual but sustained with respect to drugs.[121]

The established drug treatment for polyuric bedwetting is desmopressin, a synthetic analog of the pituitary hormone arginine vasopressin, which reduces urine production by increasing water absorption.[119,120] It is available in tablet or fast-melting oral lyophilisate form. Desmopressin should be taken 1 hour before going to sleep. Treatment begins with a 0.2-mg desmopressin tablet or 120 mg of the melt tablet. If the starting dose does not lead to a clinical response, after 14 days the dose can be increased up to 0.4 or 240 mg. If treatment is successful, it can continue to be prescribed in 3-month blocks.[119] The sudden discontinuation of desmopressin results in a high recurrence of enuresis.[122] Desmopressin is considered a safe drug. The rare and most severe side effect of oral desmopressin therapy is the risk of "water intoxication" (if medication intake coincides with drinking large volumes) with symptoms of vomiting, headache, decreased consciousness, possible seizures, and hyponatremia. Therefore, fluid intake in the evening should be restricted to 250 mL, and nighttime drinking is not recommended. This complication seems to be more frequent during therapy with intranasal formulation of desmopressin.[123] Desmopressin is mostly indicated in children with nocturnal polyuria and normal bladder reservoir function and in those in whom alarm therapy has failed or who are thought to be unlikely to comply with alarm therapy.[124] It is frequently used as a stopgap (sleepovers and school camps) rather than cure for long term. About 30% of children with enuresis are full responders, and 40% have a partial response to desmopressin.[124] However, the long-lasting curative effect is low.[125]

The tricyclic antidepressant imipramine has anticholinergic, antispasmodic, and local anesthetic effects, and possibly a central nervous system effect on voiding, and has been approved for use in treating nocturnal enuresis in children aged 6 years and older.[126] It is effective in about 40% of patients with enuresis but only 25% of them experience complete dryness once the medication is withdrawn.[127] Side effects encompass cardiac arrhythmias, hypotension, hepatotoxicity, central nervous system depression, interaction with other drugs, and the danger of intoxication by accidental overdose. Therefore, screening for a long QT syndrome with electrocardiogram before starting treatment is recommended.

Anticholinergic drugs are used for SE, mainly for nonmonosymptomatic cases.[117–120] They are thought to act by increasing the functional bladder capacity and enabling patients affected to achieve better control over micturition. The anticholinergic drug most frequently used is represented by oxybutynin (0.1–0.3 mg/kg/d), although it has considerable risk of side effects (flushing, blurred vision, constipation, tremor, decreased salivation, and decreased ability to sweat) because of its relatively nonspecific affinity for several cholinergic receptor isoforms. The fourth International Consultation on Incontinence[128] recommended the use of propiverine (0.8–1 mg/kg/d) as first-line medication for nonmonosymptomatic SE (level of evidence 1, grade of recommendation B/C). Recent studies have shown the efficacy and safety of other anticholinergic drugs, such as trospium chloride, soli-fenacin,[129] and tolterodine[130] in children.

Although anticholinergic monotherapy could be ineffective, it can improve treatment response when combined with other established treatments, such as imipramine, desmopressin, or enuresis alarms, particularly in treatment-resistant cases.[131] Indeed, a recent meta-analysis demonstrated that the combination therapy, comprising desmopressin plus an anticholinergic agent, was more effective compared with desmopressin monotherapy for the treatment of SE in children.[132]

CLINICS CARE POINTS

- For parasomnia treatment every priming or triggering factor (i.e. inadequate sleep routines, co-existing sleep disorders, drugs) should be investigated and avoided.
- Disorders of arousal (DOA) are often relatively benign and transitory, and pharmacological therapy is usually unnecessary.
- No properly powered randomised controlled studies evaluating the efficacy of behavioural or pharmacological interventions for DOA exists; thus, no drug has yet been approved.
- The treatment of rapid eye movement sleep behaviour disorder is mainly symptomatic and usually consists of clonazepam and melatonin.

REFERENCES

1. American Academy of Sleep Medicine. International classification of sleep disorders-third edition (ICSD-3). Darien (Illinois); 2014.
2. Stallman HM, Kohler M. Prevalence of sleepwalk ing: a systematic review and meta-analysis. PLoS One 2016;11(11):e0164769.
3. Derry CP, Harvey AS, Walker MC, et al. NREM arousal parasomnias and their distinction from nocturnal frontal lobe epilepsy: a video EEG anal ysis. Sleep 2009;32(12):1637–44.
4. Howell MJ. Parasomnias: an updated review. Neurotherapeutics 2012;9(4):753–75.
5. Zadra A, Desautels A, Petit D, et al. Somnambu lism: clinical aspects and pathophysiological hy potheses. Lancet Neurol 2013;12(3):285–94.
6. Siclari F, Khatami R, Urbaniok F, et al. Violence in sleep. Brain 2010;133(12):3494–509.
7. Lopez R, Jaussent I, Scholz S, et al. Functional impairment in adult sleepwalkers: a case-control study. Sleep 2013;36(3):345–51.
8. Harris M, Grunstein RR. Treatments for somnambu lism in adults: assessing the evidence. Sleep Med Rev 2009;13(4):295–7.
9. Attarian H, Zhu L. Treatment options for disorders of arousal: a case series. Int J Neurosci 2013; 123(9):623–5.
10. Arnulf I, Zhang B, Uguccioni G, et al. A scale for assessing the severity of arousal disorders. Sleep 2014;37(1):127–36.
11. Attarian H. Treatment options for parasomnias. Neurol Clin 2010;28(4):1089–106.
12. Tinuper P, Bisulli F, Provini F. The parasomnias: mech-anisms and treatment: the parasomnias: mecha- nisms and treatment. Epilepsia 2012;53:12–9.

13. Kotagal S. Treatment of dyssomnias and parasom nias in childhood. Curr Treat Options Neurol 2012;14(6):630–49.
14. Galbiati A, Rinaldi F, Giora E, et al. Behavioural and cognitive-behavioural treatments of parasomnias. Behav Neurol 2015;2015:786928.
15. Guilleminault C, Kirisoglu C, Bao G, et al. Adult chronic sleepwalking and its treatment based on polysomnography. Brain 2005;128(Pt 5):1062–9.
16. Cochen De Cock V. Sleepwalking. Curr Treat Options Neurol 2016;18(2):6.
17. Rudolph U, Mohler H. GABA-based therapeutic approaches: GABAA receptor subtype functions. Curr Opin Pharmacol 2006;6(1):18–23.
18. Dolder CR, Nelson MH. Hypnosedative-induced complex behaviours: incidence, mechanisms and management. CNS Drugs 2008;22(12): 1021–36.
19. Mason TBA, Pack AI. Sleep terrors in childhood. J Pediatr 2005;147(3):388–92.
20. Allen RM. Attenuation of drug-induced anxiety dreams and pavor nocturnus by benzodiazepines. J Clin Psychiatry 1983;44(3):106–8.
21. Schenck CH, Milner DM, Hurwitz TD, et al. A polysomnographic and clinical report on sleep-related injury in 100 adult patients. Am J Psychiatry 1989;146(9):1166–73.
22. Schenck CH, Mahowald MW. Long-term, nightly benzodiazepine treatment of injurious parasomnias and other disorders of disrupted nocturnal sleep in 170 adults. Am J Med 1996;100(3):333–7.
23. Goldbloom D, Chouinard G. Clonazepam in the treatment of neuroleptic-induced somnambulism. Am J Psychiatry 1984;141(11):1486.
24. Schenck CH, Mahowald MW. A polysomnographically documented case of adult somnambulism with long-distance automobile driving and frequent nocturnal violence: parasomnia with continuing danger as a noninsane automatism? Sleep 1995; 18(9):765–72.
25. Remulla A, Guilleminault C. Somnambulism (sleep walking). Expert Opin Pharmacother 2004;5(10): 2069–74.
26. Reid WH, Haffke EA, Chu CC. Diazepam in intractable sleepwalking: a pilot study. Hillside J Clin Psychiatry 1984;6(1):49–55.
27. Berlin RM, Qayyum U. Sleepwalking: diagnosis and treatment through the life cycle. Psychosomatics 1986;27(11):755–60.
28. Kavey NB, Whyte J, Resor SR, et al. Somnambu lism in adults. Neurology 1990;40(5):749–52.
29. Kierlin L, Littner MR. Parasomnias and antidepressant therapy: a review of the literature. Front Psychiatry 2011;2:71.
30. Cooper AJ. Treatment of coexistent night-terrors and somnambulism in adults with imipramine and diazepam. J Clin Psychiatry 1987;48(5):209–10.
31. Balon R. Sleep terror disorder and insomnia treated with trazodone: a case report. Ann Clin Psychiatry 1994;6(3):161–3.
32. Wilson SJ, Lillywhite AR, Potokar JP, et al. Adult night terrors and paroxetine. Lancet 1997; 350(9072):185.
33. Frölich Alfred Wiater Gerd Lehmkuhl J. Successful treatment of severe parasomnias with paroxetine in a 12-year-old boy. Int J Psychiatry Clin Pract 2001; 5(3):215–8.
34. Lillywhite AR, Wilson SJ, Nutt DJ. Successful treat ment of night terrors and somnambulism with par oxetine. Br J Psychiatry 1994;164(4):551–4.
35. Kawashima T, Yamada S. Paroxetine-induced somnambulism. J Clin Psychiatry 2003;64(4):483.
36. Xie Z, Chen F, Li WA, et al. A review of sleep dis orders and melatonin. Neurol Res 2017;39(6):559–65.
37. Jan JE, Freeman RD. Melatonin therapy for circadian rhythm sleep disorders in children with mul tiple disabilities: what have we learned in the last decade? Dev Med Child Neurol 2004;46(11): 776–82.
38. Jan JE, Freeman RD, Wasdell MB, et al. A child with severe night terrors and sleep-walking responds to melatonin therapy. Dev Med Child Neurol 2004;46(11):789.
39. Ozcan O, Donmez YE. Melatonin treatment for childhood sleep terror. J Child Adolesc Psychopharmacol 2014;24(9):528–9.
40. Bruni O, Ferri R, Miano S, et al. l-5-Hydroxytryptophan treatment of sleep terrors in children. Eur J Pediatr 2004;163(7):402–7.
41. Sasayama D, Washizuka S, Honda H. Effective treatment of night terrors and sleepwalking with ra-melteon. J Child Adolesc Psychopharmacol 2016;26(10):948.
42. Winkelman JW, Johnson EA, Richards LM. Sleep-related eating disorder. Handb Clin Neurol 2011; 98:577–85.
43. Inoue Y. Sleep-related eating disorder and its asso ciated conditions: clinical implication of SRED. Psychiatry Clin Neurosci 2015;69(6):309–20.
44. Howell MJ, Schenck CH. Restless nocturnal eating: a common feature of Willis-Ekbom Syndrome (RLS). J Clin Sleep Med 2012;8(4):413–9.
45. Auger RR. Sleep-related eating disorders. Psychiatry (Edgmont) 2006;3(11):64.
46. Brion A, Flamand M, Oudiette D, et al. Sleep-related eating disorder versus sleepwalking: a controlled study. Sleep Med 2012;13(8): 1094–101.
47. Chiaro G, Caletti MT, Provini F. Treatment of sleep-related eating disorder. Curr Treat Options Neurol 2015;17(8):361.
48. Howell MJ, Schenck CH. Treatment of nocturnal eating disorders. Curr Treat Options Neurol 2009; 11(5):333–9.

49. Provini F, Albani F, Vetrugno R, et al. A pilot double-blind placebo-controlled trial of low-dose prami pexole in sleep-related eating disorder. Eur J Neurol 2005;12(6):432–6.
50. Santin J, Mery V, Elso MJ, et al. Sleep-related eating disorder: a descriptive study in Chilean pa tients. Sleep Med 2014;15(2):163–7.
51. Schenck CH, Hurwitz TD, O'Connor KA, et al. Additional categories of sleep-related eating disorders and the current status of treatment. Sleep 1993; 16(5):457–66.
52. Miyaoka T, Yasukawa R, Tsubouchi K, et al. Suc cessful treatment of nocturnal eating/drinking syndrome with selective serotonin reuptake in-hibitors. Int Clin Psychopharmacol 2003;18(3):175–7.
53. Martinez-Salio A, Soler-Algarra S, Calvo-Garcia I, et al. Nocturnal sleep-related eating disorder that responds to topiramate. Rev Neurol 2007;45(5): 276–9 [in Spanish].
54. Winkelman JW. Treatment of nocturnal eating syndrome and sleep-related eating disorder with topir amate. Sleep Med 2003;4(3):243–6.
55. Winkelman JW. Efficacy and tolerability of open-label topiramate in the treatment of sleep-related eating disorder: a retrospective case series. J Clin Psychiatry 2006;67(11):1729–34.
56. Wilkes JJ, Nelson E, Osborne M, et al. Topiramate is an insulin-sensitizing compound in vivo with direct effects on adipocytes in female ZDF rats. Am J Physiol Endocrinol Metab 2005;288(3): E617–24.
57. Zapp AA, Fischer EC, Deuschle M. The effect of agomelatine and melatonin on sleep-related eating: a case report. J Med Case Rep 2017; 11(1):275.
58. Comella CL, Nardine TM, Diederich NJ, et al. Sleep-related violence, injury, and REM sleep behavior disorder in Parkinson's disease. Neurology 1998;51(2):526–9.
59. McCarter SJ, St Louis EK, Boswell CL, et al. Factors associated with injury in REM sleep behavior disorder. Sleep Med 2014;15(11):1332–8.
60. Olson EJ, Boeve BF, Silber MH. Rapid eye movement sleep behaviour disorder: demographic, clin-ical and laboratory findings in 93 cases. Brain J Neurol 2000;123(Pt 2):331–9.
61. Postuma RB, Gagnon J-F, Tuineaig M, et al. Antidepressants and REM sleep behavior disorder: isolated side effect or neurodegenerative signal? Sleep 2013;36(11):1579–85.
62. Aurora RN, Zak RS, Maganti RK, et al. Best practice guide for the treatment of REM sleep behavior disorder (RBD). J Clin Sleep Med 2010;6(1):85–95.
63. Schenck CH, Bundlie SR, Ettinger MG, et al. Chronic behavioral disorders of human REM sleep: a new category of parasomnia. Sleep 1986;9(2): 293–308.
64. Li SX, Lam SP, Zhang J, et al. A prospective, natu ralistic follow-up study of treatment outcomes with clonazepam in rapid eye movement sleep behavior disorder. Sleep Med 2016;21:114–20.
65. McCarter SJ, Boswell CL, St Louis EK, et al. Treat ment outcomes in REM sleep behavior disorder. Sleep Med 2013;14(3):237–42.
66. Terzaghi M, Sartori I, Rustioni V, et al. Sleep disor ders and acute nocturnal delirium in the elderly: a comorbidity not to be overlooked. Eur J Intern Med 2014;25(4):350–5.
67. Kunz D, Mahlberg R. A two-part, double-blind, placebo-controlled trial of exogenous melatonin in REM sleep behaviour disorder. J Sleep Res 2010; 19(4):591–6.
68. Kunz D, Bes F. Melatonin as a therapy in REM sleep behavior disorder patients: an open-labeled pilot study on the possible influence of melatonin on REM-sleep regulation. Mov Disord 1999;14(3): 507–11.
69. Boeve BF, Silber MH, Ferman TJ. Melatonin for treatment of REM sleep behavior disorder in neuro-logic disorders: results in 14 patients. Sleep Med 2003;4(4):281–4.
70. Nomura T, Kawase S, Watanabe Y, et al. Use of ramelteon for the treatment of secondary REM sleep behavior disorder. Intern Med 2013;52(18): 2123–6.
71. Esaki Y, Kitajima T, Koike S, et al. An open-labeled trial of ramelteon in idiopathic rapid eye movement sleep behavior disorder. J Clin Sleep Med 2016; 12(5):689–93.
72. St. Louis EK, McCarter SJ, Boeve BF. Ramelteon for idiopathic REM sleep behavior disorder: impli cations for pathophysiology and future treatment trials. J Clin Sleep Med 2016;12(05): 643–5.
73. Bonakis A, Economou N-T, Papageorgiou SG, et al. Agomelatine may improve REM sleep behavior dis order symptoms. J Clin Psychopharmacol 2012; 32(5):732–4.
74. Fantini ML, Gagnon J-F, Filipini D, et al. The effects of pramipexole in REM sleep behavior disorder. Neurology 2003;61(10):1418–20.
75. Sasai T, Matsuura M, Inoue Y. Factors associated with the effect of pramipexole on symptoms of idio pathic REM sleep behavior disorder. Parkinsonism Relat Disord 2013;19(2):153–7.
76. Schmidt MH, Koshal VB, Schmidt HS. Use of pra mipexole in REM sleep behavior disorder: results from a case series. Sleep Med 2006;7(5):418–23.
77. Kumru H, Iranzo A, Carrasco E, et al. Lack of effects of pramipexole on REM sleep behavior disorder in Parkinson disease. Sleep 2008;31(10): 1418–21.
78. McCarley RW. Neurobiology of REM and NREM sleep. Sleep Med 2007;8(4):302–30.

79. Fernandez HH, Wu C-K, Ott BR. Pharmacotherapy of dementia with Lewy bodies. Expert Opin Pharmacother 2003;4(11):2027–37.
80. Terzaghi M, Rustioni V, Manni R, et al. Agrypnia with nocturnal confusional behaviors in dementia with Lewy bodies: immediate efficacy of rivastigmine. Mov Disord 2010;25(5):647–9.
81. Brunetti V, Losurdo A, Testani E, et al. Rivastigmine for refractory REM behavior disorder in mild cogni tive impairment. Curr Alzheimer Res 2014;11(3): 267–73.
82. Di Giacopo R, Fasano A, Quaranta D, et al. Rivastigmine as alternative treatment for refractory REM behavior disorder in Parkinson's disease. Mov Disord 2012;27(4):559–61.
83. Massironi G, Galluzzi S, Frisoni GB. Drug treatment of REM sleep behavior disorders in dementia with Lewy bodies. Int Psychogeriatr 2003;15(4):377–83.
84. Ringman JM, Simmons JH. Treatment of REM sleep behavior disorder with donepezil: a report of three cases. Neurology 2000;55(6):870–1.
85. Yeh S-B, Yeh P-Y, Schenck CH. Rivastigmine-induced REM sleep behavior disorder (RBD) in a 88-year-old man with Alzheimer's disease. J Clin Sleep Med 2010;6(2):192–5.
86. Babson KA, Sottile J, Morabito D. Cannabis, cannabinoids, and sleep: a review of the literature. Curr Psychiatry Rep 2017;19(4):23.
87. Chagas MHN, Eckeli AL, Zuardi AW, et al. Cannabi- diol can improve complex sleep-related behaviours associated with rapid eye movement sleep behav iour disorder in Parkinson's disease patients: a case series. J Clin Pharm Ther 2014; 39(5):564–6.
88. Anderson KN, Shneerson JM. Drug treatment of REM sleep behavior disorder: the use of drug ther apies other than clonazepam. J Clin Sleep Med 2009;5(3):235–9.
89. Bonakis A, Howard RS, Ebrahim IO, et al. REM sleep behaviour disorder (RBD) and its associa tions in young patients. Sleep Med 2009;10(6):641–5.
90. Jung Y, St Louis EK. Treatment of REM sleep behavior disorder. Curr Treat Options Neurol 2016;18(11):50.
91. Moghadam KK, Pizza F, Primavera A, et al. Sodium oxybate for idiopathic REM sleep behavior disor der: a report on two patients. Sleep Med 2017;32: 16–21.
92. Shneerson JM. Successful treatment of REM sleep behavior disorder with sodium oxybate. Clin Neuropharmacol 2009;32(3):158–9.
93. Detweiler MB, Pagadala B, Candelario J, et al. Treatment of post-traumatic stress disorder nightmares at a Veterans Affairs medical center. J Clin Med 2016;5(12):E117.
94. Jeffreys M, Capehart B, Friedman MJ. Pharmacotherapy for posttraumatic stress disorder: review with clinical applications. J Rehabil Res Dev 2012;49(5):703–15.
95. Miller KE, Brownlow JA, Woodward S, et al. Sleep and dreaming in posttraumatic stress disorder. Curr Psychiatry Rep 2017;19(10):71.
96. George KC, Kebejian L, Ruth LJ, et al. Meta-analysis of the efficacy and safety of prazosin versus placebo for the treatment of nightmares and sleep distur bances in adults with posttraumatic stress disorder. J Trauma Dissociation 2016;17(4): 494–510.
97. Kung S, Espinel Z, Lapid MI. Treatment of night mares with prazosin: a systematic review. Mayo Clin Proc 2012;87(9):890–900.
98. Raskind MA, Peterson K, Williams T, et al. A trial of prazosin for combat trauma PTSD with night- mares in active-duty soldiers returned from Iraq and Afghanistan. Am J Psychiatry 2013;170(9): 1003–10.
99. Hudson SM, Whiteside TE, Lorenz RA, et al. Prazo sin for the treatment of nightmares related to post traumatic stress disorder: a review of the literature. Prim Care Companion CNS Disord 2012;14(2).
100. Khachatryan D, Groll D, Booij L, et al. Prazosin for treating sleep disturbances in adults with posttraumatic stress disorder: a systematic review and meta-analysis of randomized controlled trials. Gen Hosp Psychiatry 2016;39:46–52.
101. Cameron C, Watson D, Robinson J. Use of a synthetic cannabinoid in a correctional population for posttraumatic stress disorder-related insomnia and nightmares, chronic pain, harm reduction, and other indications: a retrospective evaluation. J Clin Psychopharmacol 2014;34(5):559–64.
102. Fraser GA. The use of a synthetic cannabinoid in the management of treatment-resistant nightmares in posttraumatic stress disorder (PTSD). CNS Neurosci Ther 2009;15(1):84–8.
103. Jetly R, Heber A, Fraser G, et al. The efficacy of nabilone, a synthetic cannabinoid, in the treatment of PTSD-associated nightmares: a preliminary randomized, double-blind, placebo-controlled cross over design study. Psychoneuroendocrinology 2015;51:585–8.
104. Roitman P, Mechoulam R, Cooper-Kazaz R, et al. Preliminary, open-label, pilot study of add-on oral D9-tetrahydrocannabinol in chronic post-traumatic stress disorder. Clin Drug Investig 2014;34(8): 587–91.
105. Guilleminault C, Raynal D, Takahashi S, et al. Evaluation of short-term and long-term treatment of the narcolepsy syndrome with clomipramine hydrochloride. Acta Neurol Scand 1976;54(1):71–87.
106. Hishikawa Y, Ida H, Nakai K, et al. Treatment of narcolepsy with imipramine (tofranil) and desme- thylimipramine (pertofran). J Neurol Sci 1966;3(5): 453–61.

107. Mitler MM, Hajdukovic R, Erman M, et al. Narco lepsy. J Clin Neurophysiol 1990;7(1):93–118.
108. Koran LM, Raghavan S. Fluoxetine for isolated sleep paralysis. Psychosomatics 1993;34(2): 184–7.
109. Schrader H, Kayed K, Bendixen Markset AC, et al. The treatment of accessory symptoms in narcolepsy: a double-blind cross-over study of a selective serotonin re-uptake inhibitor (femoxetine) versus placebo. Acta Neurol Scand 1986;74(4): 297–303.
110. Abad VC, Guilleminault C. New developments in the management of narcolepsy. Nat Sci Sleep 2017;9:39–57.
111. Frese A, Summ O, Evers S. Exploding head syndrome: six new cases and review of the literature. Cephalalgia 2014;34(10):823–7.
112. Sharpless BA. Exploding head syndrome. Sleep Med Rev 2014;18(6):489–93.
113. Sachs C, Svanborg E. The exploding head syndrome: polysomnographic recordings and therapeutic suggestions. Sleep 1991;14(3):263–6.
114. Chakravarty A. Exploding Head syndrome: report of two new cases. Cephalalgia 2008;28(4): 399–400.
115. Jacome DE. Exploding head syndrome and idiopathic stabbing headache relieved by nifedipine. Cephalalgia Int J Headache 2001;21(5):617–8.
116. Palikh GM, Vaughn BV. Topiramate responsive exploding head syndrome. J Clin Sleep Med 2010; 6(4):382–3.
117. Harari MD. Nocturnal enuresis: nocturnal enuresis. J Paediatr Child Health 2013;49(4):264–71.
118. Jain S, Bhatt GC. Advances in the management of primary monosymptomatic nocturnal enuresis in children. Paediatr Int Child Health 2016;36(1):7–14.
119. Kuwertz-Broking E, von Gontard A. Clinical man agement of nocturnal enuresis. Pediatr Nephrol 2018;33(7):1145–54.
120. Caldwell PHY, Deshpande AV, Gontard AV. Man agement of nocturnal enuresis. BMJ 2013; 347(oct29 11):f6259.
121. Glazener CMA, Evans JHC, Peto RE. Alarm interventions for nocturnal enuresis in children. Cohrane Database Syst Rev 2005;2:CD002911.
122. Hjalmas K, Arnold T, Bower W, et al. Nocturnal enuresis: an international evidence based management strategy. J Urol 2004;171(6 Pt 2): 2545–61.
123. Robson WLM, Leung AKC, Norgaard JP. The comparative safety of oral versus intranasal desmopressin for the treatment of children with nocturnal enuresis. J Urol 2007;178(1):24–30.
124. Neveus T, Eggert P, Evans J, et al. Evaluation of and treatment for monosymptomatic enuresis: a standardization document from the International Children's Continence Society. J Urol 2010;183(2): 441–7.
125. Glazener CM, Evans JH. Desmopressin for nocturnal enuresis in children. Cochrane Database Syst Rev 2002;3:CD002112.
126. Neveus T. Nocturnal enuresis-theoretic back ground and practical guidelines. Pediatr Nephrol 2011;26(8):1207–14.
127. Caldwell PHY, Sureshkumar P, Wong WCF. Tricyclic and related drugs for nocturnal enuresis in children. Cochrane Database Syst Rev 2016;1: CD002117.
128. International Consultation on Incontinence, Abrams P, Cardozo L, et al, editors. Incontinence. 4th edition. Paris: Health Publication; 2009.
129. Hoebeke P, De Pooter J, De Caestecker K, et al. Solifenacin for therapy resistant overactive bladder. J Urol 2009;182(4 Suppl):2040–4.
130. Raes A, Hoebeke P, Segaert I, et al. Retrospective analysis of efficacy and tolerability of tolterodine in children with overactive bladder. Eur Urol 2004; 45(2):240–4.
131. Deshpande AV, Caldwell PHY, Sureshkumar P. Drugs for nocturnal enuresis in children (other than desmopressin and tricyclics). Cochrane Database Syst Rev 2012;12:CD002238.
132. Yu J, Yan Z, Zhou S, et al. Desmopressin plus anticholinergic agent in the treatment of nocturnal enuresis: a meta-analysis. Exp Ther Med 2017; 14(4):2875–84.

Precision Medicine for Idiopathic Hypersomnia

Isabelle Arnulf, MD, PhD[a,b,*], Smaranda Leu-Semenescu, MD[a], Pauline Dodet, MD[a]

KEYWORDS

• Hypersomnia • Long sleep time • Drowsiness • GABA • Modafinil • Sodium oxybate

KEY POINTS

- Idiopathic hypersomnia (IH) is characterized by excessive daytime sleepiness despite normal, undisturbed sleep of normal or prolonged duration.
- New studies insist on the lack of sensitivity, specificity, and reproducibility of multiple sleep latency tests, and the interest in measuring excessive sleep duration on prolonged protocols.
- Cerebrospinal fluid (CSF) analysis suggests that some patients with resistant central hypersomnia may produce during wakefulness an endogenous peptide-binding GABA-A receptors.
- Functional brain imaging supports this concept, with low activity of the medial prefrontal cortex during wakefulness in patients with IH.
- Retrospective and recent placebo-controlled studies illustrate the respective benefit of modafinil, sodium oxybate, pitolisant, mazindol, flumazenil, and clarithromycin in IH treatment.

INTRODUCTION

Idiopathic hypersomnia (IH) is a rare sleep disorder characterized by excessive daytime sleepiness (without sleep onset in rapid eye movement [REM] periods [SOREMPs]), despite normal, undisturbed sleep, of normal or prolonged duration. However, this simple definition broadly covers various clinical profiles of patients, which may be captured by different methods of sleep monitoring, and that illustrate the interest of precision medicine in this disorder. Furthermore, IH definitions have suffered from their contrast with narcolepsy type 1, in which several pathognomonic features, including cataplexy, SOREMps, and cerebrospinal fluid (CSF) hypocretin-1 deficiency define a more homogeneous disorder. To date, there are no definitive biological markers and causes for IH. In addition, the clinical phenotypes and sleep abnormalities (eg, multiple sleep latency test [MSLT] vs long-term monitoring) are heterogeneous. In the past decade, several cohorts have highlighted the lack of sensitivity and long-term reproducibility of the MSLT in patients with IH (and with narcolepsy type 2) and have developed other methods of sleep monitoring to assess patient symptoms more objectively and to define normative values. An important step in identifying the etiology of central hypersomnolence disorders (apart from hypocretin-1 deficiency), was reached when the Atlanta, Georgia, group found indirect evidence that an endogenous hypnotic neurotransmitter when secreted, stimulates GABA-A receptors in some patients with IH (mostly those refractory to stimulants). In addition, functional brain imaging suggests that the prefrontal medial cortex of patients with IH is "asleep" when they would otherwise be characterized as awake. Subsequently, there have been formal, placebo-controlled evaluations of modafinil, clarithromycin, and low sodium oxybate in IH, and retrospective series showing the benefit of sodium oxybate, mazindol, flumazenil, and the new prohistamine stimulant, pitolisant, in IH.

Sleep Med Clin 14 (2019) 333-350 https://doi.org/10.1016/j.jsmc.2019.05.007 1556-407X/19/© 2019 Elsevier Inc.

[a] Service des pathologies du sommeil, Hopital Pitie-Salpetriere, 83 boulevard de l'Hopital, Paris 75013, France;
[b] Sorbonne University, Paris, France
* Corresponding author.
E-mail address: isabelle.arnulf@aphp.fr

Sleep Med Clin 17 (2022) 379–398
https://doi.org/10.1016/j.jsmc.2022.06.016
1556-407X/22/

In many textbooks, IH is often described as "what it is not" (eg, it is not narcolepsy, a mild chronic sleep insufficiency, especially in long sleepers, an upper airway resistance syndrome, a mood disorder with excessive sleepiness, a posttraumatic hypersomnia, a non-REM [NREM] parasomnia with daytime sleepiness). Because IH is a diagnosis of exclusion, these conditions should be first ruled out. The association of IH symptoms with chronic fatigue syndrome/myalgia, attention deficit hyperactivity disorder, and mood disorders raises the potential for overlap with these disorders and the need for more objective measures. In this article, we discuss IH alone and presume that the other hypersomnia disorders have been ruled out by experienced sleep specialists.

HISTORY

Abnormal hypersomnia has been recognized under various terms (idiopathic narcolepsy, NREM narcolepsy, functional, mixed, or harmonious hypersomnia) since the nineteenth century. Bedrich Roth[1] (Prague, Czech Republic) is considered to be the father of the disorder, having described, since the 1940s, a large series of patients suffering from non-narcoleptic daytime sleepiness with sleep drunkenness. Although some patients in this first series likely suffered from sleep apnea, many of them had clinical features suggestive of IH with long sleep time. In the International Classification of Sleep Disorders (ICSD), the disorder was coined as "idiopathic central nervous system hypersomnolence" in 1979. The condition, named "idiopathic hypersomnia" in 2001,[2] was split between IH with versus without long sleep time in 2005,[3] and later merged together in 2013.[4] There has been more recent debate to split the condition again, to merge narcolepsy type 2 and IH without long sleep time together and to isolate IH with long sleep time as a separate entity. This "coming and going" movement illustrates the difficulty to define clinical phenotypic clusters in IH, although data driven, unsupervised clustering goes in this recent direction. Indeed, studies on IH remain scarce, especially if one compares with the number of publications on narcolepsy, a rare disorder, and on Kleine–Levin syndrome, a much rarer syndrome (but has some pathognomonic clinical features).

EPIDEMIOLOGY

The exact prevalence of IH is unknown, but it is slightly less frequent in expert centers than narcolepsy, suggesting a prevalence of 1 to 2 affected persons for 10,000 inhabitants. The disorder mostly starts during adolescence and early adulthood (**Table 1**). Several series of patients with IH in expert sleep centers indicate that IH affects women (75%) more than men and more frequently persons of European origin (see **Table 1**). The familial appearance of this disorder is observed more frequently than in narcolepsy, but no formal study of familial aggregation has been published to date. The IH rarity can be compared with daytime sleepiness associated with long sleep in epidemiologic studies. In the general population, 1.6% of adults reported sleeping more than 9 hours per 24 hours with concomitant distress or daytime impairment.[5] This sample contained more women, more young (18–24 year old) and older (>65 year old) subjects, and more unemployed and retired persons than workers in the general population. Cerebrovascular diseases, disease of the central nervous system (mostly mood disorders, 12 times more frequent), heart diseases, and diseases of the musculoskeletal system were on average twice more prevalent in this subcategory. This epidemiologic study highlights the differential diagnoses of IH. The prevalence of *Diagnostic and Statistical Manual of*

Table 1
Symptoms in idiopathic hypersomnia

1. Excessive Daytime Sleepiness • Continuous drowsiness/fogginess without naps • Single vs repeated daytime naps • Brief (eg, <30–60 min) vs prolonged naps • Restorative vs nonrestorative naps • Irresistible (eg, sleep attacks) vs resistible sleep episodes • Hyperactive counterstrategy	2. Nighttime Sleep • Normal vs long (>10 h) duration (during unrestrained conditions) • High vs normal or low sleep efficiency • Dream recall: absent ("black out"), normal, excessive • Sleep inertia: none, mild, or severe (sleep drunkenness)
3. Associated symptoms • Automatic behaviors • Trouble focusing • Sleep-related hallucinations • Sleep paralysis • Orthostatic hypotension • Raynaud phenomenon • Headaches	4. Epidemiology • Rare neonatal forms • Mostly young adult onset • Women > men • More evening chronotype

Mental Disorders, Fourth Edition hypersomnia disorder in this sample was 0.5% (0.4%-0.6%),[5] which suggests that IH is underdiagnosed.

CLINICAL ASPECTS THE SPECTRUM OF SLEEPINESS IN IDIOPATHIC HYPERSOMNIA

Although all patients with IH are sleepy, the quality of daytime sleepiness varies among them. Sleepiness ranges from frequent, brief, irresistible, and restorative naps (as in narcolepsy) to continuous drowsiness, culminating in rare, prolonged, and nonrestorative naps (see **Table 1**). Many patients with IH, particularly those with long sleep time, describe rare if any daytime sleep attacks.[6] When naps are taken, 87% of patients with IH report a nap duration longer than 60 minutes; 52% to 78% consider their naps unrefreshing, to the point that many patients avoid the situation to prevent severe postnapping inertia. Patients with IH often report suffering from continuous nonimperative sleepiness, which leads them to never feel fully awake during the daytime, to feel "foggy" and lack alertness. In patients with sleep drunkenness, this drowsiness is maximal on awakening and may transiently fade in the evening.[6] Consequently, many patients with IH are more alert in the evening than in the morning.[6] Although the descriptions of sleepiness seem different in IH than in narcolepsy type 1, both groups have on average similar scores on the Epworth sleepiness scale (ESS),[7] and benefit to a similar degree from stimulants such as modafinil, sodium oxybate, and mazindol.[7–9]

Maintaining a hyperactive state can help patients with IH to resist sleepiness.[6] This can include any increased motor activity (eg, standing, walking while learning, speaking continuously) or performing several activities at the same time (eg, writing while listening, listening to an audiobook when doing housework).[6] Some patients with IH have a rapid, continuous speech during their medical appointment, as if they need to be excited to maintain sufficient alertness. On average, patients describe that they cannot sustain attention for more than 1 hour (vs almost 4 hours in controls), suggesting a cognitive fatigability.[6] This lack of attention can produce automatic behaviors (see **Table 1**). In our clinical practice, however, they are often extremely organized, making "to do lists" (possibly to compensate for sleepiness and forgetfulness) and reacting rapidly and precisely to questions and requests, in sharp contrast to the frequent procrastination and disorganization observed in patients with narcolepsy or attention deficit hyperactivity disorder. Eventually, autonomic symptoms, including orthostatic hypotension, headache, and Raynaud phenomenon are reported by half of the patients with IH.

Sleep Duration in Idiopathic Hypersomnia

The profile of the major sleep episode in IH varies from a normal (eg, 7–8 hours) sleep duration, rarely with frequent awakenings, to a prolonged (eg, 10–15 hours) sleep duration with a high sleep efficiency, which seems more specific to IH. In ICSD-2,[3] IH was divided into 2 types, with and without long sleep time, defined by whether the usual sleep duration was more or less than 10 hours per night. The 2 types were later merged in ICSD-3, because the committee considered that there was not enough data yet to demonstrate that these were different entities. However, a recent clustering analysis in a series of patients in Prague (Czech Republic) found 2 clearly different clusters, with differing nocturnal sleep times, and no clinical difference between patients with IH without long sleep time and those with narcolepsy type 2.[10] The cutoff of 10 hours of nocturnal sleep for "long sleep time" has not been determined by specific analysis, but is derived from the sleep duration defining a long sleeper (a person needing more than 10 hours of sleep to feel alert during daytime). In the IH series, the frequency of patients usually sleeping more than 10 hours varies from 19% to 58% (**Table 2**). The term "long sleep time" in IH refers only to the main sleep period and does not include any daytime napping periods. Some patients with IH will sleep 9 hours during the night and 3 hours during the day, far exceeding this limit of 10 hours when the 24-h day is considered. During weekdays, sleep duration for patients with IH is often constrained by the working schedule, and does not exceed 7 to 9 hours, whereas sleep rebounds of 10 to 18 hours may occur during the weekend and vacations. Most patients with IH feel that they sleep very deeply through the night. Frequent sleep disruption is atypical in IH, although common in narcolepsy.[2] In patients with IH, sleep mentation also varies, from a complete blackout with no memory of anything between the sleep onset and offset, to vivid dreams (25% of patients[11]) and "being tired of dreaming too much." Sleep-related hallucinations (4%–43% of patients) and sleep paralysis (10%–40%) are reported in IH series.

Sleep Drunkenness Is A Major Feature in Idiopathic Hypersomnia

The ability to wake up in the morning for patients with IH varies from an easy awakening (as in narcolepsy) to major sleep inertia characterized by a

Table 2
Demographic and clinical features in various series of patients with idiopathic hypersomnia

Measure	IH (Mixed)	IH without LST	IH with LST
Demographic features			
Age at onset, y	17 ± 9[11]; 17.5–18[12]; 20 [16][13]; 22 ± 9[8]; 22 ± 12[7]	16[14]; 19 ± 7[15]; 22[16]; 22 ± 13[17]; 29 ± 10[10]	16[14]; 21 ± 9[10]; 24[16]
Age at diagnosis, y	29 ± 12[8]; 33 ± 13[7]; 34 ± 12[11]; 34 ± 13[18]; 34 [16][13]; 35[16]	32[14]; 34 ± 13[18]	27[14]; 34 ± 13[18]
Sex ratio, female/male	38[12]; 51[11]; 64[18]; 64[16] 65[13]; 74[7]; 77[19]; 78[8]	42[17]; 44[16]; 49[15]; 60[10,18];82[14];	63[16]; 68[18]; 73[10]; 79[14]
European origin, %	93[16]; 100[18]	—	—
Body mass index, kg/m^2	24 ± 5[7],[18]; 25 [4][11]; 25.4 [6.2][13]; 25–26[12]	22[14]; 25.2 ± 3.6[20]; 26 ± 5[18]	22[14]; 23 ± 4[18]
Circadian score	48 ± 13[18]; 49 ± 8[19]	53 ± 10[18]	44 ± 14[18]
Daytime symptoms			
Score on the Epworth sleepiness scale at diagnosis, 0–24	14–15[16]; 15 ± 4[18]; ± 3[11]; 16 ± 4[7,8]; ± 4[19]; 17 [7][13]	± 6.7[21]; 14.1 ± 3.2[22]; 15 ± 4[7,18]; 16[14]; 14 ± 3[15]; 15 ± 4[18]; 16 ± 3[11]; ± 4.3[10] 16 ± 3.2[10]; 16.5 ± 4.4[20]; 16.5[14]; 16 ± 4[16] 17 ± 4[11]; 18 ± 4[7,16]	
Nap frequency/wk	2.7 ± 2.6[6]	—	—
Average nap duration, h	1.2 ± 0.5[18]; 1.5 ± 0.9[13]	—	—
Total daytime sleep, min	90 ± 56[18]	89 ± 73[17]	
Sleep attacks, %	54[16]	56[16]; 80[10]	75[16]; 27[10]
Long (>30 min) naps, %	51[16]	—	—
Nap longer than 60 min, %	87[11]	—	—

Refreshing short naps, %	25[6]	56[16]	0[16]
Nonrefreshing naps, %	52[6]; 72[13]; 77[16]; 78[11]	8[10]; 45[6]	48[6]; 72[10]
Attention complaint, %	55[6]	—	—
Memory complaint, %	79[6]	—	—
Automatic behaviors, %	58[6]; 61[16]	63[16]	38[16]
Nighttime symptoms			
Usual sleep duration, h	8 [1][13]; 8.4 ± 1.9[16]; 9 ± 2[11]	—	—
Usual sleep time > 10 h, %	19[13]; 30[11]; 58[7]	0[11]	100[11]
Sleep paralysis, %	10[13]; 28[18]; 40[16]	14[14]; 2 2[22]; 29[18]; 44[16]	19[14]; 23[18]; 25[16]; 27[18]
Hypnagogic hallucination,%	4[13]; 4.5[11]; 24[18]; 43[16]	4[11]; 25[18,22]; 30[14]; 56[16]	5[11]; 23[18]; 27[14]; 38[16]
Difficulty waking up in the morning, %	66[13]; 100[8]	11[16]; 40[10]; 60[14]	75[16]; 77[14]; 96[10]
Sleep drunkenness, %	37[18]; 55[11]; 66[13]	0[10]; 11[16]; 23[18]; 46[11]	36[16]; 50[18]; 70[11]; 58.3[10]
Time to get going in the morning, min	42[16]	7 ± 6[16]	72 ± 62[16]
Comorbidities			
Migraine, %	7–12[16]; 8[11]	—	—
Minor depression, %	14[11]	—	—
HAD depression score	7.1 ± 5 (>controls)[18]	7.5 ± 4.6[18]	6.8 ± 5.4[18]
Orthostatic hypotension, headache, Raynaud, %	46[6]; 50[16]		
Allergy, %	12[23]	—	—
Autoimmune disease, %	4[23]	—	—
Inflammatory disease, %	7[23]	—	—
Heavy alcohol drinker, %	9[24]	—	—
Tobacco smoker, %	20[24]	—	—
Substance use, %	2[24]	—	—

Measures are mean ± SD or %, except for x-y which indicate median or mean values from 2 different IH groups.
Abbreviations: HAD, hospital anxiety and depression rating scale; IH, idiopathic hypersomnia; LST, long sleep time (>10 h).

"sleep drunkenness," which can be the main complaint of the patients with IH. Sleep drunkenness is conceptualized as a state intermediate to sleep and wake. It seems to be an exacerbation of the normal sleep inertia observed in the normal population, especially during postdeprivation sleep rebound, and in delayed sleep phase syndrome.[25] With sleep drunkenness, patients may not awaken without several successive, strong alarm clocks, and still may immediately return to sleep. Confusion, slowness, incoordination, and aggressiveness are described. Many patients with IH with sleep drunkenness report being slow during the first hour after awakening, with a poor sense of time. Parents of teenagers with IH report having to shake the patient or pull them away from the bed, as if they would "try to wake up a dead person." The disability associated with sleep drunkenness contributes to tardiness at work or even losing their job. Many patients need to be awakened by another person, making them dependent on others to keep their work schedule. Mothers with IH have significant difficulties awakening when their baby cries, needing some assistance for performing their parental duties during the night. Sleep drunkenness, however, is not a consistent finding in IH, with the symptom reported by 37% to 100% of patients, depending on series and on the presence of the "long sleep time" phenotype (see **Table 2**). The symptom is independent of sleep time and the presence or absence of slow-wave sleep at the end of the night.[18] Patients with unipolar depression also report difficulties waking up, but compared with IH, this is associated with anhedonia and decreased motivation. The severity of sleep drunkenness makes it more specific to IH. Note that rare patients with narcolepsy with long sleep time (a disorder cumulating symptoms and signs of narcolepsy and of IH with long sleep time) also report sleep drunkenness.[14]

SLEEP TESTS MULTIPLE SLEEP LATENCY TEST IS NORMAL IN MOST CASES OF IDIOPATHIC HYPERSOMNIA WITH LONG SLEEP TIME

A striking example for which the MSLT was normal in spite of obviously excessive sleep time was reported by Voderholzer and colleagues.[26] This 16-year-old boy had a 4-year history of severely increased sleep need, daytime fatigue, and great difficulty waking after 9 hours of nighttime sleep, with hypotonia and dizziness in the morning, and no cataplexy or sleep attacks during daytime. His mean daytime sleep latency was 11 minutes (a normal value) despite previously sleeping for 27 hours during 36 hours of monitoring. During longer-term monitoring, he slept 19 hours 22 minutes per 24 hours (from 11 PM to 6:30 PM the next day, with a 97% sleep efficiency). This extreme case illustrates the contrast between a measure of daytime sleep-onset propensity (MSLT) and a measure of ad libitum sleep (long-term sleep monitoring). Ad libitum sleep, measured over 24 to 48 hours, may better capture the sleep needs of people in absence of sleep restriction. By definition, the MSLT should be performed after unrestricted sleep (which would allow recognizing the long sleepers), but many sleep laboratories set up a maximal waking time (from 6:30 AM to 8 AM) for organization purposes and because the first MSLT should start after a minimum time of 90 minutes (ie, between 8 AM and 9:30 AM).

To determine the sensitivity of the MSLT (mean sleep latency [MSL] <8 minutes) in patients with IH, one has to compare it to a reference standard in reaching the IH diagnosis. Studies have used different approaches, including a clinical assessment of IH with careful exclusion of competing diagnoses,[11] or a clinical assessment combined with objective criterion, including either a minimal sleep time during ad libitum long-term monitoring,[14,18] or an abnormal potentiation of the GABA-A receptor in CSF.[27] In other cases, when the MSL for an MSLT is set as abnormal if < 8 minutes, patients without this criterion are generally classified as suffering from "subjective hypersomnia."[17] The Cambridge (United Kingdom) group showed that among 72 patients who had a typical clinical phenotype of IH, including those without long sleep time, 49% did not fulfill the criteria of an MSL less than 8 minutes.

The Paris (France) group defined patients suffering from IH with long sleep time as sleeping more than 11 hours during ad libitum monitoring of 19 hours (second night and second day) following a habituation first night and a first day with MSLT.[18] In the group with total sleep time longer than 10 hours, as many as 71% did not fulfill the criteria of an MSL less than 8 minutes, of which only 17% had borderline (between 8 and 10 minutes) sleep latencies.[18] When considering all patients with IH (with and without long sleep time), the MSL was less than 8 minutes in 61%, still leaving 39% of patients with IH with normal mean sleep latencies.[18] In the Bologna group (Italy), it was not possible to infer the frequency of normal MSL in patients with IH, because those with mean sleep latencies >8 minutes were ruled out as suffering from "subjective hypersomnia."[17] The Montpellier (France) group used a 2-step procedure to set up a minimal sleep time per 32 hours of ad libitum monitoring (first night followed by a day and a second night) leading to a lower limit of 19 hours of sleep per 32 hours in 37 patients with frank clinical symptoms of IH and MSL <10 minutes.[14] Among 90 patients with clear-cut or probable IH, 29 (67.8%) did not fulfill the criteria of an MSL <8 minutes, despite more than 19 hours of sleep during the 36-h procedure. Repeating the MSLT using a modified procedure by interrupting each nap after 1 minute of sleep, which should preserve sleep pressure and decrease the sleep-onset latency, in the same group still resulted in 48 (42%) patients with an MSL >8 minutes.

The Atlanta group identified a new biological marker in the CSF suggestive of potentiating the GABA-A receptor function. In 7 patients with drug-resistant hypersomnia and various initial diagnoses (including long sleeper, narcolepsy type 2, and Kleine–Levin syndrome), the activity at the GABA receptor was increased, despite an MSL greater than 8 minutes in 5 (71%) of 7 patients.[27] In 16 patients with nonnarcoleptic, drug-resistant hypersomnia and GABA-A receptor potentiation, 6 (37.5%) of 16 had a normal MSL at the MSLT.[28]

The Importance of Measuring Excessive Sleep Duration

These results highlight the importance of measures outside the MSLT to capture the IH sleep characteristics. The word *hypersomnia* comes from the Greek root *"hyper"* for "excessive" and the Latin root *"somnius"* for sleep. Thus, the word means "excessive sleep duration," not excessive daytime sleepiness. In IH, excessive need for sleep is best expressed in unrestricted conditions, such as during the weekend, holidays, and in the sleep laboratory, with on average 3 additional hours slept than during weekdays.[6] The duration of spontaneous nighttime sleep time can be measured during unrestrained polysomnography; however, this would not include the daytime sleep time performed during naps. Hence, several groups have developed procedures aimed at assessing the maximum sleep time that can be produced in unrestrained (often boring) conditions, over periods lasting 24 to 48 hours.

To avoid potential postsleep deprivation rebound, the 3 main procedures include the classic recommendation to visit the sleep laboratory after 1 to 2 weeks without sleep deprivation, as assessed by sleep log or actigraphy. However, patients with IH with long sleep time hardly sleep more than 7 to 9 hours during weekdays when they work, still leaving them sleep-deprived relative to their daily sleep needs, unless tests are performed after 1 week of vacation with unrestrained sleep. The increased homeostatic need for sleep in patients with IH can be partly alleviated by the 48-hour procedure developed in Paris (France), which includes a habituation night followed by the 5-nap MSLT test, during which the patients often sleep, although the MSL is longer than in patients with narcolepsy. Whether home-based studies can replace in-laboratory procedures is questionable, as normative measures have not been established for these conditions.

So far, 3 different procedures have been developed to capture excessive need for sleep (**Fig. 1**, **Table 3**).[14,17,18] One of the procedures (Bologna, Italy) does not include normative measures.[17] The shorter procedure is the Paris (France) procedure (48 hours) and the longest (82hours, in 2 separated periods of 24 hours and 58 hours, respectively) is the Montpellier (France) procedure.

The Paris procedure lasts a total of 48 hours in the sleep laboratory and is routinely used to evaluate central hypersomnolence in most French expert centers for hypersomnia.[18,29,30] In addition to measures obtained during standard full polysomnography, the procedure characterizes the "narcoleptic" phenotype (ie, rapidity to fall asleep during the MSLT and identification of SOREMPs), and the "sleep excess" phenotype (measured by the time slept during the second night and day). Patients undergo first nighttime polysomnography interrupted at 6:30 AM, followed by 5 MSLT starting at 8 AM, and a second night and day ad libitum monitoring, with uninterrupted naps in the morning

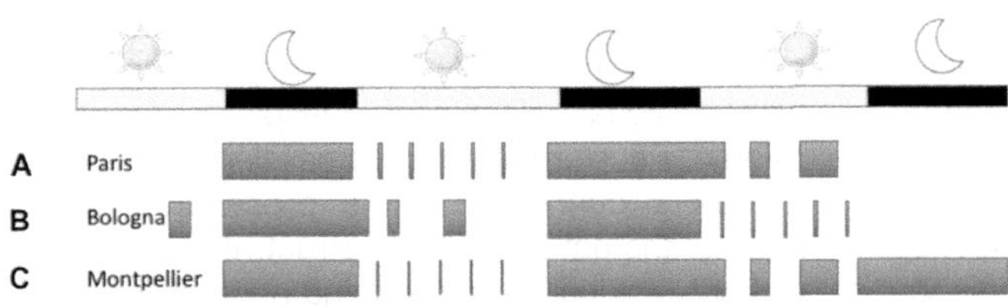

Fig. 1. The various prolonged monitoring procedures are used to diagnose IH, when the multiple sleep latency is normal or borderline. A is the Paris (France) procedure, B is the Bologna (France) procedure and C is the Montpellier (France) procedure. Daytime is presented as a yellow bar topped by a sun, night as a dark bar topped by a half-moon, over 3 consecutive days and nights (*upper line*). Blue bars represent sleep periods, either as long sleep episodes (nighttime sleep and long, unrestricted daytime naps) or as brief and restricted naps corresponding to the multiple sleep latency test (presented here as 5 successive brief naps opportunities, lasting 20–34 min in Paris and Bologna and 1 min in Montpellier).

Table 3
Extended sleep-monitoring procedures

Procedure	Protocol
Paris procedure[18,29,30](48-h protocol)	Main protocol

	• Night 1: Full polysomnography until 6:30 AM
	• Day 1: 5-nap multiple sleep latency test (MSLT) starting at 8 AM
	• Night 2: ad libitum polysomnography
	• Day 2: ad libitum polysomnography until 5 PM
	• Dinner at 7 PM on the first night
	• TV, computer, and visits from friends prohibited
	• Books, newspapers, watches, and daylight allowed
	• 2nd night of ad libitum sleep
	  ○ Patient's sleep is not interrupted o Patient decides when to sleep and
	  ○ switch off lights o Patient decides when to wake up the next day
	  ○ Patients recommended to take 2 naps in a darkened room o One in the morning
	  ○ One in the afternoon
	  ○ Stopped after 30 min if patient cannot fall asleep
	  ○ Continued if they do fall asleep until the patient wakes up.
	• Meals provided

Bologna procedure[17]	Main protocol
(60-h protocol)	• Ad libitum sleep for the first 48 h • MSLT on the 3rd day Notes • Patient may move around, read, and watch TV Amount of daytime sleep is determined by the patient
Montpellier procedure[14]	Main protocol

(80-h protocol)	• Night 1: Full polysomnography
	• Day 1: 5-nap MSLT
	• If borderline sleep latency on the MSLT:
	• Night 2: Full polysomnography
	• Day 2: modified 5-nap MSLT (patient is awoken after 1 min of sleep)
	• Night 3, Day, 3, Night 4: 32-h bed rest procedure - ad libitum sleep Notes
	• Amount of daytime sleep is determined by the patient 32-h rest procedure conducted in darkness
	  ○ Daylight, TV, computer, newspapers, phones, watches, and visits from family and friends prohibited
	  ○ Dim light at 10 lux

and afternoon, stopped at 5 PM, which provides an 18-h-long to 20-h-long opportunity to sleep (see **Fig. 1**A). In 75 patients with IH undergoing the Paris procedure, the sleep time obtained during the 18-h long-term monitoring in the sleep laboratory was very similar to the usual sleep time during holidays and weekends in patients, suggesting that the procedure is not a completely artificial measure, disconnected from the real world, but is an objective measure.[6] When measures in patients with IH are contrasted with those of age-matched and sex-matched healthy controls, the cutoff of 11 hours of sleep time has the best sensitivity (72%) and specificity (97%). In contrast, a lower cutoff of 10 hours has a sensitivity of 55% and a specificity of 77%; and a higher cutoff of 11 hours 30 minutes is highly specific (100%) but poorly sensitive (53%).[30] Only 1 in 20 patients with residual sleepiness despite adequately treated sleep apnea syndrome slept more than 11 hours during the same procedure, versus none of the patients with obstructive sleep apnea without residual sleepiness and none of the older controls.[30] Notably, up to 18% of patients with narcolepsy slept longer than 11 hours during the long-term procedure. This form of narcolepsy "with long sleep time" was characterized by less-prevalent cataplexy and was more severe in terms of clinical impairment (with more frequent sleep drunkenness and nonrefreshing naps) compared with patients with narcolepsy without long sleep time.[29]

The Bologna (Italy) procedure lasts 60 hours in total (see **Fig. 1**B), and includes an ad libitum monitoring of sleep during the first 48 hours, followed by an MSLT on the third day.[17] Daytime sleep is not imposed in darkness but is dictated by patient preference. The investigators did note that patients with narcolepsy type 1 slept longer during the daytime than those with narcolepsy type 2 or with IH without long sleep time.

The Montpellier procedure starts with standard polysomnography followed by an MSLT (see **Fig. 1**C).[16]Then, depending on the clinical assessment and if there is a borderline sleep latency during the MSLT, patients are scheduled for a second procedure lasting 58 hours, beginning with standard polysomnography and followed by a modified MSLT (naps are interrupted after 1 minute of sleep, to avoid decreasing the homeostatic sleep pressure). Sleep is then monitored during a 32-hour bed rest procedure in darkness, including a second night, a second day, and then a third night. Subjects are invited to sleep as long as possible, ad libitum. The investigators determined the sleep duration during the 32-h bed rest period in 32 patients with typical IH symptoms and mean sleep latencies of less than 10 minutes during the first MSLT, and compared it with 21 healthy controls. A cutoff of 19 hours sleep/32 hours of monitoring reached the highest sensitivity (92%) and specificity (86%) to distinguish both groups. When confining the analysis to the first 24 hours of the 32-h bed rest, a surrogate cutoff of 12 hours of sleep has the highest sensitivity (100%)/specificity (86%).

Each procedure has its advantages (measuring ad libitum, unrestrained sleep during 24–48 hours, ease of implementation) and disadvantages (long duration of testing, availability of normative measures, control of zeitgebers, costs). The 3 laboratories have a long-lasting, unpublished experience with their procedure in other cases (eg, the 48-h procedure is applied to 20 patients per week in the Paris laboratory for more than 10 years, leading to more than 8000 patients having followed it), which provides some robustness in the diagnosis. The cutoffs identified across these procedures, interestingly approximate the cutoffs of 11 to 12 hours during ad libitum sleep that was identified in the ICSD-2 as an alternative criterion of IH with long sleep time in absence of an MSLT less than 8 minutes. Thus, more recent, controlled studies seem to have reached similar conclusions to prior clinical experience from old, uncontrolled studies in expert centers.[31]

MECHANISMS

Triggers

The cause of IH remains unknown. Excessive sleep duration associated with daytime drowsiness can be observed in posttraumatic hypersomnia,[32] post-viral hypersomnia, and various hypersomnias associated with neurologic disorders (including tumors of the diencephalon, Prader–Willi syndrome,[33] inflammatory disorders), making it important to rule out these causes (eg, to perform brain MRI, identify head trauma within the last year before hypersomnia onset, and assess for recent viral conversion) before reaching the diagnosis of IH. The onset of IH is usually progressive, making it difficult to identify a trigger. Severe hypersomnia can suddenly occur in the context of a viral infection (eg, Epstein–Barr virus, cytomegalovirus), but the symptoms usually improve after a few months. However, some patients remain sleepy for years. Similarly, some patients have hypersomnia since birth or for decades, but seek medical advice when their life factors change (eg, raising young children, changing job schedule), which can jeopardize the previous adjustment to what was not considered yet as a disorder.

An abnormal sleep structure?

Many patients with IH sense that their sleep is not normal. In sharp contrast with this feeling, the sleep architecture in IH is classically normal or even "supernormal," with a lower arousal index and higher sleep efficiency than many controls (**Table 4**).[18] The general profile of the sleep architecture in IH is to see NREM and REM sleep in the expected proportions (**Fig. 2**).[34] In various groups of patients with IH, the percentage of N3 has been found to be unchanged,[16,18] decreased,[35] or increased.[11] Notably, some patients with IH display persistent N3 episodes at the end of the night, which is atypical of normal sleepers. The REM sleep has been found to be unchanged,[11,16,18] or increased.[35] This normal or supernormal sleep does not explain why sleep is not restorative of adequate daytime alertness in patients with IH.

Input from functional brain imaging

Recently, the Montreal group performed brain scintigraphy in 13 patients with IH and 16 healthy controls, using single-photon emission computed tomography with ^{99m}Tc-ethyl cysteinate dimer.[19] During wakefulness, patients with IH showed regional cerebral blood flow decreases in the medial prefrontal cortex and posterior cingulate cortex and putamen, as well as increases in amygdala and temporo-occipital cortices. Lower

Table 4
Sleep measures in idiopathic hypersomnia

Measure	IH Unspecified	IH Without LST	IH with LST
Multiple sleep latency test (MSLT) and maintenance of wakefulness test (MWT)			
MSL<8 min, %	44[8]; 51[11]; 61[18]	68; 100[18]	11[14]; 29[18]
MSL, min	4.3 ± 2.1[16]; 4.8 [2.5][13]; 5.8–5.9[16]; 7.3 ± 3.2,[19] 7.8 ± 0.5[18]; 8.3 ± 3.1[11] 9.3 ± 3.8[8]	4.3 ± 1.1[16]; 5.6 ± 0.3[18] 5.9 + 1.1[17]; 6.1 ± 3.4[10] 7.9 ± 2.6[11]	3.9 ± 2.4[16]; 8.9 ± 3.5[11] 9.6 ± 0.7[18]; 9.8[14]; 10.2 ± 4[10]
SOREMP, No	0.2 + 0.4[19]	0.2 ± 0.4[10]	0.2 ± 0.4[10]
MWT latency, 20 min	12.5–13.5[16]	—	—
Nighttime polysomnography			
Sleep-onset latency, min	7 [9][13]; 12 ± 8[11]; 18–19[16]; 24 ± 21[8]; 31 ± 42[18]	7[14]; 8 ± 7[42] 9 ± 9[20]; 27 ± 27[18]	10[14]; 35 ± 51[18]
REM sleep latency, min	82 [55][13]; 82 ± 48[18]; 106 ± 59[8]	69 ± 42[20]; 74[14] 83 ± 53[18]; 97 ± 53[42]	69[14]; 81 ± 44[18]
Sleep efficiency, % of total sleep time	90 [8][13]; 91 ± 6[18]; 91 ± 15[8]; 92[16]; 93 ± 5[16]; 94 ± 4[11]	87 ± 6[20]; 89 ± 5[16] 89 ± 7[18]; 91 ± 5[42]; 94[14]	92 ± 6[18]; 92.7[14] 96 ± 2[16]
Total sleep time, min	392–420[16]; 454 [62][13] 481 ± 85[8]; 579 ± 90[18]	428 ± 63[20]; 441 ± 23[16] 446[14]; 489 ± 46[42] 517 ± 60[18]	449[14]; 490 ± 50[16]; 633 ± 76[18]
Sleep stages, % of total sleep time			
Stage N1	4 ± 2,[8] 6 [4][13]	4[14]; 11 ± 7[42]	416
Stage N2	50 ± 7[8]; 56 [10][13]	53 ± 8[42]; 56[14]	55[14]
Stage N3	8 ± 5[16]; 15 [8][13]; 18–27[16]; 21 ± 8[18]; 26 ± 8[8]	6 ± 6[16]; 9 ± 8[15]; 21[14]; 21 ± 8[18]	9 ± 6[16]; 20[14]; 21 ± 9[18]
Stage R	18 ± 7[16]; 20–21[16]; 21 ± 5[8] 22 [8][13]; 24 ± 7[18]	14 ± 7[16]; 17[14] 21 ± 5[42]; 23 ± 5[18]	20[14]; 22 ± 4[16] 24 ± 7[18]
Analysis of sleep microstructure			
Arousal index, n/h	9 ± 6[18]; 10 ± 5[8]	10 ± 7[18]	7 ± 4[18]
PLMS index, n/h	1 [4][13]; 3[16]; 3 ± 3[8]; 9 ± 13[18]	0[14]; 1 ± 4[42]; 7 ± 7[20] 11 ± 15[18]	0.3[14]; 5 ± 8[18]
Long-term sleep, ad libitum monitoring			
18 h procedure, min	695 ± 99[18]	635 ± 82[18]	747 ± 82[18]
32 h bed rest procedure, first 24h	—	646[14]	892[14]

Measures are mean ± SD or %, except for those presented asx-y, which represent means or medians from two different IH groups.

Abbreviations: IH, idiopathic hypersomnia; LST, long sleep time; MSL, mean sleep latency; PLMS, periodic leg movements during sleep; REM, rapid eye movement; SOREM, sleep onset in REM period.

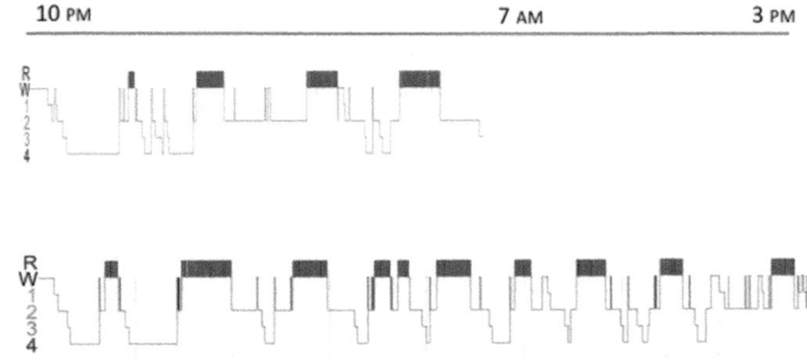

Fig. 2. Hypnogram in a patient with IH (*bottom*), measured during prolonged monitoring (here 18-h long) in Paris (France), compared with a healthy subject (*top*). Sleep is highly efficient, 9 sleep cycles are performed instead of 4, and slow-wave sleep is present even during morning sleep. Y axis: R: REM sleep; W: wakefulness; 1,2, 3, 4: Non-REM sleep N1, N2, and N3 (former 314 stages).

regional cerebral blood flow in the medial prefrontal cortex correlated with higher daytime sleepiness, as measured by the ESS and the MSL at the MSLT (**Fig. 3**). The investigators make an interesting parallel between this profile of decreased blood flow in the medial prefrontal cortex in awake patients with IH, which is also seen during NREM stage N2 sleep in healthy subjects.[36] This seminal work suggests that the wakefulness in IH contains local sleep in the medial prefrontal cortex, and compensatory efforts to promote wakefulness from the amygdala and temporo-occipital cortices.

Autoimmunity and inflammation in idiopathic hypersomnia

The rate of comorbid autoimmune disorder is low (4%) in IH, and not different from that of controls.[23] HLA-DQB1*0602 has been examined in many IH series, with frequencies varying from 16% to 31%.[7,8,11,18,37] There was no difference of HLA DQB1*0602 frequency between patients with IH with or without long sleep time,[18] and between patients with IH and healthy controls.[18] Measures of other HLA DRB1 and DQB1 alleles (low resolution) did not identify any differences between 61

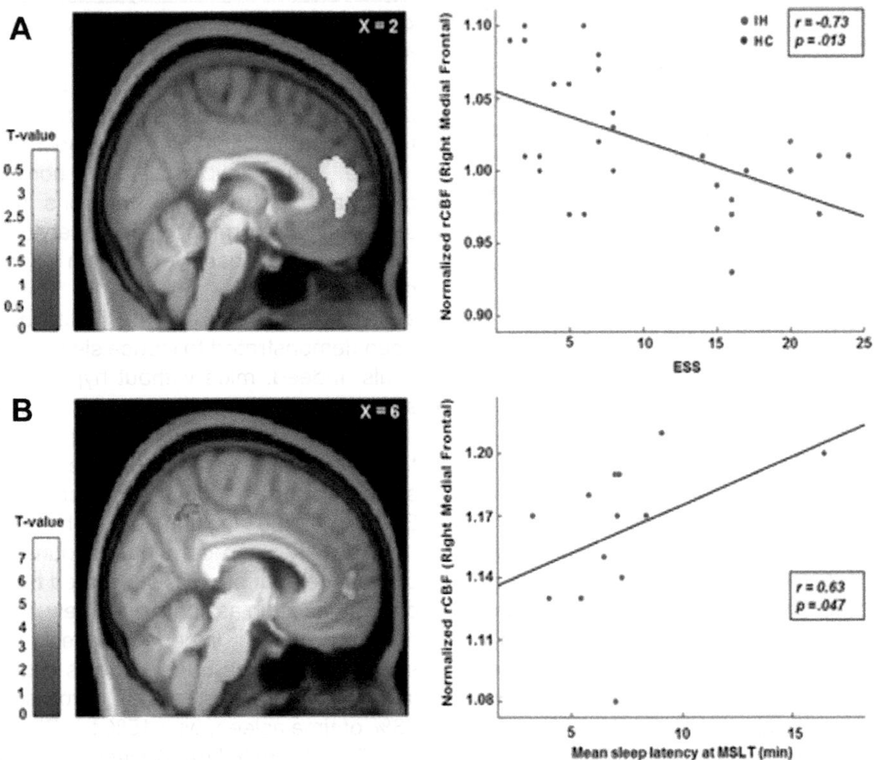

Fig. 3. Decreased regional blood flow in IH (compared with healthy controls [HC], *left*) during brain scintigraphy performed in awake subjects correlates with the level of sleepiness measured by ESS (*A*, *right*) and by measured by ESS (*A*, *right*) and by MSLT (*B*, *right*). rCBF, regional cerebral blood flow. (*From* Boucetta S, Montplaisir J, Zadra A, et al. Altered regional cerebral blood flow in idiopathic hypersomnia. Sleep 2017;40(10); with permission.)

patients with IH and 30 controls.[18] In contrast, in a series of 138 patients with IH, the prevalence of inflammatory disorders, allergies, and the incidence of family members with inflammatory disorders was increased in patients compared with controls, suggesting that inflammation may play a role in some cases of IH.[23]

Deficiency of an arousal system?

Among the arousal systems, in IH there is no deficiency in hypocretin-1 (as there is one in narcolepsy type 1) or in histamine (which is, as hypocretin, released by a single isolated group of neurons).[37] In 29 patients with IH (with or without long sleep time), the hypocretin-1 CSF levels were 307 $\pm$ 10 pg/mL.[38] In 26 patients with IH without long sleep time, the CSF hypocretin levels were 280.7 $\pm$ 14.8 pg/mL.[39] The histamine CSF levels were 161 $\pm$ 29.3 pg/mL, a measure in the range of healthy controls.[37] These levels were lower (143.3 $\pm$ 28.8 pg/mL) in untreated than treated patients (259.5 $\pm$ 94.9 pg/mL), as in narcolepsy and in other disorders associated with daytime sleepiness (including obstructive sleep apnea syndrome), suggesting that histamine is a nonspecific marker of sleepiness.[37] In 6 patients with IH, the CSF levels of melanin-concentrating hormone, which is secreted by the hypothalamus and promotes REM sleep, were 104 $\pm$ 26 pg/mL, which was not different from that of healthy controls.[40] Measures of serotonin, norepinephrine,[41] epinephrine, glutamate, acetylcholine, and their metabolites have been rarely performed in the CSF of patients with IH, with difficult to interpret results when studied.[41] The likelihood that a single bioamine deficiency would specifically affect the arousal system alone is low, as these bioamines are released by numerous neuronal systems out of the arousal networks, and are essential for many other brain functions

Production of an endogenous hypnotic factor?

Recently, the Atlanta group produced evidence that some resistant cases of hypersomnia (including IH, narcolepsy type 2, "long sleepers," and subjective hypersomnia) could result from the inappropriate release of an endogenous hypnotic substance that activates the GABA-A receptors. In support of this hypothesis, the CSF of these patients was applied to GABA-A receptors and was able to displace the normal GABA-A binding. Furthermore, some of these patients benefited from drugs blocking GABA receptors, including flumazenil (commonly used for benzodiazepine overdose) and clarithromycin (an antibiotic that antagonizes the GABA-A receptor).[27,28] The Montpellier group could not reproduce these results in a group of 15 patients with IH.[43]

Contribution of the circadian system?

The more frequent evening chronotype in IH,[18] as well as the occasional benefit of evening melatonin to reduce sleep drunkenness,[18,25] has led the Czech group to measure the profile of melatonin secretion over 24 hours in IH.[44] There was a delayed melatonin secretion in 10 patients with IH, which has not been reproduced. In 15 patients with IH, the circadian period length in peripheral skin fibroblast was longer by 0.82 hour than in controls.[45] This finding suggests a genetic contribution of the circadian system in patients with IH. However, of note is that patients with IH do not suffer from delayed sleep phase syndrome, possibly because they try not to shift their sleep onset across nights. This longer circadian period may contribute to the sleep drunkenness observed in these patients.

Animal models of idiopathic hypersomnia?

Animal models have been key for understanding the mechanisms of narcolepsy; however, they have been less helpful in the study of IH. In rodents and feline models, the main arousal systems include histamine and hypocretin neurons in the lateral hypothalamus, norepinephrine, glutamate, and dopamine neurons in the brainstem reticular formation, and acetylcholine neurons in the basal forebrain and in the pedunculopontine nucleus.[46] The selective absence of hypocretin or histamine has not been demonstrated to induce sleep excess in animals. Indeed, mice without hypocretin neurons spend as much time asleep as wild-type mice (both sleep 57% of the 24-h time period), whereas their periods of wakefulness are fragmented by sleep episodes containing occasional SOREMPs.[47] Mice lacking brain histamine have normal daily sleep duration (accounting for 57% of the time), but are less stimulated by behavioral challenges such as lights off, a new environment, or food delivery.[48] In contrast, a lesion of the dorsal norepinephrine bundle in cats causes a long-lasting, harmonious, severe hypersomnia with 78% of time asleep, with 15% to 27% REM sleep and 73% to 85% NREM sleep.[49] Lesions of the dopamine neurons in the ventral periaqueductal gray matter cause a 20% increase of the daily total sleep time in rats, with proportional increases of NREM and REM sleep.[50]

TREATMENT

Among drugs, only low sodium oxybate has been approved for IH in US.58 Other treatment options are based on consensus from professional sleep societies, and, depending on the country, advice from expert centers, as in France.[51] Many advances in the treatment of narcolepsy have benefited IH, but without the same extent of improvements in symptoms (eg, long, unrefreshing naps and of sleep drunkenness) in patients with IH (**Table 5**).

Preventive naps

In sharp contrast with narcolepsy, naps (even when brief) are rarely beneficial in IH. Rather, they are often followed by sleep drunkenness and fail to restore adequate alertness. The MSLT is a good test to evaluate their benefit. If naps are beneficial during the MSLT, then they can be recommended as part of a care plan (eg, at school, university, and work). However, knowing that the naps were unrefreshing during the MSLT (eg, "it took me a while to fall asleep and then I was awakened by the nurse, which was horrible") is helpful so that this strategy is not included in the treatment plan.

Reduction and adaptation of working time

There are several adjustments that may help patients remain functional at work despite suffering from IH. Accommodations by the employer to allow a patient with IH to begin work at a later hour (eg, to sleep an extra hour in the morning, or not to risk being fired because of lateness), or to work from home (eg, 1 day teleworking for every 2 days at the work place) can be helpful to patients, as we recently demonstrated during COVID-19 pandemic associated lockdown.[60] Living close to the workplace will reduce the fatigue linked to commuting time and early awakening. Some patients have developed hyperactivity as a counterstrategy to boost their alertness, such as always being active, speaking frequently, standing, or not resting.[6] Although these activities can be useful counter strategies, patients with IH may need additional rest days separate from vacations, otherwise they may be at risk of exhaustion.

Managing to wake up in the morning

Alarm clocks, phone calls, bright lights, dawn-simulation lights, noises, and pets seem insufficient to assist patients with IH with sleep drunkenness in waking[6] (except in those who have an anxious personality in our experience). Being awoken (and shaken) by another person (parent, spouse, roommate) is efficient, but makes patients with IH more dependent on others to achieve adequate awakening.[6] This is particularly problematic for mothers with IH to wake up to prepare their children for school, forcing some families to teach their children to be more autonomous in their morning preparation. Some patients prepare their clothes, take a shower and shave in the evening to save the time on morning awakening.

Reducing Sleep Drunkenness

No drug has been approved for sleep drunkenness. The French expert consensus statement mentions that melatonin at 3 mg (or 2 mg slow-release melatonin) at sleep onset may be useful in some patients with IH to reduce sleep drunkenness.[51] Sodium oxybate (whether as a single dose at sleep onset or split into an evening and a night dose) substantially mitigated sleep drunkenness in a case series from our center.[8] The recent large placebo-controlled study of low sodium oxybate in IH showed a frank effect on sleep drunkenness as assessed in the idiopathic hypersomnia severity scale and using an analogic visual scale.[58] Other strategies include prescribing a dose of a stimulant at bedtime, or awakening the patients 1 hour before their usual wakeup time and having them ingest the medication or use a transdermal formulation.[25] Improvement in sleep drunkenness has been reported in individual cases with transdermal and subcutaneous flumazenil, a nicotine patch, and etilefrine (the latter in a patient with comorbid hypotension).[25] Bright light therapy rarely dissipates sleep inertia.[6]

Increasing daytime alertness

Modafinil The various drugs prescribed for IH are shown in **Table 5**. Modafinil was approved from 1994 to 2010 in Europe for IH, until approval was revoked due to the lack of trials by pharmaceutical companies. The mean doses were 367 ± 140 mg in the United States,[13] 400 mg in the United Kingdom,[11] 318 ± 192 mg in France,[7] and 200 mg (fixed dose) in Germany.[12]

In an open, retrospective series in 104 patients with IH and 126 patients with narcolepsy type 1, modafinil was the first-line treatment in 96% to 99% of patients.[7] Similar changes in the ESS were reported between patients with IH and patients with narcolepsy (−2.6 ± 5.1 vs −3 ± 5.1) and a similar benefit as estimated by the patients and clinicians; however, the change in the ESS was lower in patients with IH with long sleep time compared with those without long sleep time. Seventy-two percent of patients with IH reported a benefit of modafinil on their symptoms, similar

Table 5
Drugs used in idiopathic hypersomnia

Reference	No. Patients	Type of Trial	Benefit	Level of Evidence
Modafinil				
Bastuji and Jouvet[52], 1988	18	Observational open	Less frequent daily naps in 89%	III
Anderson et al[11], 2007	39	Observational open	ESS reduction > 4 in 62% Mean ESS reduction: −6 ± 5.4	III
Ali et al[13], 2009	25	Observational open	72% have a complete (ESS reduction = −9), and 16% a partial response to modafinil	III
Lavault et al[7], 2011	104	Observational, open, compared with narcolepsy type 1	Over a period of 4.7 y long, mean ESS reduction: −2.6 ± 5.1 in IH, vs −3 ± 5.1 in the narcolepsy group (ITT analysis). Mean efficacy on the analogic visual scale: 6.9/10 in IH, vs 6.5/10 in the narcolepsy group	IIb
Philip et al[53], 2014 ± 9.8 min)	14	Randomized, double-blind crossover, vs placebo	In a composite group of patients with IH and patients with narcolepsy, improved driving performance and improved MWT (from ± 9.2 min under placebo to	Ib

Mayer et al,2015[12]	33	Randomized, double-blind parallel, vs placebo	Over 3 wk, mean ESS reduction: −6 with modafinil 200 mg/d, vs −1.5 with placebo; CGI improved: −1 point; MWT: + 3 min vs 0 min but not significant	Ib
Inoue et al, 202159	71	Randomized, double-blind parallel, vs placebo	Mean ESS reduction: −5 MWT:+5 min over placebo	Ia
Methylphenidate				
Ali et al[13], 2009	40	Observational open	52% have a complete (ESS reduction = −9), and 33% a partial response to modafinil	III
Amphetamine, dextroamphetamine, methamphetamine				
Anderson et al[11], 2007	11	Observational open	54% are responders (ESS reduction > 4)	III
Ali et al[13] 2009	20	Observational open	25% are complete (ESS reduction = −9) and 10% partial responders	III
Pemoline				
Ali et al[13] 2009	7	Observational open	43% are responders	III
Mazindol				
Nittur et al[9], 2013	37	Observational open	The mean ESS reduction was −4.8 ± 4.7; 84% of patients were responders	III
Sodium oxybate				

(continued on next page)

Table 5
(continued)

Reference	No. Patients	Type of Trial	Benefit	Level of Evidence
Leu-Semenescu et al[8], 2016	46	Observational open, compared with narcolepsy	The ESS reduction was −3.5 ± 4.5, similar to its effect in narcolepsy type 1 (−3.2 ± 4.2). Sleep drunkenness was improved in 71% of these patients	IIb
Dauvilliers et al, 202258	154	Randomized, double-blind parallel, vs placebo	ESS mean change:- 6.5 Improved IHSS score	Ia
Pitolisant				
Leu-Semenescu et al[54], 2014	65	Observational open	36% of patients were responders (ESS reduction > 3)	III
Flumazenil				
Trotti et al[55], 2016	36	Observational open	68% of patients were responders (mean ESS reduction = 5)	III
Clarithromycin				
Trotti et al[56], 2014	53	Observational open	34% of patients chose to use it in the long term	III
Trotti et al[28], 2015	23, with 10 IH	Randomized, double-blind crossover, vs placebo	ESS reduction = −3.9 between clarithromycin and placebo, with −5.4 in the IH group with long sleep time; Improved QoL; unchanged PVT	II

Abbreviations: CGI, clinical general impression; ESS, Epworth sleepiness score; IH, idiopathic hypersomnia; ITT, intention to treat; MWT, maintenance of wakefulness test; PVT, psychomotor vigilance test; QoL, quality of life.

to patients with narcolepsy type 1.[7] In a randomized, double-blind, placebo-controlled study in 33 patients with IH without long sleep time in Germany, the ESS decreased in patients treated with modafinil.[12] Compared with placebo, modafinil decreased sleepiness significantly but did not significantly improve MSL in the maintenance of wakefulness test. The clinical general impression improved significantly from baseline to the last visit on treatment. In a recent Japanese multicenter double-blind randomized study in the parallel group of 73 patients with IH, the ESS decreased and the MWT latency increased under modafinil 200 mg/d.[59] In a randomized, placebo-controlled crossover trial of modafinil 400 mg/d in 13 patients with narcolepsy and 14 patients with IH, modafinil treatment was associated with improved driving simulation results.[53] In this study, MSL on the maintenance of wakefulness test greatly improved from 19.7 $\pm$ 9.2 minutes with placebo to 30.8 $\pm$ 9.8 minutes with modafinil, but results were not separated by diagnosis. The safety of modafinil was similar between IH and in narcolepsy groups.[7] For these reasons, modafinil is considered first-line treatment in IH.[51]

Methylphenidate and amphetamines Although methylphenidate is frequently used as a second-line medication in IH, very few data are published in case series and no controlled study has been performed (see **Table 5**). Methylphenidate was the first-line treatment in IH at the Mayo Clinic (Rochester, MN) until 1998, when modafinil emerged.[13] The mean dose of methylphenidate was 50.9 $\pm$ 27.3 mg/d in 61 patients, of whom 40 took as monotherapy. Patients took 3 to 4 doses per day using the immediate release form, but many patients took a combination of immediate and slow-release forms. Twenty-one (52%) patients were considered complete responders (ESS reduction of −9 points on average), 13 (33%) patients were partial responders (ESS reduction of −6 points on average), and 2 (5%) patients did not respond to the drug. In total, 95% of patients were responders to methylphenidate versus 88% to modafinil (*P* = .29).[13]

The use of dextroamphetamine (35.7 $\pm$ 44.4 mg/d), methamphetamine (36 $\pm$ 17 mg/d), and combination of amphetamine and dextroamphetamine (79.3 $\pm$ 30.6 mg/d) in IH has been reported in the United Kingdom[11] and in the United States,[13] alone or in combination with modafinil or methylphenidate, with 25% to 52% of responders, depending on the criteria used to define responders (see **Table 5**). Pemoline (66.9 $\pm$ 36.6 mg/d) was used in 7 patients, with 3 (43%) responders.[13] Mazindol is a pseudo-amphetamine that has been developed for losing weight in obese children and was efficacious in open trials in narcolepsy and in cataplexy.[9] In 37 patients with IH resistant to 2 drugs, the ESS fell from 17 $\pm$ 4.4 to 12.5 $\pm$ 5.1 under treatment with mazindol (maximum dose in patients 3.6 $\pm$ 1.2 mg).[9] The benefit was similar if not larger than in patients with narcolepsy. The last company producing mazindol stopped its production in 2016 for insufficient sales.

Prohistamine drugs Pitolisant is a new anti-H3 agonist that blocks the presynaptic reuptake of histamine and increases its release in the brain, which was developed and approved in narcolepsy.[57] Our group has used this medication in 65 patients with IH resistant to 3 other medications and observed a beneficial, alerting effect in one-third of the patients (see **Table 5**).[54] The side effects were rare and benign. They included gastralgia, increased appetite, headache, insomnia, and anxiety.

Sodium oxybate Sodium oxybate (which stimulates GABA-A receptors in the brain) is approved as a treatment for narcolepsy. Daytime sleepiness is reduced when using 2 doses per night, reduces cataplexy, and improves dyssomnia. The rationale for using sodium oxybate in IH was not obvious at first, as patients with IH sleep well (instead of suffering from dyssomnia) and are difficult to awaken. However, in a single-center, open-label trial of sodium oxybate in our center of 46 patients with IH with no benefits from modafinil, methylphenidate, and amphetamine (see **Table 4**), sodium oxybate resulted in similar benefits as observed in narcolepsy, even when using a lower dose (a single dose at bedtime).[8] The side effects were similar to those observed in narcolepsy, but more frequent in the IH group. Half of the patients with IH stopped sodium oxybate because of disabling nausea and dizziness. Recently, a large, placebo-controlled randomized study in parallel groups of low sodium oxybate was conducted on 154 patients with IH worldwide. It demonstrated a major benefit of low sodium oxybate 2.5 to 9 g/night on ESS (median change: −6.5 points) and IHSS score (−12 points). Side effects were of the same type and frequency as in narcolepsy.[58]

Reducing daytime drowsiness

Flumazenil Following the discovery of a possible, endogenous peptide enhancing GABA-A transmission in the CSF of several patients with IH, the Atlanta group developed strategies aimed at blocking the GABA-A receptors to counteract the action of such a hypnotic peptide. The first candidate was flumazenil, which is commonly used as an antidote for benzodiazepine intoxication. Intravenous flumazenil has a short half-life, and intravenous continuous infusions of flumazenil (0.38–2 mg) were needed in their first trial to improve the psychomotor vigilance test (PVT) in a series of 7 patients with various (IH, narcolepsy type 2, long sleepers, Kleine–Levin syndrome) hypersomnias.[27] The same group developed sublingual and transdermal forms of flumazenil to avoid the immediate destruction of the drug by the liver. Among 36 patients with IH with treatment-refractory sleepiness, 23 (64%) were initial responders to flumazenil (−5 points on ESS).[55] In the full group of treated patients (which included patients with narcolepsies, IH, subjective hypersomnolence, and sleep apnea with hypersomnolence), flumazenil responders were more often women and subjects with sleep inertia.[55] The most common side effect was dizziness. Approximately one-third of initial responders discontinued flumazenil for various reasons (eg, tolerance, price).[55]

Clarithromycin These investigators have also looked for oral drugs that have anti-GABA effects. The antibiotic, penicillin, is known to block the GABA receptors and may induce a seizure for this effect. The group found that another common antibiotic, clarithromycin, used as a single morning dosage of 500 to 1000 mg/d, reduced subjective sleepiness (but did not change PVT) in a randomized, crossover, double-blind, placebo-controlled study in patients with IH with CSF evidence of endogenous GABA-A receptor activating peptide (see **Table 5**).[28] Clarithromycin may induce a bad taste and may expose to changes in vaginal and gut flora (mitigated by the use of probiotics), but it is easily available and inexpensive to try to determine if there is a short-term and long-term benefit for a patient with IH. In a longer-term study of clarithromycin in 53 patients with IH, 64% reported initial improvement in subjective sleepiness, and 38% elected to continue clarithromycin therapy for the long term.[56]

SUMMARY

IH is a devastating and poorly studied disorder, affecting women more often than men. The disorder has not received sufficient medical attention. However, recent advances in precision medicine suggest that the disorder can be better characterized in many patients with the use of prolonged protocols rather than the MSLT. The development of home-based monitoring systems, measuring appropriate surrogates of sleep, may be a future approach to support< the IH diagnosis. Standardized approaches to medication treatment have developed. The identification of a benzodiazepine-like endogenous peptide in some patients with IH with stimulant-refractory sleepiness paves the way for treating these patients with benzodiazepine antagonists such as flumazenil and clarithromycin. The clear benefit of modafinil and low sodium oxybate in 2 large randomized placebo-controlled studies in IH demonstrates that the disorder is treatable. Because the prevalence of IH is close to that of narcolepsy, this should motivate pharmaceutical companies to develop drugs targeted at this disorder.

CLINICS CARE POINTS

- Normal or borderline MSLT results do not rule out IH.
- Patients suspected of IH who report prolonged sleep time should be monitored continuously sleep night and day for diagnosis purposes
- Many patients with IH prefer avoiding naps because of the postnapping inertia
- Adapted schedules allowing patients with IH to sleep longer and arrive later in the morning to help adjusting to the disorder.
- Teleworking is highly beneficial in IH and should be applied whenever possible
- Modafinil and low-sodium oxybate have demonstrated substantial benefits in IH, including sleep drunkenness.

DISCLOSURE

The authors declare that they have no conflicts of interest related to this article. The authors are members of the National Reference Center for Rares Hypersomnias, which receives annuities from the French Health Ministry to electively diagnose and treat these patients, as well as to develop medical and social awareness for these disorders, consensus, cohorts, and retrospective studies. National Reference Center for Rare Hypersomnias, Pitie-Salpetriere University Hospital, APHP, and Sorbonne University, 483 Boulevard de l'Hopital, Paris 75013, France.

REFERENCES

1. Roth B. Narcolepsy and hypersomnia. Basel (Switzerland): Karger; 1980.
2. American Sleep Disorders Association. The international classification of sleep disorders. Diagnosis

and coding manual 1990. American Academy of Sleep Medicine (Ed) Rochester (MN).

3. American Academy of Sleep Medicine. The international classification of sleep disorders revised. Chicago: American Academy of Sleep Medicine; 2005.
4. American Academy of Sleep Medicine. The interna tional classification of sleep disorders. 3rd edition. Darien (IL): American Academy of Sleep Medicine; 2014.
5. Ohayon M, Reynolds CI, Dauvilliers Y. Excessive sleep duration and quality of life. Ann Neurol 2013; 73:785–94.
6. Vernet C, Leu-Semenescu S, Buzare M, et al. Sub jective symptoms in idiopathic hypersomnia: beyond excessive sleepiness. J Sleep Res 2010; 19(4):525–34.
7. Lavault S, Dauvilliers Y, Drouot X, et al. Benefit and risk of modafinil in idiopathic hypersomnia vs. nar colepsy with cataplexy. Sleep Med 2011;12(6): 550–6.
8. Leu-Semenescu S, Louis P, Arnulf I. Benefits and risk of sodium oxybate in idiopathic hypersomnia versus narcolepsy type 1: a chart review. Sleep Med 2016;17:38–44.
9. Nittur N, Konofal E, Dauvilliers Y, et al. Mazindol in narcolepsy and idiopathic and symptomatic hyper somnia refractory to stimulants: a long-term chart re view. Sleep Med 2013;14(1):30–6.
10. Sonka K, Susta M, Billiard M. Narcolepsy with and without cataplexy, idiopathic hypersomnia with and without long sleep time: a cluster analysis. Sleep Med 2015;16(2):225–31.
11. Anderson KN, Pilsworth S, Sharples LD, et al. Idiopathic hypersomnia: a study of 77 cases. Sleep 2007;30:1274–81.
12. Mayer G, Benes H, Young P, et al. Modafinil in the treatment of idiopathic hypersomnia without long sleep time—a randomized, double-blind, placebo-controlled study. J Sleep Res 2015;24:74–81.
13. Ali M, Auger R, Slocumb N, et al. Idiopathic hyper somnia: clinical features and response to treatment. J Clin Sleep Med 2009;5:562–8.
14. Evangelista E, Lopez R, Barateau L, et al. Alternative diagnostic criteria for idiopathic hypersomnia: a 32-hour protocol. Ann Neurol 2018;83(2):235–47.
15. Ozaki A, Inoue Y, Hayashida K, et al. Quality of life in patients with narcolepsy with cataplexy, narcolepsy without cataplexy, and idiopathic hypersomnia without long sleep time: comparison between patients on psychostimulants, drug-naive patients and the general Japanese population. Sleep Med 2012;13(2):200–6.
16. Bassetti C, Aldrich M. Idiopathic hypersomnia. A se ries of 42 patients. Brain 1997;120(8):1423–35. Pubmed Partial Issue.
17. Pizza F, Moghadam K, Vandi S, et al. Daytime continuous polysomnography predicts MSLT results in hypersomnias of central origin. J Sleep Res 2013; 22:32–40.
18. Vernet C, Arnulf I. Idiopathic hypersomnia with and without long sleep time: a controlled series of 75 pa tients. Sleep 2009;32(6):753–9.
19. Boucetta S, Montplaisir J, Zadra A, et al. Altered regional cerebral blood flow in idiopathic hypersomnia. Sleep 2017;40(10).
20. Pizza F, Ferri R, Poli F, et al. Polysomnographic study of nocturnal sleep in idiopathic hypersomnia without long sleep time. J Sleep Res 2013;22:185–96.
21. Vignatelli L, D'Alessandro R, Mosconi P, et al. Health-related quality of life in Italian patients with narcolepsy: the SF-36 health survey. Sleep Med 2004;5:467–75.
22. Sasai T, Inoue Y, Komada Y, et al. Comparison of clinical characteristics among narcolepsy with and without cataplexy and idiopathic hypersomnia without long sleep time, focusing on HLA- DRB1*1501/ DQB1*0602 finding. Sleep Med 2008;10:961–6.
23. Barateau L, Lopez R, Arnulf I, et al. Comorbidity between central disorders of hypersomnolence and immune-based disorders. Neurology 2017;88: 93–100.
24. Barateau L, Jaussent I, Lopez R, et al. Smoking, alcohol, drug use, abuse and dependence in narcolepsy and idiopathic hypersomnia: a case-control study. Sleep 2016;39(3):573–80.
25. Trotti L. Waking up is the hardest thing I do all day: sleep inertia and sleep drunkenness. Sleep Med 2017;35:78–84.
26. Voderholzer U, Backhaus J, Hornyak M, et al. A 19-h spontaneous sleep period in idiopathic central ner vous system hypersomnia. J Sleep Res 1998;7: 101–3.
27. Rye DB, Bliwise DL, Parker K, et al. Modulation of vigilance in the primary hypersomnias by endogenous enhancement of GABAA receptors. Sci Transl Med 2012;4(161):161ra151.
28. Trotti LM, Saini P, Bliwise D, et al. Clarithromycin in g-aminobutyric acid-related hypersomnolence: a ran domized, crossover trial. Ann Neurol 2015;78: 454–65.
29. Vernet C, Arnulf I. Narcolepsy with long sleep time: a specific entity? Sleep 2009;32(9):1229–759.
30. Vernet C, Redolfi S, Attali V, et al. Residual sleepiness in obstructive sleep apnoea: phenotype and related symptoms. Eur Respir J 2011;38(1):98–105.
31. Billiard M, Merle C, Carlander B, et al. Idiopathic hy persomnia. Psychiatry Clin Neurosci 1998;52(2): 125–9.
32. Imbach LL, Valko PO, Li T, et al. Increased sleep need and daytime sleepiness 6 months after traumatic brain injury: a prospective controlled clinical trial. Brain 2015;138(Pt 3):726–35.
33. Ghergan A, Coupaye M, Leu-Semenescu S, et al. Prevalence and phenotype of sleep disorders in 60

adults with Prader-Willi syndrome. Sleep 2017;40. https://doi.org/10.1093/sleep/zsx1162. Pubmed Exact.
34. American Academy of Sleep Medicine. International classification of sleep disorders. In: Diag nostic and coding manual. 2nd edition. Westchester (IL): Amer ican Academy of Sleep Medicine; 2005.
35. Sforza E, Gaudreau H, Petit D, et al. Homeostatic sleep regulation in patients with idiopathic hyper somnia. Clin Neurophysiol 2000;111(2):277–82.
36. Dang-Vu T, Desseilles M, Laureys S, et al. Cerebral correlates of delta waves during non-REM sleep re visited. Neuroimage 2005;28:14–21.
37. Kanbayashi T, Kodama T, Kondo H, et al. CSF hista mine contents in narcolepsy, idiopathic hypersomnia and obstructive sleep apnea syndrome. Sleep 2009; 32(2):181–7.
38. Mignot E, Lammers GJ, Ripley B, et al. The role of cerebrospinal fluid hypocretin measurement in the diagnosis of narcolepsy and other hypersomnias. Arch Neurol 2002;59(10):1553–62.
39. Kanbayashi T, Inoue Y, Chiba S, et al. CSF hypocretin-1 (orexin-A) concentrations in narcolepsy with and without cataplexy and idiopathic hyper somnia. J Sleep Res 2002;11(1):91–3.
40. Peyron C, Valentin F, Bayard S, et al. Melanin concentrating hormone in central hypersomnia. Sleep Med 2011;12:768–72.
41. Montplaisir J, de Champlain J, Young SN, et al. Nar colepsy and idiopathic hypersomnia: biogenic amines and related compounds in CSF. Neurology 1982;32(11):1299–302.
42. Takei Y, Komada Y, Namba K, et al. Differences in findings of nocturnal polysomnography and multiple sleep latency test between narcolepsy and idio-pathic hypersomnia. Clin Neurophysiol 2012;123: 137–41.
43. Dauvilliers Y, Evangelista E, Lopez R, et al. Absence of g-aminobutyric acid-a receptor potentiation in central hypersomnolence disorders. Ann Neurol 2016;80:259–68.
44. Nevsimalova S, Blazejova K, Illnerova H, et al. A contribution to pathophysiology of idiopathic hy persomnia. Suppl Clin Neurophysiol 2000;53:366–70.
45. Materna L, Halfter H, Heidbreder A, et al. Idiopathic hypersomnia patients revealed longer circadian period length in peripheral skin fibroblasts. Front Neurol 2018;9:424.
46. Saper CB, Scammell TE, Lu J. Hypothalamic regula tion of sleep and circadian rhythms. Nature 2005; 437(7063):1257–63.
47. Hara J, Beuckmann CT, Nambu T, et al. Genetic ablation of orexin neurons in mice results in narco lepsy, hypophagia, and obesity. Neuron 2001; 30(2):345–54.
48. Parmentier R, Ohtsu H, Djebbara-Hannas Z, et al. Anatomical, physiological, and pharmacological characteristics of histidine decarboxylase knock-out mice: evidence for the role of brain histamine in behavioral and sleep-wake control. J Neurosci 2002;22(17):7695–711.
49. Petitjean F, Sakai K, Blondaux C, et al. Hypersomnia by isthmic lesion in cat. II. Neurophysiological and pharmacological study. Brain Res 1975;88(3): 439–53 [in French].
50. Lu J, Jhou T, Saper C. Identification of wake-active neurones in the ventral periaqueductal gray matter. J Neurosci 2006;26(1):193–202.
51. Lopez R, Arnulf I, Drouot X, et al. French consensus. Management of patients with hypersomnia: which strategy? Rev Neurol (Paris) 2017;173:8–18.
52. Bastuji H, Jouvet M. Successful treatment of idio pathic hypersomnia and narcolepsy with modafinil. Prog Neuropsychopharmacol Biol Psychiatry 1988; 12:695–700.
53. Philip P, Chaufton C, Taillard J, et al. Modafinil im proves real driving performance in patients with hy- persomnia: a randomized double-blind placebo-controlled crossover clinical trial. Sleep 2014;37(3): 483–7.
54. Leu-Semenescu S, Nittur N, Golmard J, et al. Effects of pitolisant, a histamine H3 inverse agonist, in drug-resistant idiopathic and symptomatic hypersomnia: a chart review. Sleep Med 2014;15:681–7.
55. Trotti LM, Saini P, Koola C, et al. Flumazenil for the treatment of refractory hypersomnolence: clinical experience with 153 patients. J Clin Sleep Med 2016;12(10):1389–94.
56. Trotti L, Saini P, Freeman A, et al. Improvement in daytime sleepiness with clarithromycin in patients with GABA-related hypersomnia: clinical experi ence. J Psychopharmacol 2014;28(7):697–702.
57. Dauvilliers Y, Bassetti C, Lammers GJ, et al. Pitoli-sant versus placebo or modafinil in patients with nar-colepsy: a double-blind, randomised trial. Lancet Neurol 2013;12:1068–75.
58. Dauvilliers Y, Arnulf I, Foldvary-Schaefer N, Morse AM, Šonka K, Thorpy MJ, et al. Safety and efficacy of lower-sodium oxybate in adults with idio-pathic hypersomnia: a phase 3, placebo-controlled, double-blind, randomised withdrawal study. Lancet Neurol 2022;21:53–65.
59.. Inoue Y, Tabata T, Tsukimori N. Efficacy and safety of modafinil in patients with idiopathic hypersomnia without long sleep time: a multicenter, randomized, double-blind, placebo-controlled, parallel-group comparison study. Sleep Med 2021;80:315–21.
60.. Nigam M, Hippolyte A, Dodet P, Gales A, Maranci JB, Al Youssef S, Leu-Semenescu S, Arnulf I. Sleeping through a pandemic: impact of COVID-19-related restrictions on narcolepsy and idiopathic hypersomnia. J Clin Sleep Med 2022; 18:255–63.

Drugs Used in Narcolepsy and Other Hypersomnias

Gert Jan Lammers, MD, PhD[a,b,*]

KEYWORDS

- Narcolepsy • Idiopathic hypersomnia • Nonpharmacologic treatment • Pharmacologic treatment
- Stimulants • Sodium oxybate • Pitolisant

KEY POINTS

- State-of-the-art treatment of narcolepsy and hypersomnias of central origin consists of a combination of facilitating acceptance of the disorder, lifestyle advice, and pharmacologic treatment.
- The goal of pharmacologic treatment must be improved performance and avoidance of side effects.
- Even when optimally treated, excessive daytime sleepiness will never completely disappear. In contrast, cataplexy, hypnagogic hallucinations, and sleep paralysis may completely disappear.

INTRODUCTION

Hypersomnolence may have various expressions and lead to a variety of complaints, including a subjective feeling of sleepiness, difficulty in sustaining attention, impaired performance, memory complaints, automatic behavior, unintended naps, irritability, and/or an increased amount of sleep. Regarding sleep, usually 1 of 2 distinctive phenotypes is predominantly present: an inability to stay awake during the day or an increased need for sleep. This distinction may not only guide the underlying diagnosis but also predict efficacy of certain (pharmacologic) treatment interventions. By definition, the complaint is present each and every day.

Narcolepsy with cataplexy is a typical example of a disorder characterized by an inability to stay awake during the day, usually accompanied by an inability to stay asleep at night but without a significant increase in the hours spent asleep during the 24 hours of the day. The classic form of idiopathic hypersomnia (IH) is the typical example of an increased need for sleep: there is an irresistible need for an increased number of hours spent asleep during the night and, despite this increase, there are complaints of sleepiness during the day. This latter phenotype is more difficult to treat.

It must be kept in mind that by far the most prevalent cause of excessive daytime sleepiness (EDS) is sleep deprivation. Complaints caused by sleep deprivation are neither quantitatively nor qualitatively different from complaints caused by sleep disorders, which may cause diagnostic challenges. In case of doubt, patients must always be first advised to extend sleep to assess whether sleep deprivation is the likely cause of their complaints. It is also important to realize that if a sleep disorder is the cause for EDS, sleep apnea is a much more prevalent cause than narcolepsy or IH because of its much higher prevalence.

THE COMPLAINTS TO BE TREATED

The key problem of most patients who suffer from narcolepsy or IH is their inability to remain fully

Sleep Med Clin 13 (2018) 183-189 https://doi.org/10.1016/j.jsmc.2018.02.009 1556-407X/18/© 2018 Elsevier Inc.

[a] Department of Neurology, Leiden University Medical Center, Albinusdreef 2, Leiden 2333 AA, the Netherlands; [b] Sleep-Wake Centers of Stichting Epilepsie Instellingen Nedereland (SEIN), Achterweg 5, Heemstede 2103 SW, the Netherlands
* Department of Neurology, Leiden University Medical Center, Albinusdreef 2, Leiden 2333 AA, the Netherlands.
E-mail address: G.J.Lammers@LUMC.nl

Sleep Med Clin 17 (2022) 399–405
https://doi.org/10.1016/j.jsmc.2022.06.005
1556-407X/22/© 2022 Elsevier Inc.

alert and/or even awake during longer periods of the day, relentlessly present each and every day of their life.[1,2] In narcolepsy with cataplexy in addition, the strict physiologic boundaries of specific components of wake and sleep stages are fluid. This fluidity leads to partial expressions, particularly identifiable in rapid eye movement (REM) sleep, explaining such symptoms as cataplexy, hypnagogic hallucinations (HHs), and sleep paralysis (SP).[2] The loss of state boundaries leads to more symptoms that are not always mentioned in textbooks, such as automatic behavior, memory complaints, and dream delusions.

COMORBIDITY

Patients who suffer from narcolepsy with cataplexy clearly bear a risk of becoming obese, and those who suffer from narcolepsy and IH have an increased chance of developing complaints of fatigue and psychiatric comorbidities, such as anxiety and depression.[2,3]

It may be important to treat these comorbidities as well; however, that is beyond the scope of this article.

BURDEN

It is not difficult to imagine that narcolepsy and IH have a severe negative impact on daily functioning and the experienced quality of life. It is even more detrimental when it starts during childhood because of the additional negative impact on social development and achievements at school.[2,4]

EPIDEMIOLOGY

Narcolepsy with cataplexy has an estimated prevalence of 25 to 50 per 100,000 population. The incidence is estimated to be 0.74 to 1.37 per 100,000 person-years.[5–7] There are no reliable prevalence or incidence estimations of narcolepsy without cataplexy and IH, but the prevalence is probably lower than for narcolepsy with cataplexy.

The age of onset is usually between 15 and 35 years, but it may start at any age. There is a trend for a diagnosis at younger age and, probably, also for an earlier symptom onset during the last decade.

CURRENTLY AVAILABLE TREATMENTS

Before starting treatment, it is of paramount importance that patients and their relatives are informed about the consequences of their chronic disease and learn to accept the diagnosis, which greatly facilitates the implementation of the behavioral modifications and decreases the burden of the disease. Accepting the diagnosis implies implementing behavioral or lifestyle modifications. Initiating pharmacologic treatment only after the implementation of lifestyle changes will prevent medication being used to compensate for a lack of lifestyle adjustment and will optimize treatment response. Only when medication is added to lifestyle adjustments can optimal and long-term improvement be established.

In addition, a supportive social environment (eg, family members, friends, employer, colleagues, patient group organizations, and support groups) is highly valuable.

TREATMENT GOALS

Unfortunately, there is currently only symptomatic treatment of narcolepsy and IH. Although symptomatic, it may lead to profound improvement. There are 2 known effective treatment modalities: behavioral modification and pharmacologic therapy. As a rule, both are needed to achieve sufficient improvement.[2]

Therapy for EDS as expression of narcolepsy or IH should focus on the key problem: improving sustained attention and, therefore, performance, and reducing the chance for involuntary sleep attacks or naps. Because treatment is symptomatic, EDS complaints will never completely disappear. It should be explained to patients that the treatment goal is to improve the quality and duration of wakefulness during the day. Patients must be warned that there will usually remain a high chance of falling asleep in sedentary situations.

When initiating treatment of cataplexy, HHs, and SP, the intention should be to let them disappear. To reach this, pharmacologic treatment is almost always needed. HHs may sometimes be less prevalent when falling asleep in the supine position is avoided.

Behavioral Modification

Patients should be advised to live a regular life, go to bed at the same hour each night, and get up at the same time each morning as much as possible. Scheduled daytime naps, usually less than 20 minutes, may temporarily alleviate and prevent daytime sleepiness, and a short nap just before certain activities demanding a high degree of attention may facilitate the proper completion. The optimal frequency, duration, and timing of these naps must be established on an individual basis. In most narcoleptic patients, longer naps have no better or longer lasting refreshing properties. Moreover, it is more difficult and inconvenient to wake up after a longer nap because, in most instances, deep sleep will occur. However, some patients only do well with longer naps. Unfortunately, there are few published studies regarding this important topic.[8]

Many particularly narcoleptic patients experience an influence from diet. These patients feel better when avoiding (large amounts of) carbohydrates during the day. Unfortunately, there also are few scientific data regarding this observation.[9] Alcohol consumption should preferably be avoided.

Pharmacologic Therapy

Despite these behavioral measures, most patients will need adjuvant pharmacologic treatment. A variety of substances can be used. This observation already indicates that no drug is efficacious in all. Because most drugs predominantly act on either EDS or cataplexy, combinations are often needed to control both symptoms in those who suffer from narcolepsy with cataplexy. The only available drug that may improve all major symptoms of narcolepsy is sodium oxybate (SXB). Combinations of SXB with, for example, stimulants may have a synergistic effect for the amelioration of EDS and, therefore, may be preferred over monotherapy.

What Should Be Kept in Mind When Making a Choice for a Certain Drug or Combinations of Drugs in an Individual Patient, and How to Evaluate Its Efficacy?

- EDS will never be completely alleviated, whereas cataplexy, HHs, and SP may completely disappear in some patients.
- Improvement of daytime performance is a much more important treatment goal than reduction of the total amount of daytime sleep.
- Long-term improvement of nocturnal sleep can only be reached with SXB.
- History taking from both the patients and partners or relatives is the best way to guide and adjust therapy.
- Individual differences in efficacy, side effects, and tolerability of drugs seem to be extensive. Knowledge about the efficacy of a drug as assessed in groups is, therefore, of relative importance for making a choice in an individual.
- Pharmacokinetic aspects, that is, short-acting and fast-acting versus slow-acting and long-acting drugs, may be more important than the expected efficacy.

Treatment of Excessive Daytime Sleepiness

Stimulants still are the mainstay of the treatment of EDS.[10,11] Stimulants enhance release and inhibit the reuptake of catecholamines and, to a lesser extent, serotonin in the central nervous system and the periphery. Stimulants are also weak inhibitors of monoamine oxidase; these include dextroamphetamine (5–60 mg/d; usually in 1–3 doses per day), methylphenidate (10–60 mg/d; usually in 2–4 doses per day), and mazindol (1–6 mg/d; usually in 1–2 doses per day). Side effects and tolerance are drawbacks in the use of stimulants. The most important side effects include irritability, agitation, headache, and peripheral sympathetic stimulation. These side effects are usually dose related. Although addiction does not seem to be a problem in narcolepsy or presumably in IH, some patients tend to increase their dosage because they prefer high alertness.[12] Tolerance develops in about one-third of patients.[12,13] Mazindol has been withdrawn from the market in most countries owing to observed uncommon but severe side effects in related drugs that suppress appetite, in particular fenfluramines. The side effects were pulmonary hypertension and valvular regurgitation.[14] Because some patients respond better to mazindol than to any other drug, it may be considered, provided treatment is closely monitored.

Modafinil (100–400 mg/d; usually in 1 or 2 doses) is usually grouped with stimulants but is chemically unrelated to amphetamine.[11] Modafinil blocks the dopamine reuptake, but the mode of action is not yet fully explained. The efficacy is probably equal to that of the stimulants, although direct comparisons are lacking. The clinical impression of most experts in the field is that during treatment with modafinil all the described side effects, as well as tolerance, of stimulants may occur but are less frequent and less severe in general. More specific side effects of modafinil are headache and nausea. However, they usually disappear after 2 to 3 weeks of treatment. Although the experts are probably right, this opinion is not very relevant for deciding for a certain stimulant or modafinil in an individual patient: the interindividual differences in experienced response and side effects are too widespread to guide treatment only on opinions regarding efficacy on a group level. When prescribed to women of childbearing age, it must be kept in mind that there is interaction with oral contraceptives. Dose adjustment is required.

The European Medicines Agency (EMA) completed a remarkable review of the safety and effectiveness of modafinil in 2010.[15] The EMA's Committee for Medicinal Products for Human Use concluded that the benefits of modafinil-containing medicines continue to outweigh their risks but that their use should be restricted to the treatment of adults suffering from narcolepsy. It is not exactly clear on which data this advice was based, or why apparently narcolepsy was generally considered to be a more relevant or more invalidating disorder than IH. Moreover, it contained no risk evaluation when replacing modafinil with another stimulant.[15] Because of these unanswered questions, most national and international guidelines, including in Europe, still recommend the use of modafinil in IH.[16–18]

Armodafinil is the *R*-enantiomer of modafinil and has very similar effects; it is not available in most European countries. Caffeine may alleviate sleepiness but has a weak effect: the alerting effect of 6 cups of strong coffee is comparable with that of 5 mg of dexamphetamine.

Long-acting agents (modafinil, armodafinil, dexamphetamine, methylphenidate, controlled release) are generally better tolerated than the short-acting ones. The quick and short-acting agents can be used to good effect when targeted at social events or difficult periods during the day. For this reason, combinations of stimulants may be tailored to the circumstances. Unfortunately, there are no studies assessing the advantages or disadvantages of combinations of stimulants.

Pitolisant, a selective histamine-3 receptor antagonist, has recently been approved by the EMA. Pitolisant was the first histamine-3 receptor antagonist to reach the market. It is an advantage to have an additional option for the treatment of EDS with a different and selective mode of action when compared with stimulants. The dose range is 9 to 36 mg. Published studies show efficacy, particularly regarding improvement of EDS, and also regarding improvement of cataplexy.[19,20] On a group level, the efficacy for EDS is comparable to that of modafinil; the same holds true for side effects.[19] Because of the different mode of action, it can be combined with other stimulants and with SXB. However, scientific data regarding combination with other stimulants are currently lacking. Pitolisant is not registered for the treatment of IH, although there are encouraging results in a published study with subjects suffering from IH.[21]

Pitolisant shares with modafinil the disadvantage of interaction with oral contraceptives, requiring dose adjustment of the oral contraceptives. However, recently, new studies have been initiated to assess whether the interaction is indeed clinically relevant.

SXB, the sodium salt of gamma-hydroxybutyrate (GHB), is a hypnotic and, therefore, prescribed for use during the night, with a shown beneficial effect on nocturnal sleep, EDS, and cataplexy.[22–24] SXB is a naturally occurring substance in the human brain, and GHB receptors have been identified in the brain. However, the therapeutic effect of SXB seems to be mediated by the gamma-aminobutyric acid (GABA)-B receptor. Because of its very short half-life, 2 separate doses are required during the night. The usual starting dose is 2.25 g twice a night. The dose must be gradually increased, keeping in mind that the optimal daytime effects after a dose increase will reveal after weeks. Therefore, it usually takes several months to reach an optimal situation. Moreover, a relevant improvement of EDS is, in most patients, achieved only with higher doses (6–9 g/night).[24] Efficacy for nocturnal sleep and/or cataplexy usually already occurs on lower dosages. The effect on EDS of higher doses seems to be similar to that of modafinil, and side effects are, if present, usually mild.[24] The combination of both of these substances is even more effective.[24] The most frequent side effect is nausea, and the most disabling are enuresis, sleep walking, and uncommon but possible mood disturbance, including depression. Lowering the dose usually ends the enuresis and sleep walking. Mood disturbance may be a reason to discontinue the medication. Weight loss may also occur.[25]

In follow-up studies, there is no indication that tolerance develops and abrupt cessation does not induce rebound cataplexy. However, long-term clinical experience shows that a substantial proportion of patients may develop (some) tolerance for the sleep-promoting effects, although efficacy for the other symptoms remains.

SXB should not be used in conjunction with other sedatives or alcohol. If patients have consumed alcohol in the evening, they should omit 1 or both doses afterward. In patients with comorbid obstructive sleep apnea syndrome (OSAS), treatment should be closely monitored because SXB may worsen OSAS. Cotreatment with continuous positive airway pressure may be indicated.[26]

Unfortunately, there may be concern for misuse. Although potential threats related to misuse may result in hesitation in patients to take, and in physicians to prescribe, the substance, it is important to realize that when the drug is properly used it is safe and bears no risk for dependence, at least when used in the treatment of narcolepsy. There are few data for the use in IH, and it is not registered for the treatment of IH.[17,27]

Treatment of Cataplexy

Most studies concerning the treatment of the REM dissociation phenomena focused on cataplexy. Amelioration of cataplexy is generally associated with improvement of HHs and SP.[11] SXB and tricyclic antidepressants are the most effective treatments. The different tricyclic antidepressants all inhibit the reuptake of norepinephrine and serotonin and are potent REM sleep inhibitors. The most commonly used ones are clomipramine in a low dose (10–50 mg/d) and imipramine, also in a relatively low dose.[11] As with stimulants, side effects are a drawback. Side effects are largely due to the anticholinergic properties. The most frequently reported are dry mouth, increased sweating, sexual dysfunction (impotence, delayed orgasm, and erection and ejaculation dysfunction), weight gain, tachycardia, constipation, blurred vision, and urinary retention. However, very low doses, up to 20 mg, are often remarkably effective and are seldom accompanied by significant side effects. Therefore, many clinicians consider clomipramine to be the treatment of choice. The most relevant drawback, even with low doses, is the occurrence of tolerance. Moreover, tricyclic antidepressants should never be stopped abruptly because of the risk of severe aggravation of cataplexy, which may lead to a status cataplecticus.

Many alternative antidepressants have been studied, especially selective serotonin reuptake inhibitors, and more selective noradrenergic reuptake inhibitors, such as fluoxetine, zimelidine, viloxazine, femoxetine, fluvoxamine, and paroxetine. These antidepressants should be prescribed in the same dosages as used in the treatment of depression and, therefore, their side effect profile seems not favorable compared with the side effects with low dosages of clomipramine. All these substances seem to act mainly via less selective desmethyl metabolites. In recent years, venlafaxine and atomoxetine have become very popular in the treatment of cataplexy, although there are no randomized placebo-controlled studies available. Acute withdrawal of these substances will also lead to rebound cataplexy.

SXB is the best studied drug in the treatment of cataplexy and is probably the most potent inhibitor in most patients.[23] SXB has never been compared with any antidepressant, so it is difficult to know whether it is really most effective in most patients. However, the relatively mild side effect profile, as well as the broader action on the other symptoms of narcolepsy, such as disturbed nocturnal sleep and EDS, makes it a favorable option.

Several drugs may theoretically be expected to aggravate cataplexy but only prazosin, an alpha 1 antagonist, is reliably documented to treat arterial hypertension.

In recent studies, the recently registered histamine-3 antagonist pitolisant was also showed to be effective in the treatment of cataplexy. However, its exact place in the treatment of cataplexy needs to be established.

Treatment of Disturbed Nocturnal Sleep

Disturbed nocturnal sleep can be a major complaint of patients. Unfortunately, treatment options are limited because SXB is the only drug with a proven long-term effect on nocturnal sleep.[22] Short-term beneficial effects of benzodiazepines have been described. Although nocturnal sleep may (temporarily) be improved with benzodiazepines, improvement of EDS is not the rule. The efficacy of baclofen, another GABA-B receptor agonist, has not been convincingly proved.[28] However, there are anecdotal reports of its efficacy. Occasionally, patients report on improvement when using cannabis or cannabidiol oil but there are no scientific studies performed with these substances or for this indication.

Treatment in Children

Treatment of children suffering from narcolepsy does not differ significantly from treatment in adulthood, although hardly any treatment studies have focused on children. Behavioral problems as expressions of narcolepsy only occur at young age. There are indications that treatment of EDS may have a positive impact on behavior, but studies focusing on this important symptom are urgently needed.

RECOMMENDATIONS FOR THE INITIATION OF PHARMACOLOGIC TREATMENT

Patients should continue the scheduled daytime naps and always start with 1 medication at a time. It is usually best to treat the most invalidating symptoms first. If this clearly is EDS, one should start with a stimulant; if it clearly is cataplexy and/or HHs, one should start with a low dose of clomipramine. If both disturbed nocturnal sleep and/or cataplexy are severe, SXB may be considered as the first choice. Treatment should always start with a low dose and the dose should be increased based on history taking, keeping in mind the tradeoff between efficacy and side effects. The exact place of pitolisant has to be determined. It may very well become a first-line drug in a subgroup of patients.

FUTURE PHARMACOLOGIC TREATMENTS

Idiopathic Hypersomnia

There are studies reporting on subjective improvement of EDS with clarithromycin, a negative allosteric modulator of the GABA-A receptor.

However, its use is still controversial.[17] These studies need replication and, preferably, evidence for objective improvement and long-term safety.[17]

Flumazenil, an antagonist of benzodiazepine-binding domain in GABA-A receptors, improved subjective sleepiness and reaction time in a single-blind trial.[29] Also, its use is controversial. A phase 2, dose-finding study of pentylenetetrazole (BTD-001-NCT02512588), another GABA-A antagonist for EDS in IH, is currently running.[17]

One observational study has shown SXB to be a potential effective treatment of IH.[27]

Narcolepsy

Because narcolepsy with cataplexy is presumed to be an autoimmune disorder, various immune-modulating treatments have been proposed. Some have been applied in individual cases in which the diagnosis was made shortly after symptom onset, up to now without real convincing or promising results. Although these therapies may potentially prevent progression of the disorder and/or rescue cells that are attacked but not yet destroyed, the timing of such treatment is very difficult. Application after the appearance of cataplexy may already be too late because cataplexy probably occurs when more than 80% of the hypocretin (also named orexin) cells are lost. Initiation in an earlier phase is difficult because there currently are no clinical signs or laboratory findings that reliably predict the evolution of narcolepsy without cataplexy to narcolepsy with cataplexy. Another problem is that immune-modulating therapies may have serious side effects. With the currently available nonimmunologic treatments known to be safe and effective in most patients, and a normal life expectancy for those who suffer from narcolepsy, it is difficult from an ethical perspective to initiate studies with risk-bearing immune-modulating therapies. Last, but not least, clinicians can currently only speculate about the autoimmune mechanisms involved in the development of narcolepsy. Therefore, it is impossible to make a rational choice for a specific immune-modulating therapy.

The most effective symptomatic treatment of narcolepsy would be expected to be treatment with hypocretin. Unfortunately, this is not as easy as may be expected. In a normal situation, hypocretin is locally produced in the brain and, as far as is known, only acts in the brain. When applied as a drug, it can hardly pass the blood-brain barrier. Nasal application has been suggested as an alternative, but this route may only be effective if active transport of hypocretin can be facilitated. Without such facilitation, the mucosa surface of the human nose will probably be too small to allow the uptake of enough hypocretin to induce a clinically significant effect. At present, hypocretin agonists are the most promising substances. Phase 3 trials are about to start.

The following are alternative symptomatic treatments currently under study:

- A new psychostimulant JZP-110 (solriamfetol), a dopaminergic and noradrenergic phenylalanine derivative: First results in narcolepsy are encouraging.[30] Several phase 3 studies will be completed soon.
- Long-acting SXB: A phase 3 study is currently being performed.
- Low-sodium formulation of SXB: A phase 3 study is currently running.
- In an animal study, it has been shown that modafinil, when coadministered with a connexin inhibitor, flecainide, is more effective than when administered alone.[31] Follow-up studies are expected.

SUMMARY

Lifestyle adjustment, in combination with symptomatic pharmacologic treatment, allows most patients, particularly those with an inability to stay awake, to live a relatively normal life. New pharmacologic substances show encouraging results in phase 2 and 3 studies to improve the current situation. More dedicated studies in IH, particularly in those who suffer from an increased need for sleep, are needed.

CLINICS CARE POINTS

- Always start treatment with lifestyle advices including short scheduled daytime naps before starting pharmacological treatment. This makes people aware of the impact of these changes and particularly the daytime naps.
- Pharmacological treatment should not replace lifestyle advices.
- Improvement of daytime performance is a much more important treatment goal than reduction of the total amount of daytime sleep.

DISCLOSURE

G.J. Lammers is a consultant or member of the international advisory boards on narcolepsy of UCB International, Jazz Pharmaceuticals, and Bioprojet Pharma.

REFERENCES

1. American Academy of Sleep Medicine. The international classification of sleep disorders. 3rd edition. Darien (IL): American Academy of Sleep Medicine; 2014.
2. Overeem S, Mignot E, van Dijk JG, et al. Narcolepsy: clinical features, new pathophysiologic insights, and future perspectives. J Clin Neurophysiol 2001;18: 78–105.
3. Ruoff CM, Reaven NL, Funk SE, et al. High rates of psychiatric comorbidity in narcolepsy: findings from the burden of narcolepsy disease (BOND) study of 9,312 patients in the United States. J Clin Psychiatry 2017;78(2):171–6.
4. Postiglione E, Antelmi E, Pizza F, et al. The clinical spectrum of childhood narcolepsy. Sleep Med Rev 2018;38:70–85.
5. Silber MH, Krahn LE, Olson E, et al. The epidemi- ology of narcolepsy in Olmsted County, Minnesota: a population-based study. Sleep 2002;25:197–202.
6. Longstreth WT, Koepsell TD, Ton TG, et al. The epidemiology of narcolepsy. Sleep 2007;30:13–26.
7. Wijnans L, Lecomte C, de Vries C, et al. The incidence of narcolepsy in Europe: before, during, and after the influenza A(H1N1) pandemic and vaccination campaigns. Vaccine 2013;31(8):1246–54.
8. Mullington J, Broughton R. Scheduled naps in the management of daytime sleepiness in narcolepsy-cataplexy. Sleep 1993;16:444–56.
9. Bruck D, Armstrong S, Coleman G. Sleepiness after glucose in narcolepsy. J Sleep Res 1994;3:171–9.
10. Wise MS, Arand DL, Auger RR, et al. Treatment of narcolepsy and other hypersomnias of central origin. Sleep 2007;30:1712–27.
11. M Billiard, C Bassetti, Y Dauvilliers, et al. EFNS guidelines on management of narcolepsy. Eur J Neurol 2006;13(10):1035–48.
12. Parkes JD, Dahlitz M. Amphetamine prescription. Sleep 1993;16:201–3.
13. Mitler MM, Aldrich MS, Koob GF, et al. Narcolepsy and its treatment with stimulants. ASDA standards of practice. Sleep 1994;17:352–71.
14. Ryan DH, Bray GA, Helmcke F, et al. Serial echocardiography and clinical evaluation of valvular regurgitation before, during, and after treatment with fenfluramine or dexfenfluramine and mazindol or phentermine. Obes Res 1999;7:313–22.
15. Available at: http://www.ema.europa.eu/docs/en_GB/document_library/Referrals_document/Modafinil_31/WC500105597.pdf. Accessed March 26, 2018.
16. Lopez R, Arnulf I, Drouot X, et al. French consensus. Management of patients with hypersomnia: which strategy? Rev Neurol (Paris) 2017;173(1–2):8–18.
17. Evangelista E, Lopez R, Dauvilliers Y. Update on treatment for idiopathic hypersomnia. Expert Opin Investig Drugs 2018;27(2):187–92.
18. Mayer G, Benes H, Young P, et al. Modafinil in the treatment of idiopathic hypersomnia without long sleep time—a randomized, double-blind, placebo-controlled study. J Sleep Res 2015;24:74–81.
19. Dauvilliers Y, Bassetti C, Lammers GJ, et al, HARMONY I study group. Pitolisant versus placebo or modafinil in patients with narcolepsy: a double-blind, randomised trial. Lancet Neurol 2013;12(11): 1068–75.
20. Szakacs Z, Dauvilliers Y, Mikhaylov V, et al, HARMONY-CTP study group. Safety and efficacy of pitolisant on cataplexy in patients with narcolepsy: a randomised, double-blind, placebo-controlled trial. Lancet Neurol 2017;16(3):200–7.
21. Leu-Semenescu S, Nittur N, Golmard J-L, et al. Effects of pitolisant, a histamine H3 inverse agonist, in drug-resistant idiopathic and symptomatic hypersomnia: a chart review. Sleep Med 2014;15:681–7.
22. Black J, Pardi D, Hornfeldt CS, et al. The nightly use of sodium oxybate is associated with a reduction in nocturnal sleep disruption: a double-blind, placebo-controlled study in patients with narcolepsy. J Clin Sleep Med 2010;6(6):596–602.
23. U.S. Xyrem Multicenter Study Group. Sodium oxybate demonstrates long-term efficacy for the treatment of cataplexy in patients with narcolepsy. Sleep Med 2004;5:119–23.
24. Black J, Houghton WC. Sodium oxybate improves excessive daytime sleepiness in narcolepsy. Sleep 2006;29:939–46.
25. Schinkelshoek MS, Smolders IM, Donjacour CE, et al. Decreased body mass index during treatment with sodium oxybate in narcolepsy type 1. J Sleep Res 2019;28(3). [Epub ahead of print].
26. Feldman NT. Clinical perspective: monitoring sodium oxybate-treated narcolepsy patients for the development of sleep-disordered breathing. Sleep Breath 2010;14(1):77–9.
27. Leu-Semenescu S, Louis P, Arnulf I. Benefits and risk of sodium oxybate in idiopathic hypersomnia versus narcolepsy type 1: a chart review. Sleep Med 2016;17:38–44.
28. Brown MA, Guilleminault C. A review of sodium oxy bate and baclofen in the treatment of sleep disorders. Curr Pharm Des 2011;17(15):1430–5.
29. Trotti LM, Saini P, Koola C, et al. Flumazenil for the treatment of refractory hypersomnolence: clinical experience with 153 patients. J Clin Sleep Med 2016;12:1389–94.
30. Ruoff C, Swick TJ, Doekel R, et al. Effect of oral JZP-110 (ADX-N05) on wakefulness and sleepiness in adults with narcolepsy: a phase 2b study. Sleep 2016;39(7):1379–87.
31. Duchene A, Perier M, Zhao Y, et al. Impact of astroglial connexins on modafinil pharmacological properties. Sleep 2016;39(6):1283–92.

Pharmacologic and Nonpharmacologic Treatment of Restless Legs Syndrome

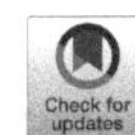

Galia V. Anguelova, MD, MSc, PhD, Monique H.M. Vlak, MD, PhD, Arthur G.Y. Kurvers, MD, Roselyne M. Rijsman, MD, PhD*

KEYWORDS

- Restless legs syndrome • Therapy • Treatment • Pharmacologic • Nonpharmacologic • Augmentation

KEY POINTS

- There is limited evidence for nonpharmacologic treatment in primary restless legs syndrome (RLS): pneumatic compression, near-infrared light spectroscopy, and transcranial magnetic stimulation.
- In moderate-to-severe RLS, pharmacologic treatment may be considered, starting with iron suppletion if applicable.
- There is strong evidence for both $\alpha 2\delta$ ligands and dopamine agonists in the therapy for RLS; however, an $\alpha 2\delta$ ligand may be preferred considering the risk of augmentation with dopaminergic treatment and current clinical consensus.
- When single-drug therapy with an $\alpha 2\delta$ ligand or dopamine agonist is insufficient, a combination of both may be considered or oxycodone/naloxone.
- To treat augmentation, a low dose or longer-acting dopaminergic drug may be chosen, or a switch to an $\alpha 2\delta$ ligand or oxycodone/naloxone may be considered.

INTRODUCTION

Restless legs syndrome (RLS) is a sleep-related disorder defined by an urgency to move the legs, usually combined with uncomfortable or unpleasant sensations, which occurs or worsens during rest, usually in the evening or at night, and disappears with the movement of the legs.[1] It occurs in 5% to 15% of European and North American adults, 2% to 3% with moderate-to-severe symptoms, twice as often in women as in men, and has a mean onset age between 30 and 40 years.[1] RLS can be classified as idiopathic or primary, and secondary to comorbid conditions (eg, renal disease, polyneuropathy).[1] The pathophysiology of RLS is still unclear. However, dopaminergic dysfunction and iron deficiency have been suggested to play an essential role, possibly interacting with each other as well.[1] Glutamate, adenosine, and opiate systems are also considered to play a role in the pathophysiology.[1] This article provides an updated practical guide for the treatment of primary RLS in adults. Iron deficiency is included in our definition of primary RLS because of its essential role in the pathophysiology. Treatment of periodic limb movements was beyond the focus of this article. The available evidence is reviewed for pharmacologic and nonpharmacologic treatment options.

Sleep Med Clin 13 (2018) 219-230 https://doi.org/10.1016/j.jsmc.2018.02.005 1556-407X/18/

Center for Sleep and Wake Disorders, Haaglanden Medical Center, The Hague, the Netherlands
* Corresponding author. Center for Sleep and Wake disorders, Haaglanden Medical Center, PO 432, The Hague 2501 CK, the Netherlands.
E-mail address: r.rijsman@haaglandenmc.nl

Sleep Med Clin 17 (2022) 407–419
https://doi.org/10.1016/j.jsmc.2022.06.006
1556-407X/22/

METHODS

This article was written in continuation of the 2016 RLS guidelines by the American Academy of Neurology (AAN).[2] The authors performed a PubMed search for articles on the treatment of primary RLS using Medical Subject Headings (MeSHs) terms and keywords with a start date of January 1, 2015, because the AAN guideline included articles published until the July 15, 2015.[2] Our initial search was performed on October 15, 2017 and a revision was last performed on October 15, 2021. Details on the latest search strategy are given in **Box 1**.

The titles and abstracts of the eligible articles were screened. The authors only included studies that met the following criteria: (1) original article; (2) on the treatment of primary RLS (including iron deficiency-related RLS); (3) in adult humans; (4) published in English. Case reports were excluded. We focused primarily on the effect on RLS symptoms and periodic limb movements. A standardized tool to report RLS symptom severity is the International Restless Legs Syndrome Study Group rating scale (IRLS), which measures symptoms in the past week with 10 items each graded from 0 to 4 with increasing severity (with a maximum score of 40).[2] Because international guidelines no longer recommend the use of pergolide for RLS, we did not include new studies on pergolide alone. Acupuncture, Chinese herbs, meditation, music, and prayer were considered outside the scope of our review.

Additional articles found in the references of articles identified through our database search were also reviewed if considered relevant according to the criteria mentioned earlier. Relevant articles were classified according to their risk of bias (increasing from I to IV) and subsequent recommendations were made according to the criteria described by the AAN guideline (level A, B, C, and U in decreasing order of evidence level).[2] Studies published after the 2016 AAN guideline are discussed in detail. For studies already described in the 2016 AAN guideline, we refer to the AAN guideline.

RESULTS

Pharmacologic Treatment Options

Table 1 shows the pharmacologic agents effective in RLS treatment with at least evidence level C with their initial and usual daily dose, pharmacokinetics, specific considerations, and side effects.

Dopamine Precursors

Levodopa

Levodopa was one of the first drugs studied for treating RLS. There are four class III studies showing a benefit of levodopa (100–200 mg) on RLS severity (level C).[2] Also a possible effect on the periodic limb movement index (PLMI) was found based on three class III studies (level C).[2] Augmentation (discussed later) is a major problem with long-term daily use of levodopa in RLS. It occurs in 40% to 60% of patients after 6 months of follow-up, but augmentation rates as high as 71% have been reported.[3]

Non-ergot-derived dopamine agonists pramipexole

Pramipexole is a dopamine agonist which is excreted by the kidney. There is level A evidence that pramipexole improves RLS symptoms based on three class I studies and six class II studies.[2] Improvement of PLMI was seen in three class II studies giving level B evidence.[2] Two open-label studies reported that efficacy on RLS symptoms continues up to 1 year.[4,5] A study comparing pramipexole with dual-release levodopa/benserazide found that both drugs are effective in reducing RLS symptoms and PLMI, but levodopa had a higher rate of augmentation (21%) compared with pramipexole (6%).[6]

Ropinirole

Ropinirole was effective in improving RLS symptoms for up to 6 months according to two class I studies and up to 1 year according to two class I studies (level B).[2] Ropinirole also improves PLMI according to two class I studies (level A).[2] Ropinirole is a dopamine agonist primarily metabolized by the liver, mainly via the cytochrome P(CYP) 1A2 enzyme but also via CYP3A. Substances that inhibit and promote those enzymes can interact with ropinirole.[7]

Rotigotine

Rotigotine is a dopaminergic agonist delivered through a transdermal patch allowing a continuous release and thus maintaining stable concentrations that mimic physiologic striatal dopamine receptor function.[8–10] Because of the transdermal delivery, rotigotine is especially useful in patients with daytime symptoms, patients with swallowing difficulties, and patients undergoing surgery.[11] Rotigotine has been shown to reduce RLS symptoms for up to 6 months in two class I and two class II studies (level A) and reduce PLMI in one class I study (level B).[2] Our search strategy identified one new class I study that has been published since the AAN guideline in 2016.[12] This study randomized 150 patients to receive an optimal dose of rotigotine (1–3 mg) or placebo (randomization 2:1). Although rotigotine was effective in improving IRLS scores at 4 weeks of treatment, there was no superiority compared with placebo (least square mean with 95% confidence intervals [CIs] from an analysis of covariance model −0.27, 95% CI −3.0–2.4;

Box 1
PubMed search strategy

- Dopamine agonists ("Dopamine Agonists"[MeSH] OR "Dopamine Agonists" [Pharmacological Action] OR (dopamin* AND agonist*) OR "Levodopa"[MeSH] OR levodopa*[tiab] OR "pramipexole" [Supplementary Concept] OR pramipexol*[tiab] OR "ropinirole" [Supplementary Concept] OR ropinirol* [tiab] OR "rotigotine" [Supplementary Concept] OR Rotigotin*[tiab] OR "Pergolide"[MeSH] OR Pergolid*[tiab] OR "cabergoline" [Supplementary Concept] OR Cabergolin*[tiab]) AND ("Restless Legs Syndrome"[MeSH] OR "rls"[ti] OR rls'*[ti] OR (restles*[ti] AND leg*[ti]) OR restless leg*[tiab] OR ekbom*[tiab]) NOT ("Animals"[MeSH] NOT "Humans"[MeSH]) AND 2017/10:3000/01 [dp]
- α2δ ligands (alpha-2-delta[tiab] OR alpha2delta[tiab] OR α2δ[tiab] OR α-2-δ[tiab] OR "gabapentin" [Supplementary Concept] OR gabapentin*[tiab] OR "Pregabalin"[MeSH] OR pregabalin*[tiab] OR "1-(((alpha-isobutanoyloxyethoxy)carbonyl)aminomethyl)-1-cyclohexaneacetic acid" [Supplementary Concept] OR "Cyclohexanecarboxylic Acids"[MeSH] OR "gamma-Aminobutyric Acid"[MeSH]) AND ("Restless Legs Syndrome"[MeSH] OR "rls"[ti] OR rls'*[ti] OR (restles*[ti] AND leg*[ti]) OR restless leg*[tiab] OR ekbom*[tiab]) NOT ("Animals"[MeSH] NOT "Humans"[MeSH]) AND 2017/10:3000/01 [dp]
- Specific *N*-methyl-D-aspartate receptor agonists and drugs acting on AMPA-receptors ("traxoprodil mesylate" [Supplementary Concept] OR Traxoprodil*[tiab] OR "ifenprodil" [Supplementary Concept] OR Ifenprodil*[tiab] OR "aniracetam" [Supplementary Concept] OR Aniracetam*[tiab] OR "Kynurenic Acid"[MeSH] OR Kynurenic acid*[tiab] OR Kynurenate[tiab] OR "perampanel" [Supplementary Concept] OR Perampanel*[tiab] OR "tezampanel" [Supplementary Concept] OR Tezampanel*[tiab]) AND ("Restless Legs Syndrome"[MeSH] OR "rls"[ti] OR rls'*[ti] OR (restles*[ti] AND leg* [ti]) OR restless leg*[tiab] OR ekbom*[tiab]) NOT ("Animals"[MeSH] NOT "Humans"[MeSH]) AND 2017/10:3000/01 [dp]
- Opioids ("Analgesics, Opioid"[MeSH] OR "Analgesics, Opioid" [Pharmacological Action] OR "Narcotics" [Pharmacological Action] OR Opiate[tiab] OR opioid*[tiab] OR "Tramadol"[MeSH] OR tramadol[tiab] OR tramdol[tiab] OR "Morphine"[MeSH] OR morphin*[tiab] OR "Oxycodone"[MeSH] OR Oxycodon*[tiab] OR "Fentanyl"[MeSH] OR Fentanyl[tiab] OR "Naloxone"[MeSH] OR Naloxon*[tiab] OR "Methadone"[MeSH] OR Methadon*[tiab] OR "Ketamine"[MeSH] OR Ketamin*[tiab] OR "Tilidine"[MeSH] OR Tilidine[tiab]) AND ("Restless Legs Syndrome"[MeSH] OR "rls"[ti] OR rls'*[ti] OR (restles*[ti] AND leg*[ti]) OR restless leg*[tiab] OR ekbom*[tiab]) NOT ("Animals"[MeSH] NOT "Humans"[MeSH]) AND 2017/10:3000/01 [dp]
- Iron ("Iron"[MeSH] OR "ferric carboxymaltose" [Supplementary Concept] AND ferric carboxymal-tose [tiab] OR iron carboxymaltose[tiab] OR "ferrous sulfate" [Supplementary Concept] OR ferrous sulfate [tiab] OR iron sulfate[tiab] OR ferric sulfate[tiab] OR ferrous sulphate[tiab] OR iron sulphate[tiab] OR ferric sulphate[tiab] OR "ferric oxide, saccharated" [Supplementary Concept] OR iron-saccharate[tiab] OR iron sucrose[tiab] OR "saccharated iron oxide"[tiab] OR ferric saccha-rate[tiab] OR ferri saccharate [tiab] OR "ferric gluconate" [Supplementary Concept] AND "Bioferrico" [Supplementary Concept] OR ferric gluconate[tiab] OR iron gluconate[tiab] OR ferrous gluconate[tiab] OR ferrigluconate[tiab] OR "Iron-Dextran Complex"[MeSH] OR Iron Dextran[tiab] OR ferridextran[tiab] OR "Ferrosoferric Oxide"[MeSH] OR Ferrosoferric Oxide[tiab] OR ferumoxy-tol[tiab] OR ferriferrous oxide[tiab] OR "iron isomaltoside 1000" [Supplementary Concept] OR iron isomaltoside[tiab]) AND ("Restless Legs Syndrome"[MeSH] OR "rls"[ti] OR rls'*[ti] OR (rest-les*[ti] AND leg*[ti]) OR restless leg*[tiab] OR ekbom* [tiab]) NOT ("Animals"[MeSH] NOT "Humans"[MeSH]) AND 2017/10:3000/01 [dp]
- Other medication ("Melatonin"[MeSH] OR melatonin*[tiab] OR "Glucosamine"[MeSH] OR Glucosamine[tiab] OR 2-Amino-2-Deoxyglucose[tiab] OR Hespercorbin[tiab] OR dona[tiab] OR xicil[tiab] OR "Magnesium"[MeSH] OR magnesium*[tiab] OR "Creatine"[MeSH] OR creatin*[tiab] OR "coenzyme Q10" [Supplementary Concept] OR coenzyme Q10[tiab] OR co-enzyme Q10[tiab] OR "CoQ 10"[tiab] OR "CoQ10"[tiab] OR ubidecarenone[tiab] OR ubiquinone[tiab] OR Bio-Quinone Q10 [tiab] OR ubisemiquinone radical[tiab] OR Q-ter[tiab] OR ubisemiquinone[tiab] OR "Dipyridamole"[-MeSH] OR dipyridamol*[tiab] OR dipyramidol*[tiab] OR dipirid*[tiab] OR dipyrid*[tiab] OR apodipyridamol*[tiab] OR apo-dipyridamol*[tiab] OR cerebrovasc*[tiab] OR persantin*[tiab] OR curantil* [tiab] OR curantyl*[tiab] OR kurantil*[tiab] OR miosen*[tiab] OR novo-dipiradol*[tiab] OR novodipiradol*[tiab] OR antistenocardin*[tiab] OR cléridium*[tiab] OR "Nortriptyline"[MeSH] OR nortriptylin* [tiab] OR nortri-ptylin*[tiab] OR Desitriptylin*[tiab] OR Desmethylamitriptylin*[tiab] OR Allegron* [tiab] OR Paxtibi*[tiab] OR Nortrilen*[tiab] OR Pamelor*[tiab] OR Norfenazin*[tiab]) AND ("Restless Legs Syndrome"[MeSH] OR "rls"[ti] OR rls'*[ti] OR (restles*[ti] AND leg*[ti]) OR restless leg*[tiab] OR ekbom*[tiab]) NOT ("Animals"[MeSH] NOT "Humans"[MeSH]) AND 2017/10:3000/01 [dp]

- Benzodiazepines ("Benzodiazepines"[MeSH] OR Benzodiazepin*[tiab] OR "Clonazepam"[MeSH] OR clonazepam*[tiab] OR "zolpidem" [Supplementary Concept] OR zolpidem*[tiab]) AND ("Restless Legs Syndrome"[MeSH] OR "rls"[ti] OR rls'*[ti] OR (restles*[ti] AND leg*[ti]) OR restless leg*[tiab] OR ekbom*[tiab]) NOT ("Animals"[MeSH] NOT "Humans"[MeSH]) AND 2017/10:3000/01 [dp]
- Antiepileptics("Anticonvulsants" [Pharmacological Action] OR "Anticonvulsants"[MeSH] OR anticonvuls*[tiab] OR anti-convuls*[tiab] OR antiepileptic*[tiab] OR anti-epileptic*[tiab] OR "Carbamazepine"[MeSH] OR Carbamazepin*[tiab] OR "etiracetam" [Supplementary Concept] OR etiracetam [tiab] OR Levetiracetam[tiab] OR "Valproic Acid"[MeSH] OR Valproic acid*[tiab] OR Tegretol[tiab] OR Carbazepin[tiab] OR Epitol[tiab] OR Finlepsin[tiab] OR Neurotol[tiab] OR Amizepine[tiab] OR Keppra[tiab] OR Propylisopropylacetic Acid[tiab] OR 2 Propylpentanoic Acid[tiab] OR Divalproex [tiab] OR Depakene[tiab] OR Depakine[tiab] OR Convulsofin[tiab] OR Depakote[tiab] OR Vupral [tiab] OR Divalproex Sodium[tiab] OR Valproate[tiab] OR Ergenyl[tiab] OR Dipropyl Acetate[tiab]) AND ("Restless Legs Syndrome"[MeSH] OR "rls"[ti] OR rls'*[ti] OR (restles*[ti] AND leg*[ti]) OR restless leg*[tiab] OR ekbom* [tiab]) NOT ("Animals"[MeSH] NOT "Humans"[MeSH]) AND 2017/10:3000/01 [dp]

Nonpharmacologic treatment options

- Sleep hygiene ("Sleep Hygiene"[MeSH] OR sleep hygiene[tiab] OR sleep habit*[tiab]) AND ("Restless Legs Syndrome"[MeSH] OR "rls"[ti] OR rls'*[ti] OR (restles*[ti] AND leg*[ti]) OR restless leg*[tiab] OR ekbom*[tiab]) NOT ("Animals"[MeSH] NOT "Humans"[MeSH]) AND 2017/10:3000/01 [dp]
- Caffeine, alcohol, tobacco and cannabis use ("coffee"[MeSH Terms] OR "Caffeine"[MeSH] OR coffee [tiab] OR Caffeine[tiab] OR "Alcohol Drinking"[MeSH] OR "alcoholic beverages"[MeSH Terms] OR alcohol*[tiab] OR "Cannabis"[MeSH] OR "Medical Marijuana"[MeSH] OR Cannabi*[tiab] OR Marijuana*[tiab] OR Marihuana*[tiab] OR Hemp[tiab] OR Hemps[tiab] OR Hashish*[tiab] OR Bhang* [tiab] OR Ganja*[tiab] OR cannador*[tiab] OR charas[tiab]) AND ("Restless Legs Syndrome"[MeSH] OR "rls"[ti] OR rls'*[ti] OR (restles*[ti] AND leg*[ti]) OR restless leg*[tiab] OR ekbom*[tiab]) NOT ("Animals"[MeSH] NOT "Humans"[MeSH]) AND 2017/10:3000/01 [dp]
- Mental activity ("Mental Processes"[MeSH] OR "mental activity"[tiab] OR "Reading"[MeSH] OR reading[tiab] OR read[tiab] OR card game*[tiab] OR brain teaser*[tiab] OR chess[tiab] OR computer work[tiab]) AND ("Restless Legs Syndrome"[MeSH] OR "rls"[ti] OR rls'*[ti] OR (restles*[ti] AND leg* [ti]) OR restless leg*[tiab] OR ekbom*[tiab]) NOT ("Animals"[MeSH] NOT "Humans"[MeSH]) AND 2017/10:3000/01 [dp]
- Physical activity (including yoga) (Aerobic*[tiab] OR "Exercise Therapy"[MeSH] OR "Exercise"[MeSH] OR exercise[tiab] OR "Yoga"[MeSH] OR yoga[tiab] OR "Resistance Training"[MeSH] OR resistance training[tiab] OR "Weight Lifting"[MeSH] OR Weight lifting[tiab] OR weight bearing[tiab] OR "Bicy-cling"[MeSH] OR bicycl*[tiab] OR cycling[tiab] OR cycle[tiab]) AND ("Restless Legs Syndrome"[-MeSH] OR "rls"[ti] OR rls'*[ti] OR (restles*[ti] AND leg*[ti]) OR restless leg*[tiab] OR ekbom*[tiab]) NOT ("Animals"[MeSH] NOT "Humans"[MeSH]) AND 2017/10:3000/01 [dp]
- Pneumatic compression ("Intermittent Pneumatic Compression Devices"[MeSH] OR ((Pneumatic[tiab] OR mechanical[tiab]) AND compression[tiab]) OR IPC[tiab]) AND ("Restless Legs Syndrome"[MeSH] OR "rls"[ti] OR rls'*[ti] OR (restles*[ti] AND leg*[ti]) OR restless leg*[tiab] OR ekbom*[tiab]) NOT ("Animals"[MeSH] NOT "Humans"[MeSH]) AND 2017/10:3000/01 [dp]
- Tactile stimulus (including hot baths, massage and vibratory pads) ("Vibration"[MeSH] OR vibrat* [tiab] OR pad[tiab] OR pads[tiab] OR "Balneology"[MeSH] OR "Hydrotherapy"[MeSH] OR "HotTemperature"[MeSH] OR "Hot Springs"[MeSH] OR bath*[tiab] OR "Massage"[MeSH] OR massage*[tiab] OR bodywork*[tiab]) AND ("Restless Legs Syndrome"[MeSH] OR "rls"[ti] OR rls'*[ti] OR (restles*[ti] AND leg*[ti]) OR restless leg*[tiab] OR ekbom*[tiab]) NOT ("Animals"[MeSH] NOT "Humans"[MeSH]) AND 2017/10:3000/01 [dp]
- Current or magnetic stimulus ("Transcranial Direct Current Stimulation"[MeSH] OR tsDCS*[tiab] OR tDCS*[tiab] OR ((transcranial[tiab] OR cathodal[tiab] OR anodal[tiab] OR electric*[tiab]) AND stimul*[tiab]) OR "Transcutaneous Electric Nerve Stimulation"[MeSH] OR TENS[tiab] OR tsDCS[tiab] OR ((Percutaneous[tiab] OR Transcutaneous[tiab] OR transdermal[tiab] OR cutaneous[tiab]) AND (Electric[tiab] OR electrical[tiab] OR electrostimulation[tiab] OR stimul*[tiab])) OR ("Transcranial Magnetic Stimulation"[MeSH] OR Transcranial Magnetic Stimulation*[tiab] OR rTMS[tiab] OR TMS [tiab] OR "Cortical Excitability"[MeSH] OR Cortical Excitability[tiab])) AND ("Restless Legs Syndrome"[MeSH] OR "rls"[ti] OR rls'*[ti] OR (restles*[ti] AND leg*[ti]) OR restless leg*[tiab] OR ekbom* [tiab]) NOT ("Animals"[MeSH] NOT "Humans"[MeSH]) AND 2017/10:3000/01 [dp]
- Light stimulus ("Infrared Rays"[MeSH] OR near-infrared light[tiab] OR NIR[tiab] OR near-infrared ray* [tiab] OR "Phototherapy"[MeSH] OR phototherap*[tiab] OR light therap*[tiab] OR phototherap*

[tiab] OR photoradiation therap*[tiab] OR heliotherap*[tiab] OR) AND ("Restless Legs Syndrome"[-MeSH] OR "rls"[ti] OR rls'*[ti] OR (restles*[ti] AND leg*[ti]) OR restless leg*[tiab] OR ekbom*[tiab]) NOT ("Animals"[MeSH] NOT "Humans"[MeSH]) AND 2017/10:3000/01 [dp]

- Cognitive therapy ("Adaptation, Psychological"[MeSH] OR "Cognitive Therapy"[MeSH] OR (cogniti*[ti] AND therap*[ti]) OR psychotherap*[tiab] OR "Mindfulness"[MeSH] OR mindful*[tiab]) AND ("Restless Legs Syndrome"[MeSH] OR "rls"[ti] OR rls'*[ti] OR (restles*[ti] AND leg*[ti]) OR restless leg*[tiab] OR ekbom*[tiab]) NOT("Animals"[MeSH] NOT "Humans"[MeSH]) AND 2017/10:3000/01 [dp]
- Vitamins ("Vitamins"[Pharmacological Action] OR vitamin*[tiab] OR ascorbic acid[tiab] OR cholecalciferol[tiab] OR calcitriol[tiab] OR calciol[tiab] OR "Calcium"[MeSH] OR "Calcium Carbonate"[MeSH] OR calcium[tiab] OR tocopherol[tiab] OR alpha-tocopherol[tiab] OR beta-tocopherol[tiab] OR gamma-tocopherol[tiab] OR "Vitamin D"[MeSH] OR "Vitamin B 6"[MeSH] OR "Vitamin B 12"[MeSH] OR "Vitamin B Complex"[MeSH] OR "Vitamin B Complex" [Pharmacological Action] OR "Folic Acid"[MeSH] OR folic acid[tiab] OR folvite[tiab] OR folacin[tiab] OR folate[tiab]) AND ("Restless Legs Syndrome"[MeSH] OR "rls"[ti] OR rls'*[ti] OR (restles*[ti] AND leg*[ti]) OR restless leg*[tiab] OR ekbom*[tiab]) NOT ("Animals"[MeSH] NOT "Humans"[MeSH]) AND 2017/10:3000/01 [dp]

$P = .8451$). Long-term efficacy was studied in three noncomparative extension studies that found continued efficacy for up to 5 years.[13–15]

Piribedil

There is insufficient evidence (level U) for the effectiveness of piribedil on RLS symptoms based on one open-label class IV study in which RLS symptoms improved in a group of 13 patients with a median dose of 50 mg of piribedil daily.[16]

Ergot-Derived Dopamine Agonists

Both pergolide (one class I study and two class II studies) and cabergoline (two class I studies) have been shown to be effective in treating RLS (level A).[2] However, all ergot-derived dopamine agonists have been associated with severe life-threatening side effects, including fibrosis and valvulopathy. International guidelines do not recommend the use of pergolide, which is no longer available in the United States for RLS.[2,17,18] European RLS guidelines also no longer recommend cabergoline for treating patients with RLS.[18] In the United States, cabergoline is only suggested as an option when other recommended agents have been tried first and failed, and on the condition that close clinical follow-up is provided.[17]

α2δ Ligands

Gabapentin enacarbil

Gabapentin enacarbil is a slow-release prodrug of gabapentin. It is absorbed by active transport in the gut and then converted to gabapentin. Four class I studies show that gabapentin enacarbil is effective in moderate-to-severe RLS in treating daytime symptoms (level A).[2] It is likely to be effective for at least 6 months (one class II study).[2] The IRLS score had improved by 15.5 points at 24 weeks. Relapses were less common in the active treatment arm compared with the placebo arm (9% vs 23%; $P = .02$). There is insufficient evidence based on one class III study (level U) for gabapentin enacarbil to have any significant effect on PLMI, although it is likely to improve other sleep measures based on one class I and one class III study.[2] One class I study shows reduced effects of gabapentin enacarbil in patients with RLS previously exposed to long-term treatment with dopamine agonists compared with dopamine treatment-naive patients.[19]

Pregabalin

Pregabalin is effective in the treatment of moderate-to-severe primary RLS for up to 1 year when dosed 150 to 450 mg/d (level B). This advice is based on one class I study: at 52 weeks' pregabalin significantly reduced IRLS scores compared with pramipexole.[2] Pregabalin is likely to improve PLMI (two class II studies), also likely to improve some other sleep measures (one class I study and two class II studies), and likely to improve subjective sleep (one class I study and three class II studies).[1,2] Compared with pramipexole, pregabalin is more likely to improve subjective sleep outcomes (based on two class II studies).[2]

Gabapentin

There is one class III study showing an effect of gabapentin at 6 weeks.[2] However, no long-term studies were performed (level U).[20] Unlike gabapentin enacarbil, the absorption of gabapentin is variable, which makes it more difficult to select the optimal dose.

Specific N-methyl-D-aspartate receptor agonists and drugs acting on α-amino-3-hydroxy-5-methyl-4-isoxazolepropionic acid (AMPA) receptors

α2δ Ligands reduce glutamatergic transmission. Therefore, other drugs with a similar effect are

Table 1
Pharmacologic treatment options for primary restless legs syndrome with a focus on restless legs syndrome symptoms

Medication	Level of Evidence	Initial Daily Dose (mg)	Usual Dose Range	*T1/2* (h)	T_{max}	Specific Considerations	Side Effects
Carbidopa/levodopa	C	125	25/100 mg PO	1.5	10–30 min	Occasional use	Headache, muscle cramps, confusion, somnolence, dizziness, depression, palpitations, orthostatic hypotension, and gastrointestinal symptoms
Pramipexole	A	0.125	0.125 mg PO up to 0.5–0.75 mg 2–3 h before bedtime Dose increasing every 4–7 d	8–12, regular; 24, extended release	1–3 h, regular; 6 h, extended release	Chronic therapy; can be used for patients with medications that affect hepatic enzymes	Nausea, sleepiness and insomnia, fatigue, vivid dreams, confusion, visual hallucinations, headache, postural hypotension, and impulse control disorder
Ropinirole	B	0.25(—0.5)	0.25–0.5 mg PO in the evening during the first week up to 4 mg PO	1.5–2.5, regular; 6–10, extended release	1.5 h	Chronic therapy; can be used for patients with decreased renal function	Nausea, somnolence, fatigue, depression, and impulse control disorder
Rotigotine	A	1	1–3 mg/24 h transdermal Dose increasing every 7 d	5–7	1–3 h	Chronic therapy; round-the-clock symptoms or swallowing difficulties	Allergic reactions at the application site, nausea, headache, fatigue, orthostatic hypotension, sleepiness, and impulse control disorders
Pregabalin	A	600	600–1200 mg PO	5.1–6	5–7.3 h	–	Somnolence and dizziness

Gabapentin enacarbil	B	75	150–450 mg PO	6	1 h	–	Unsteadiness and daytime sleepiness
Oxycodone/naloxone prolonged release	C	5/2.5	5/2.5–40/20 mg PO	4.1–17.2	1.3–5.3 h	To consider in refractory RLS	Fatigue, constipation, nausea, headache, hyperhidrosis, somnolence, dry mouth, pruritus, and OSAS
Ferrous sulfate	C	325	325 mg PO twice daily with 100 mg vitamin C	6	4 h	–	Nausea, sickness, and constipation
Ferric carboxymaltose	A	–	1000 mg IV	7–12	15 min–1.2 h	–	Nausea and headache

Abbreviations: IV, intravenous; OSAS, obstructive sleep apnea syndrome; PO, medication administered orally; $T_{1/2}$, elimination half-life; T_{max}, time to maximum plasma concentration.

being studied, such as AMPA-type glutamate receptor antagonists. One class IV study showed that perampanel (a selective noncompetitive AMPA-type glutamate receptor antagonist) administered 2 to 4 mg orally daily significantly improves IRLS scores after 2 months (longer follow-up is currently investigated by the same study group) and decreases PLMI and the periodic limb movement arousal index.[21]

Opioids

In one class II study, prolonged-release oxycodone/naloxone improved, for example, IRLS scores compared with placebo after 12 weeks (level C).[2] One class III crossover study showed that oxyco-done improved RLS symptoms and PLMI compared with placebo (level C).[2] There is insufficient evidence (level U) for both methadone (one class III and one class IV study), tramadol (one class IV study), and intrathecal morphine (one class IV study).[2] There was also insufficient evidence (level U) for dihydrocodeine, propoxyphene, and tilidine (two class IV studies).[2] Two studies have reported augmentation after RLS treatment with tramadol, whereas it has not been reported with other opioids.[22,23] One prospective class IV study shows a stable effect and dose of low-dose opioids (eg, methadone and oxycodon) after 1 year (level U).[24]

Iron

One class II study found that oral iron as ferrous sulfate 325 mg combined with vitamin C 100 mg twice a day was effective for treating RLS in patients with a serum ferritin level of less than or equal to 75 μg/L (level C).[25] Two class I studies found that ferric carboxymaltose 1000 mg is effective for the treatment of moderate-to-severe RLS in patients with a serum ferritin level less than 300 μg/L and a transferrin saturation of less than 45% (level A).[25] One class I study using ferric carboxymaltose 500 mg found no significant effect on RLS symptoms (level B).[26] One class I study using iron sucrose 200 mg and 1 class II study using iron sucrose 500 mg found no effect on RLS symptoms or PLMI (level B).[25] Expert consensus considered iron sucrose to be effective for the treatment of RLS but less so than ferric carboxymaltose or low-molecular-weight iron dextran.[25] There is insufficient evidence for the efficacy of low-molecular-weight iron dextran for the treatment of RLS (two class IV studies, level U).[25] Expert consensus, however, points to the substantial clinical experience that shows it to be effective. There is insufficient evidence for the efficacy of iron gluconate (one class IV study, level U).[25] No studies were available to evaluate the efficacy of ferumoxytol or isomaltoside for the treatment of RLS. Expert consensus was that 1000 mg of these formulations given intravenously as a single dose or as two divided doses is possibly effective for RLS.[25] In a class III study, oral iron 150 mg was compared with bupropion 300 mg and ropinirole 0.25 to 0.5 mg. IRLS score reduction was seen in all groups, but most in the ropinirole group.[27]

Other Medications

There is insufficient evidence (level U) for the use of clonidine (one class III study),[2] selenium (one class III study and one class IV study),[2,28] botulinum toxin A (one class III study),[2] oxcarbazepine (one class IV study),[29] carbamazepine (one class III study),[2] valproic acid (one class III study),[2] levetiracetam (one class IV study),[30] and clonazepam (two contradictory class III studies and one class IV study comparing effects with nortriptyline).[2,31]

Valerian (one class II study) is possibly ineffective (level C).[2] Since the 2016 AAN guideline, a new class III study has supported bupropion efficacy, because it improved RLS symptoms significantly at 6 weeks compared with baseline. A group of 30 patients treated with 300 mg of bupropion (initial 5 days with a 150 mg dose) was also compared with 30 patients treated with ropinirole (0.25–0.5 mg), but there was no placebo group.[27] A lower than recommended ropinirole dose was used in this study and it is unclear how randomization, blinding, and allocation concealment were performed. Therefore, this class III study should be viewed as a noninferiority study assuming ropinirole as the standard treatment, and bupropion was inferior to ropinirole. Based on this class III study and a class II study included in the AAN guideline, bupropion is possibly ineffective (level C).[2,27] Dipyridamole has recently emerged as a possible new treatment option and is possibly effective (level B) based on one Class IV open-label non-placebo-controlled clinical trial of 15 patients followed for 2 months and one double-blind placebo-controlled cross-over Class I study.[32,33] In the latter study, the authors showed in 28 patients with primary RLS an IRLS score improvement (mean $\pm$ standard deviation) of 24.1 $\pm$ 3.1 at baseline to 11.1 $\pm$ 2.3 after 2 weeks, compared with 23.7 $\pm$ 3.4 to 18.7 $\pm$ 3.2 under placebo ($P<.001$).[32] Dipyridamole was not added to **Table 1** because of the short follow-up time of the study, despite the level C evidence.

Augmentation

A well-known side effect of levodopa and dopamine agonist is augmentation. Augmentation is

Box 2
International Restless Legs Syndrome Study Group Task Force screening questions for augmentations in the clinical setting

1. Do restless legs syndrome (RLS) symptoms appear earlier than when the drug was first started?
2. Are higher doses of the drug now needed, or do you need to take the medicine earlier, to control the RLS symptoms, compared with the original effective dose?
3. Has the intensity of symptoms worsened since starting the medication?
4. Have symptoms spread to other parts of the body (eg, arms) since starting the medication?

From Garcia-Borreguero D, Silber MH, Winkelman JW, et al. Guidelines for the first-line treatment of restless legs syndrome/Willis-Ekbom disease, prevention and treatment of dopaminergic augmentation: a combined task force of the IRLSSG, EURLSSG, and the RLS-foundation. Sleep Med 2016;21:4; with permission.

characterized by an advance of the RLS symptoms compared with the onset time before starting the medication, a shorter latency of symptoms at rest, a spread of symptoms to other parts of the body, or a greater intensity of the symptoms. Another key symptom of augmentation is the paradoxic effect on RLS symptoms after changing the dose: dose increase causes symptom worsening, and dose reduction improvement. The time of onset of the paradoxic effect after dose change is considered, by expert opinion, drug dependent: several days after change of levodopa and weeks to months after change of the longer-acting dopamine agonists. These characteristics were outlined by the Max Planck Institute (MPI) diagnostic criteria in 2007.[34] Because the MPI definition criteria have shown some shortcomings in the everyday clinical setting, the International RLS Task Force has established consensus-based recommendations for screening for augmentation in the clinical setting to facilitate the identification of augmentation (**Box 2**).[35]

Augmentation is seen in all dopaminergic drugs but is most prevalent in levodopa (up to 73%) and less in dopamine agonists. Prevalence rates for

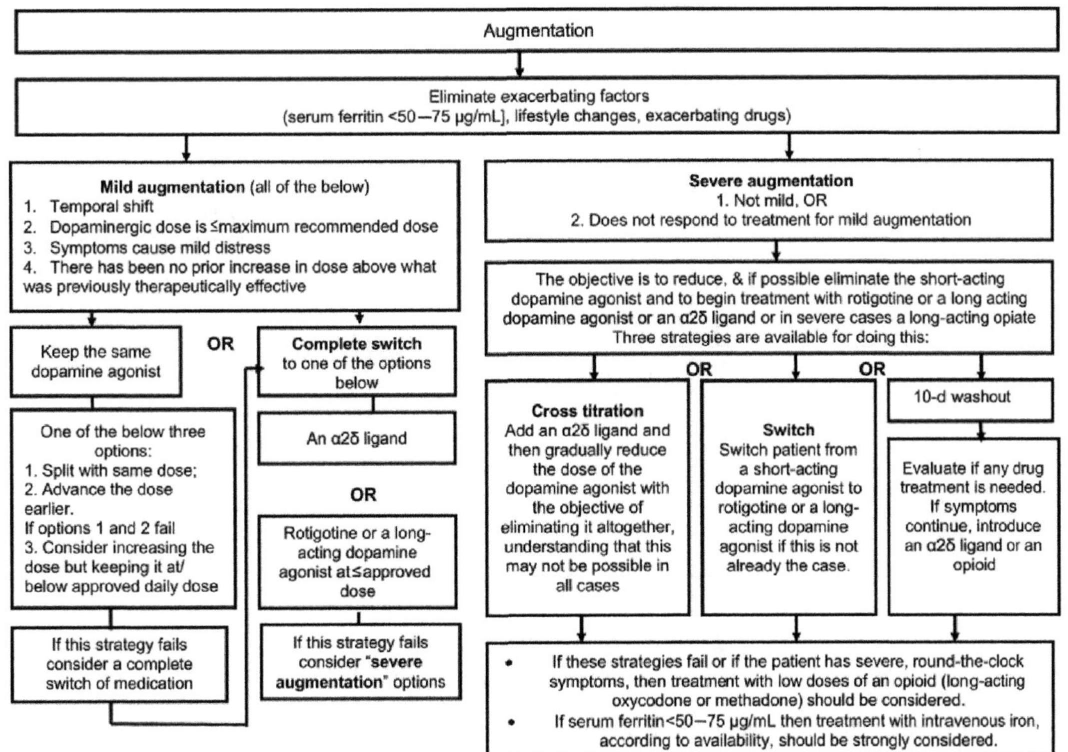

Fig. 1. Augmentation treatment algorithm. (© 2015 by the International Restless Legs Syndrome Study Group (IRLSSG). All rights reserved.)

dopamine agonist-related augmentation vary from less than 10% in the short term to 42% to 68% after approximately 10 years of treatment.[35] Approximately 76% of all patients treated with dopaminergic agents showed indications for partial or full augmentation, with a yearly incidence rate of approximately 8%.[36] The prevalence of augmentation seems to be lower in the longer-acting dopamine agonists (rotigotine and cabergo-line) compared with the short-acting dopamine agonists (ropinirole and pramipexole). Other possible risk factors for the development of augmentation are low ferritin levels, having more frequent and more severe RLS symptoms pretreatment, greater discomfort with RLS symptoms before treatment, comorbid asthma, older age, longer treatment duration, development of tolerance on dopaminergic medication, positive family history of RLS, fewer out-patient clinic visits, and lack of any neuropathy. Polysomnographic analysis does not seem useful to identify augmentation and immobilization tests might be promising.[35]

It is important to rule out augmentation mimics before diagnosing augmentation, such as the natural waxing and waning course of RLS. Other causes of RLS progression to distinguish from augmentation are iron deficiency, poor RLS medication adherence, lifestyle changes (eg, more immobile), use of RLS exacerbating medications (eg, antihistamines, selective serotonin reuptake inhibitors), and other physiologic or comorbid conditions (eg, pregnancy and renal failure). In addition, tolerance and end-of-dose exacerbation must be distinguished from augmentation, although tolerance is likely to precede augmentation and could therefore be recognized as a possible indicator to develop augmentation in the further course of the treatment. Several consensus-based measures are suggested to prevent and treat augmentation (**Fig. 1**).[35]

Nonpharmacologic Treatment Options

Evidence level B was found for the effectiveness of pneumatic compression (one class I and one class IV study)[2,37] and near-infrared light spectroscopy (NIRS) (two class II studies and one new class IV study).[2,38] Transcranial direct current stimulation (one class I study)[2] is probably ineffective (level B). Repetitive transcranial magnetic stimulation is possibly effective based on one class II study and two new class IV studies (level C).[2,39,40] Vibratory treatment is possibly ineffective in treating RLS symptoms according to two class II studies and one class IV study,[2,41] despite one recent

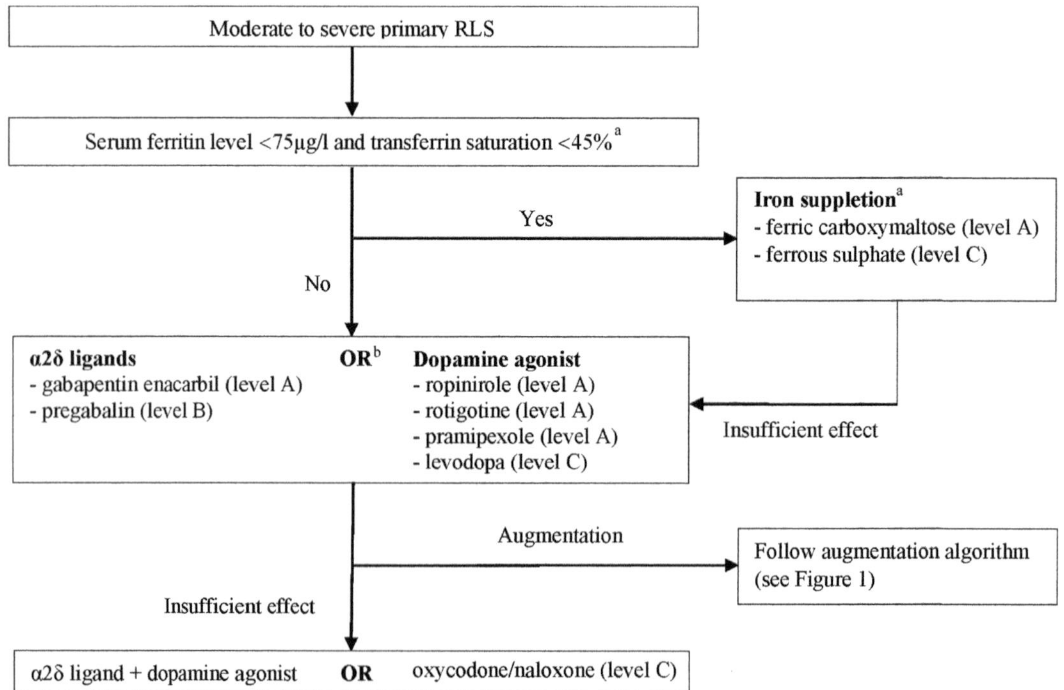

Fig. 2. Pharmacologic treatment algorithm in primary RLS. [a]Consider intravenous iron when serum ferritin level is less than 100 μg/L and transferrin saturation less than 45%.[b] The choice for an α2δ ligand or dopamine agonist may be based on considerations regarding patient characteristics (see **Table 1**), comorbidities, and the risk of augmentation with dopaminergic treatment.

class III study[42] which shows a positive effect (level C). Yoga (two Class III study)[43,44] and exercise (two Class III studies)[45,46] are possibly effective (level C). There is insufficient evidence (level U) for an effect on RLS symptoms of sleep hygiene improvement, use of caffeine, alcohol, tobacco or cannabis, mental activity, massage, hot baths (one class III study),[42] vitamin D (1 class III and 1 class IV study)[47,48] or other vitamins, aerobics/lower body training (one class III study),[46] straight leg traction (one class IV study),[49] whole-body vibration (one class III study),[50] transcutaneous spinal direct current stimulation (one class III study),[51] posterior tibial nerve stimulation (one class IV study),[52] enhanced external counterpulsation (one class IV study),[53] and cognitive behavior therapy (one class IV study).[54]

SUMMARY

For nonpharmacologic treatment options, there is some evidence for the effectiveness of pneumatic compression, NIRS, and possibly transcranial magnetic stimulation. For all other nonpharmacologic treatment options, including lifestyle changes, there is insufficient evidence.

In moderate-to-severe primary RLS, pharmacologic treatment can be considered (**Fig. 2**).[2] The first step of pharmacologic treatment is iron suppletion if applicable. Dopamine agonists and $\alpha 2\delta$ ligands are both effective for the treatment of RLS.[2] Considering the risk of augmentation with dopaminergic treatment, clinical consensus,[2,20] and recent findings of reduced effect of gabapentin enacarbil after dopaminergic treatment,[19] an $\alpha 2\delta$ ligand may be preferred to a dopamine agonist as first-line treatment.[2] The choice of treatment may also depend on comorbidity, although recommendations are mainly based on clinical consensus.[20] In patients with comorbid insomnia, painful RLS, comorbid pain syndrome, history of impulse control disorder, and comorbid anxiety, an $\alpha 2\delta$ ligand can be preferred, whereas in patients with excessive weight or comorbid depression, a dopamine agonist can be the preferred drug.[20] When prescribing dopaminergic drugs, a low dose or longer-acting version may reduce the risk of augmentation. Rotigotine could also be preferred for patients with round-the-clock symptoms or in case of swallowing difficulties. Levodopa can be considered only in patients who need occasional treatment during periods of prolonged forced immobilization or with intermittent or sporadic RLS. When single-drug therapy is insufficient, a combination of an $\alpha 2\delta$ ligand and a dopamine agonist may be considered, based on clinical consensus. In otherwise refractory primary RLS, oxycodone/naloxone may be considered.[2] If augmentation has already occurred, there are several consensus-based strategies to address (see **Fig. 1**).[35]

ACKNOWLEDGMENTS

The authors thank T. Vissers and A. van der Velden for their support with the PubMed search strategy.

DISCLOSURE

The authors declare that they have no conflict of interest. This research received no specific grant from any funding agency in the public, commercial, or not-for-profit sectors.

REFERENCES

1. Garcia-Borreguero D, Cano-Pumarega I. New concepts in the management of restless legs syndrome. BMJ (Clinical research ed.) 2017;356:j104.
2. Winkelman JW, et al. Practice guideline summary: treatment of restless legs syndrome in adults. Neurology 2016;87:2585–93.
3. Garcia-Borreguero D, Benitez A, Kohnen R, et al. Augmentation of restless leg syndrome (Willis-Ekbom disease) during long-term dopaminergic treatment. Postgrad Med 2015;127:716–25.
4. Inoue Y, et al. Long-term open-label study of pramipexole in patients with primary restless legs syndrome. J Neurol Sci 2010;294:62–6.
5. Partinen M, et al. Open-label study of the long-term efficacy and safety of pramipexole in patients with Restless Legs Syndrome (extension of the PRELUDE study). Sleep Med 2008;9:537–41.
6. Bassetti CL, et al. Pramipexole versus dual release levodopa in restless legs syndrome: a double blind, randomised, cross-over trial. Swiss Med Wkly 2011;141:w13274.
7. Kvernmo T, Härtter S, Burger E. A review of the receptor-binding and pharmacokinetic properties of dopamine agonists. Clin Ther 2006;28:1065–78.
8. Boroojerdi B, Wolff H-M, Braun M, et al. Rotigotine transdermal patch for the treatment of Parkinson's disease and restless legs syndrome. Drugs Today (Barc) 2010;46:483–505.
9. Elshoff J-P, Braun M, Andreas J-O, et al. Steady-state plasma concentration profile of transdermal rotigotine: an integrated analysis of three, open-label, randomized, Phase I Multiple dose studies* *results of study SP630 were partially presented at the 58th Annual Meeting of the American Academ. Clin Ther 2012;34:966–78.
10. Benitez A, Edens H, Fishman J, et al. Rotigotine transdermal system: developing continuous dopaminergic delivery to treat Parkinson's disease and

restless legs syndrome. Ann N Y Acad Sci 2014; 1329:45–66.
11. Högl B, Oertel WH, Schollmayer E, et al. Transdermal rotigotine for the perioperative management of restless legs syndrome. BMC Neurol 2012;12:106.
12. Garcia-Borreguero D, et al. Effects of rotigotine on daytime symptoms in patients with primary restless legs syndrome: a randomized, placebo-controlled study. Curr Med Res Opin 2016;32:77–85.
13. Oertel WH, et al. One year open-label safety and efficacy trial with rotigotine transdermal patch in moderate to severe idiopathic restless legs syndrome. Sleep Med 2008;9:865–73.
14. Oertel W, et al. Long-term safety and efficacy of rotigotine transdermal patch for moderate-to-severe idiopathic restless legs syndrome: a 5-year open-label extension study. Lancet Neurol 2011;10:710–20.
15. Högl B, et al. Treatment of moderate to severe restless legs syndrome: 2-year safety and efficacy of rotigotine transdermal patch. BMC Neurol 2010; 10:86.
16. Evidente VG. Piribedil for restless legs syndrome: a pilot study. Movement Disord 2001;16:579–81.
17. Aurora RN, et al. The treatment of restless legs syndrome and periodic limb movement disorder in adults–an update for 2012: practice parameters with an evidence-based systematic review and meta-analyses: an American Academy of Sleep Medicine Clinical Practice Guideline. Sleep 2012; 35:1039–62.
18. Garcia-Borreguero D, et al. European guidelines on management of restless legs syndrome: report of a joint task force by the European Federation of Neurological Societies, the European Neurological Society and the European Sleep Research Society. Eur J Neurol 2012;19:1385–96.
19. Garcia-Borreguero D, et al. Reduced response to gabapentin enacarbil in restless legs syndrome following long-term dopaminergic treatment. Sleep Med 2019;55:74–80.
20. Garcia-Borreguero D, et al. The long-term treatment of restless legs syndrome/Willis–Ekbom disease: evidence-based guidelines and clinical consensus best practice guidance: a report from the International Restless Legs Syndrome Study Group. Sleep Med 2013;14:675–84.
21. Garcia-Borreguero D, Cano I, Granizo JJ. Treatment of restless legs syndrome with the selective AMPA receptor antagonist perampanel. Sleep Med 2017; 34:105–8.
22. Vetrugno R, et al. Augmentation of restless legs syndrome with long-term tramadol treatment. Movement Disord 2007;22:424–7.
23. Earley CJ, Allen RP. Restless legs syndrome augmentation associated with tramadol. Sleep Med 2006;7:592–3.
24. Winkelman JW, Purks J, Wipper B. Baseline and 1-year longitudinal data from the National restless legs syndrome opioid Registry. Sleep 2021;44.
25. Allen RP, et al. Evidence-based and consensus clinical practice guidelines for the iron treatment of restless legs syndrome/Willis-Ekbom disease in adults and children: an IRLSSG task force report. Sleep Med 2018;41:27–44.
26. Cho YW, Allen RP, Earley CJ. Efficacy of ferric carboxymaltose (FCM) 500 mg dose for the treatment of Restless Legs Syndrome. Sleep Med 2018;42: 7–12.
27. Vishwakarma K, Kalra J, Gupta R, et al. A double-blind, randomized, controlled trial to compare the efficacy and tolerability of fixed doses of ropinirole, bupropion, and iron in treatment of restless legs syndrome (Willis-Ekbom disease). Ann Indian Acad Neurol 2016;19:472–7.
28. Ulfberg J, Stehlik R, Mitchell U. Treatment of restless legs syndrome/Willis-Ekbom disease with selenium. Iranian J Neurol 2016;15:235–6.
29. Jimenez-Trevino L. Oxcarbazepine treatment of restless legs syndrome: three case reports. Clin neuropharmacology 2009;32:169–70.
30. della Marca G, et al. Levetiracetam can be effective in the treatment of restless legs syndrome with periodic limb movements in sleep: report of two cases. J Neurol Neurosurg Psychiatry 2006;77. 566 LP – 567.
31. Roshi, Tandon VR, Mahajan A, et al. Comparative efficacy and safety of clonazepam versus nortriptyline in restless leg syndrome among forty Plus women: a prospective, open-label randomized study. J midlife Health 2019;10:197–203.
32. Garcia-Borreguero D, Garcia-Malo C, Granizo JJ, et al. A randomized, placebo-controlled crossover study with dipyridamole for restless legs syndrome. Movement Disord 2021;36:2387–92.
33. Garcia-Borreguero D, et al. Treatment of restless legs syndrome/Willis-Ekbom disease with the non-selective ENT1/ENT2 inhibitor dipyridamole: testing the adenosine hypothesis. Sleep Med 2018;45:94–7.
34. García-Borreguero D, et al. Diagnostic standards for dopaminergic augmentation of restless legs syndrome: report from a World association of sleep medicine – international restless legs syndrome study group consensus Conference at the Max Planck Institute. Sleep Med 2007;8:520–30.
35. Garcia-Borreguero D, et al. Guidelines for the first-line treatment of restless legs syndrome/Willis–Ekbom disease, prevention and treatment of dopaminergic augmentation: a combined task force of the IRLSSG, EURLSSG, and the RLS-foundation. Sleep Med 2016;21:1–11.
36. Allen RP, et al. Restless legs syndrome (RLS) augmentation associated with dopamine agonist

and levodopa usage in a community sample. Sleep Med 2011;12:431–9.
37. Eliasson AH, Lettieri CJ. Sequential compression devices for treatment of restless legs syndrome. Medicine 2007;86:317–23.
38. Guffey JS, et al. Using near infrared light to manage symptoms associated with restless legs syndrome. Physiother Theor Pract 2016;32:34–44.
39. Liu C, et al. Mapping intrinsic functional brain changes and repetitive transcranial magnetic stimulation neuromodulation in idiopathic restless legs syndrome: a resting-state functional magnetic resonance imaging study. Sleep Med 2015;16:785–91.
40. Lin Y-C, et al. Repetitive transcranial magnetic stimulation for the treatment of restless legs syndrome. Chin Med J 2015;128.
41. Montagna P, de Bianchi LS, Zucconi M, et al. Clonazepam and vibration in restless legs syndrome. Acta Neurol Scand 1984;69:428–30.
42. Park A, Ambrogi K, Hade EM. Randomized pilot trial for the efficacy of the MMF07 foot massager and heat therapy for restless legs syndrome. PLoS One 2020;15:e0230951.
43. Innes KE, et al. Effects of a 12-week yoga versus a 12-week educational film intervention on symptoms of restless legs syndrome and related outcomes: an exploratory randomized controlled trial. J Clin Sleep Med 2020;16:107–19.
44. Innes KE, Selfe TK, Agarwal P, et al. Efficacy of an Eight-week yoga intervention on symptoms of restless legs syndrome (RLS): a pilot study. J Altern Complement Med 2012;19:527–35.
45. Harrison EG, Keating JL, Morgan P. Novel exercises for restless legs syndrome: a randomized, controlled trial. J Am Board Fam Med 2018;31:783–94.
46. Aukerman MM, et al. Exercise and restless legs syndrome: a randomized controlled trial. J Am Board Fam Med 2006;19:487–93.
47. Wali SO, Abaalkhail B, Alhejaili F, et al. Efficacy of vitamin D replacement therapy in restless legs syndrome: a randomized control trial. Sleep Breath 2019;23:595–601.
48. Tutuncu M, Tutuncu M. The effect of vitamin D on restless legs syndrome: prospective self-controlled case study. Sleep Breath 2020;24:1101–6.
49. Dinkins EM, Stevens-Lapsley J. Management of symptoms of Restless Legs Syndrome with use of a traction straight leg raise: a preliminary case series. Man Ther 2013;18:299–302.
50. Mitchell UH, Hilton SC, Erik H, et al. Decreased symptoms without augmented skin blood flow in subjects with RLS/WED after vibration treatment. J Clin Sleep Med 2021;12:947–52.
51. Heide AC, et al. Effects of transcutaneous spinal direct current stimulation in idiopathic restless legs patients. Brain Stimulation 2014;7:636–42.
52. D Rozeman A, Ottolini T, Grootendorst DC, et al. Effect of sensory stimuli on restless legs syndrome: a randomized crossover study. J Clin Sleep Med 2021;10:893–6.
53. Rajaram S-S, Rudzinskiy P, Walters AS. Enhanced external counter pulsation (EECP) for restless legs syndrome (RLS): preliminary negative results in a parallel double-blind study. Sleep Med 2006;7:390–1.
54. Hornyak M, et al. Cognitive behavioural group therapy to improve patients' strategies for coping with restless legs syndrome: a proof-of-concept trial. J Neurol Neurosurg Psychiatry 2008;79:823–5.

Drugs Used in Circadian Sleep-Wake Rhythm Disturbances

Helen J. Burgess, PhD[a,*], Jonathan S. Emens, MD[b,c]

KEYWORDS

• Advance • Agonist • Circadian • Delay • Melatonin • Shift • Sleep

KEY POINTS

- Exogenous melatonin and other melatonin receptor agonists can be used to shift circadian timing and improve sleep in patients with sleep and circadian disturbances.
- Each medication varies in its circadian resetting and sleep-enhancing properties and safety concerns.
- The latest exogenous melatonin treatment recommendations for circadian rhythm sleep-wake disorders are reviewed.

INTRODUCTION

This article focuses on the use of melatonin and other melatonin receptor agonists as chronobiotics, that is, drugs that shift the central circadian timing (ie, reset the 24-hour biological clock) and that also have the potential to improve sleep. The article aims to provide a relevant update from a recent review of melatonin and other melatonin receptor agonists[1] and highlights the practical use of these drugs. The authors recognize that other drugs have the potential to act as chronobiotics and that different medications, including hypnotics and alerting medications, may have the potential for treating circadian rhythm sleep-wake disorders, but these are not addressed here because they remain to be tested in clinical trials examining circadian rhythm sleep-wake disorders.

This article provides a brief review of the circadian system and circadian rhythm sleep-wake disorders, followed by a summary of the relevant agents available and the safety concerns surrounding their use. The circadian phase shifting and sleep-enhancing properties of these particular chronobiotics are reviewed, along with the latest American Academy of Sleep Medicine (AASM) clinical practice guidelines regarding the use of exogenous melatonin for treating intrinsic circadian rhythm disorders.[2] The article concludes with a discussion of the use of these medications in clinical practice.

THE CIRCADIAN SYSTEM AND CIRCADIAN RHYTHM SLEEP-WAKE DISORDERS

The circadian system orchestrates the near-24-hour endogenous rhythms seen in a wide variety of physiologic variables. The molecular "gears" of the clock exist in most organ systems, and these disparate clocks are internally synchronized by a central pacemaker in the suprachiasmatic nuclei (SCN) of the hypothalamus, which is itself

Sleep Med Clin 13 (2018) 231-241 https://doi.org/10.1016/j.jsmc.2018.02.006. 1556-407X/18/© 2018 Elsevier Inc.

[a] Biological Rhythms Research Laboratory, Department of Behavioral Sciences, Rush University Medical Center, 1645 West Jackson Boulevard, Suite 425, Chicago, IL 60612, USA; [b] Department of Psychiatry, Oregon Health & Science University, VA Portland Health Care System, 3710 Southwest US Veterans Hospital, Road P3-PULM, Portland, OR 97239, USA; [c] Department of Medicine, Oregon Health & Science University, VA Portland Health Care System, 3710 Southwest US Veterans Hospital, Road P3-PULM, Portland, OR 97239, USA
* Corresponding author.
E-mail address: Helen_J_Burgess@rush.edu

Sleep Med Clin 17 (2022) 421–431
https://doi.org/10.1016/j.jsmc.2022.06.007
1556-407X/22/© 2022 Elsevier Inc.

synchronized (reset) by external time cues, primarily the light/dark cycle.[3] The timing of the clock (circadian phase) can be shifted to an earlier or later time (phase advances and phase delays, respectively) depending on when during the biological day or night a resetting stimulus is given. Circadian timing and sleep have a profound influence on mental and physical health (eg, see Refs.[4–7]), and circadian rhythm sleep-wake disorders result when wakefulness and sleep are scheduled in opposition to the timing of the biological clock (eg, attempting to sleep during the biological day). A key to understanding circadian rhythm sleep-wake disorders, and their treatment, is appreciating this difference between internal biological timing and external clock time.

The third edition of the International Classification of Sleep Disorders describes 6 circadian rhythm sleep-wake disorders that have been reviewed in depth previously.[2,8] These disorders include the extrinsic circadian rhythm sleep-wake disorders (jet lag disorder and shift work disorder) and also the intrinsic circadian rhythm sleep-wake disorders (delayed sleep-wake phase disorder), advanced sleep-wake phase disorder, irregular sleep-wake rhythm disorder, and non-24-hour sleep-wake rhythm disorder (non-24). Their primary features and possible causes are summarized in **Table 1**.

MELATONIN AND OTHER MELATONIN RECEPTOR AGONISTS

The circadian resetting effects of melatonin are well documented,[9–12] and both receptor subtypes have been shown to contribute to this effect.[13,14] Melatonin is available without a prescription in the United States both alone and in combination with other supplements, and in multiple formulations. It is estimated that 2% of US adults use exogenous melatonin, most commonly to improve sleep.[15,16] There are also melatonin formulations and other melatonin receptor agonists available via prescription in various countries, including circadin, tasimelteon, ramelteon, and agomelatine, which are summarized in **Table 2**.

TREATMENT SAFETY CONSIDERATIONS

Side effects are infrequent with exogenous melatonin, with the exception of sleepiness, but the side effects discussed in several meta-analyses are listed in **Table 2**. Because of the sleepiness side effect, patients should not drive or operate machinery after ingesting melatonin, and should test their individual response to particular doses and formulations in safe environments.

Bioavailability of melatonin can vary (eg, 1%–37%).[17] Meta-analyses have reported potential for melatonin to adversely affect people with epilepsy,[18] and for melatonin to interact with warfarin and potentially other oral anticoagulants.[18] There have also been concerns about the potential effects of melatonin on development in children,[19] and so caution is advised in the administration of melatonin to prepubertal children unless the demonstrated benefits outweigh the potential risks (eg, in children with significant developmental delay or children with non-24-hour sleep-wake schedule disorder). It is also generally recommended that women who are pregnant, trying to get pregnant, or breastfeeding do not take exogenous melatonin.[20] Exogenous melatonin (5 mg) has been found to acutely impair glucose tolerance when administered with food,[21] and further research on the effects of exogenous melatonin on glucose metabolism, and on which patients might be vulnerable to these effects,[22] is warranted. In general, large-scale randomized controlled trials are needed to evaluate the long-term safety of melatonin in children and adults.[20] Other prescription-based melatonin receptor agonists also carry their own potential side effect profiles, which are summarized in **Table 2**.

USING MELATONIN AND OTHER MELATONIN RECEPTOR AGONISTS TO SHIFT CIRCADIAN TIMING

As described in detail in our previous review,[1] both the dose and timing of exogenous melatonin administration need to be considered when attempting to reset the biological clock. The timing of melatonin administration simultaneously determines the direction and magnitude of the resulting circadian phase shift. Melatonin phase response curves (PRCs; eg, see Refs.[11,12]) are plots of average data that are similar to dose response curves, but instead of describing the effect of a drug at different doses, they describe the effect of a drug administered at different biological times. Biological timing can be determined by measuring a convenient marker of the biological clock, such as the onset of endogenous melatonin secretion assayed in plasma or saliva samples collected under dim light conditions (the dim light melatonin onset).[23–25] These PRCs indicate that exogenous melatonin typically causes phase advances when administered in the late biological afternoon and early evening (peaking about 5–7 hours before habitual bedtime), phase delays when administered late in the biological night and early morning (peaking around habitual wake time), and shifts from causing phase advances to phase delays in

Table 1
***International Classification of Sleep Disorders, Third Edition*, classification of circadian rhythm sleep-wake disorders**

Disorder	Jet Lag Disorder	Shift Work Disorder	Delayed Sleep-Wake Phase Disorder	Advanced Sleep-Wake Phase Disorder	Irregular Sleep-Wake Rhythm Disorder	Non-24-h Sleep-Wake Rhythm Disorder
Primary features	Insomnia and/or hypersomnolence with decreased total sleep time associated with transmeridian travel across ≥2 time zones	Insomnia and/or hypersomnolence with decreased total sleep time associated with work times during habitual sleep times	Sleep-wake timing is shifted ≥2 h later, sleep onset insomnia, morning somnolence, and an absence of difficulty when sleep timing is delayed	Sleep-wake timing is shifted ≥2 h earlier, evening somnolence, early morning insomnia, and an absence of difficulty when sleep timing is advanced	Irregular sleep/wake schedule with insomnia during scheduled sleep and somnolence during scheduled wake times	Sleep/wake timing that drifts progressively later (or earlier) across the 24-h d. In the blind: relapsing/remitting insomnia and somnolence while keeping a consistent sleep/wake schedule
Cause	Scheduling of sleep and wakefulness during the biological day and night, respectively, as a result of rapid transmeridian travel	Scheduling of work during the biological night with corresponding scheduling of sleep during the biological day	Altered circadian resetting (increased response to delaying evening light or decreased response to advancing morning light), altered exposure to resetting agents (eg, increased evening light exposure), and/or a long biological day (long circadian period)	Altered circadian resetting (increased response to advancing morning light or decreased response to delaying evening light), altered exposure to resetting agents (eg, increased morning light exposure), and/or a short biological day (short circadian period)	Seen in individuals with neurodegenerative or neurodevelopmental disorders	In the blind: a lack of light input to the circadian pacemaker. In the sighted: possible self-selected light/dark schedule in conjunction with factors seen in delayed sleep-wake phase disorder

Data from American Academy of Sleep Medicine. Classification of circadian rhythm sleep-wake disorders. In: International Classification of Sleep Disorders. 3rd ed. Darien, IL; 2014:191-224.

Table 2
A summary of the circadian, sleep, and possible side effects of melatonin and other melatonin receptor agonists

Drug	Approved for	Mechanism of Action	Circadian Phase Shifting Effects	Sleep Effects	Possible Side Effects
Melatonin	Available over the counter in the United States, via prescription in most other countries	MT1 and MT2 receptor agonist	Can phase advance and phase delay[11,12]	Decreases latency to sleep onset[32–34]; may increase total sleep time and sleep quality.[33] Effects may be larger when endogenous melatonin levels are low[36]	Sleepiness, dizziness, headache, blood pressure changes, gastrointestinal upset[18,20,32]
Circadin	Insomnia in adults ≥55 y old	MT1 and MT2 receptor agonist	Not clear as a prolonged-release melatonin formulation	Decreases latency to sleep onset, improves sleep quality[54]	Similar to exogenous melatonin[55]
Tasimelteon	Non-24-h sleep-wake rhythm disorder	MT1 and MT2 receptor agonist	Can phase advance[56,57]	Decreases latency to sleep onset; increases sleep efficiency when administered to enhance sleep 5 h before habitual bedtime[57]	Headache, increased liver enzyme levels, cardiac conduction changes, upper respiratory and urinary tract infections, nightmares[58]
Ramelteon	Insomnia in adults	MT1 and MT2 receptor agonist	Can phase advance[59]	Decreases latency to sleep onset; increases total sleep time, sleep efficiency, sleep quality[60]	Sleepiness, dizziness, headache, gastrointestinal upset, upper respiratory tract infections, dysmenorrhea[60]
Agomelatine	Depression	MT1 and MT2 receptor agonist, serotonin 5-HT2c receptor antagonist	Can phase advance[61,62]	Decreases latency to sleep onset in patients with major depressive disorder[63]	Liver injury[64,65]

Abbreviations: MT1, melatonin receptor 1; MT2, melatonin receptor 2.

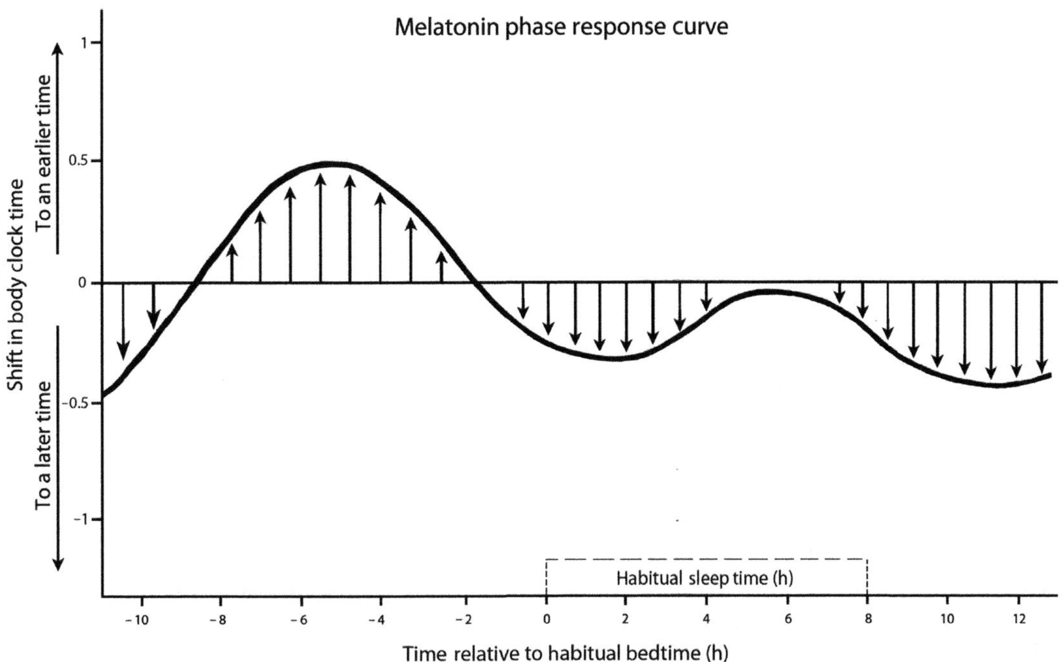

Fig. 1. A PRC rereferenced to habitual sleep timing. PRCs are usually referenced to a marker of circadian phase, but, for ease of use, the authors have rereferenced this PRC to habitual sleep timing. The melatonin PRC is adapted from a PRC generated to 3 days of a daily dose of 0.5 mg of exogenous melatonin.[12] Accordingly, we have reduced the amplitude of the melatonin PRC by a factor of 3, to better estimate the effects of a single dose. Any resulting phase shift will be a combined effect of exogenous melatonin plus concomitant light exposure.

the biological evening (**Fig. 1**). It is therefore important to point out that exogenous melatonin causes the largest phase shifts when patients are likely to be awake (assuming they are maintaining a conventional sleep/wake schedule), and so low doses that will not result in somnolence are preferred, as discussed later.

The dose of melatonin can also affect the resulting phase shift. A wide range of doses have been examined for circadian resetting,[11,12,26,27] and there is evidence that a therapeutic window exists for melatonin's chronobiotic effects: at lower doses of 0.02 to 0.30 mg, a dose response relationship has been shown,[27] whereas 0.5 and 3.0 mg doses cause similar resetting[12] and higher doses of 10 mg or more have smaller resetting effects.[26,28] This therapeutic window likely exists because increasing the dose of exogenous melatonin also increases the duration of time that circulating levels of melatonin are increased. Within the lower part of this dose range, increasing doses simply result in increased resetting effects,[27] but with higher doses more and more of the melatonin PRC is stimulated until the opposite zone begins to be stimulated and less net circadian resetting occurs. This phenomenon of exogenous melatonin "spilling over"[28] onto the opposite zone of the melatonin PRC occurs, despite a half-life of 30 to 45 minutes,[17] because even doses of 0.5 to 1.0 mg of melatonin can produce supraphysiologic levels over several hours or more.[11,29] As reviewed later, melatonin also has soporific effects, and therefore care should be taken to use the lowest dose possible when exogenous melatonin is taken during the habitual waking hours, as is often necessary for maximal circadian resetting effects.

The latest AASM clinical practice guidelines for the treatment of intrinsic circadian rhythm disorders with exogenous melatonin[2] are shown in **Table 3**. Details of the studies that formed the basis of the recommendations, including exogenous melatonin dose and timing of administration, are also summarized. Other reviews address how exogenous melatonin can be used to reduce jet lag and improve adaptation to shift work.[30,31]

USING MELATONIN AND OTHER MELATONIN RECEPTOR AGONISTS TO IMPROVE SLEEP

Melatonin is well recognized to reduce the time taken to fall asleep (sleep onset latency).[32–34]

The reports on whether melatonin can increase sleep duration and/or consolidation (eg, sleep efficiency) are mixed,[32–34] and it may not be soporific when administered during the biological night when endogenous melatonin levels are increased.[35]

Table 3
Melatonin treatment recommendations from the 2015 clinical practice guideline for treatment of intrinsic circadian rhythm sleep-wake disorders

Disorder	Number of Studies that Formed Guideline	Effective Doses and Timing Tested	Treatment Guideline
Delayed sleep-wake phase disorder	3 Adult studies 3 children studies	Adults: 0.3 mg or 3 mg fast release, 1.5–6.5 h before baseline DLMO, time pill taken advanced by 1 h after 2 wk[66] 5 mg fast release between 7 and 9 PM, treatment advanced by w 1 h after first week[67,68] Children: 0.15 mg/kg fast release 1.5–2.0 h before habitual bedtime[69] 3 or 5 mg fast release 6 or 7 PM [70,71]	Use strategically timed melatonin or other melatonin receptor agonists
Advanced sleep-wake phase disorder	No studies	NA	No recommendation
Irregular sleep-wake rhythm disorder (elderly with dementia)	1 Adult study	Null effects[72]	Do not use melatonin or other melatonin receptor agonists
Irregular sleep-wake rhythm disorder (children/adolescents with neurologic disorders)	1 Child study	2–10 mg fast release, ~30 min before planned bedtime[73]	Use strategically timed melatonin or other melatonin receptor agonists
Non-24-h sleep-wake rhythm disorder	3 Adult blind studies in patients whose circadian phase drifts later in time	10 mg 1 h before preferred bedtime[26] 0.5 mg[74] or 5 mg[75] at 9 PM	Use strategically timed melatonin or other melatonin receptor agonists

Note that a lack of recommendation does not indicate melatonin should not be used in those disorders but that the available evidence was insufficient to make a recommendation for or against treatment with melatonin and other melatonin receptor agonists.[76]

Abbreviations: DLMO, dim light melatonin onset; NA, not available.

Data from Refs.[2,48,68–76]

The soporific effects of exogenous melatonin can be larger in populations with lower levels of endogenous melatonin (eg, in hypertensive patients treated with beta-blockers[36]). Nonetheless, the sleep-enhancing effects of exogenous melatonin are usually smaller than those associated with hypnotics, and sometimes are not considered clinically meaningful.[37] The sleep-enhancing effects of melatonin may in part be mediated via binding to melatonin receptors in the periphery, which can induce thermoregulatory changes that induce sleepiness and sleep.[38] Melatonin may also reduce circadian alerting signals by binding to melatonin receptors on the SCN.[39]

PRACTICAL ASPECTS OF MELATONIN AND OTHER MELATONIN AGONIST TREATMENTS

Melatonin Preparations

The first practical consideration for clinicians is related to exogenous melatonin's classification as a dietary supplement by the US Food and Drug Administration (FDA): the purity and dose accuracy of different formulations is not necessarily assured.[40,41] In recent years, individual manufacturers have adopted improved testing procedures,[42] but ultimately clinicians may need to choose from among those formulations that have been subject to some type of outside review.[43,44] An important consideration for therapy with melatonin is the low cost (often <10 cents per pill[44]).

Melatonin Administration

As described earlier, the potential interactions between exogenous melatonin and prescription medications and/or other dietary supplements should be considered before recommending melatonin treatment. In addition, drugs metabolized by cytochrome P450 1A2 liver enzymes, including some antidepressants, caffeine, and oral contraceptives, can inadvertently increase levels of plasma melatonin after exogenous melatonin administration.[19,20] Clinicians should note that less than half of the general population are estimated to consult with their physicians about their use of supplements.[16]

Before beginning treatment, clinicians should first make sure the patient is maintaining a consistent light/dark schedule. This schedule is critical for ensuring that a correct biological time of administration is chosen and hence the desired circadian resetting effect is achieved. This schedule may also offer some benefit all on its own, because it minimizes the circadian misalignment associated with rapidly changing sleep/wake opportunities. Clinicians should be aware that exogenous melatonin, on its own, cannot overcome the resetting effect of a patient's self-selected light/dark cycle, and that it is important that the timing of melatonin and light act in concert to achieve the desired resetting effect. Evidence of this potential competition between melatonin and light can be seen in the larger resetting effects observed with exogenous melatonin administered in the laboratory (where light levels are controlled),[12] compared with administration at home.[11]

Once a patient is successfully maintaining a consistent light/dark schedule, the clinician should then administer melatonin about 5 to 6 hours before habitual bedtime to shift circadian timing to an earlier hour or at habitual wake time to shift circadian timing later. These administration times can be slowly moved an hour or less earlier or later, respectively, every few days,[45] if insomnia or somnolence symptoms have improved but sleep timing is still delayed or advanced. Just as consistent light/dark timing is critical to success, so is consistently timed administration of melatonin, and the use of alarms, such as on mobile phones, can help in this respect. In all cases, the aim is to achieve a normal and consistent relationship between the timing of sleep and the timing of the biological clock.

Non-24 in the blind is unique among the intrinsic circadian rhythm sleep-wake disorders, because the cause is clear but the treatment is more complex (for review of treatment see Ref.[46]). Non-24 arises in blind individuals because the biological clock is no longer reset by light. Most commonly, this results in circadian timing shifting ~20 minutes later every day.[47] Melatonin can arrest this drift,[26] but experiments have shown that the drift in circadian timing often does not immediately cease, and the eventual timing of the clock does not necessarily correspond with the timing of melatonin administration. As a result, clinicians should initially administer melatonin 6 hours before the desired bedtime and, as discussed earlier, slowly shift the administration time earlier or later if there are remaining symptoms that indicate a phase delay or phase advance, respectively. Less frequently, circadian timing shifts earlier each day[47] and melatonin should be administered at the desired wake time[48] (note that this is more likely to be the case in female patients[47,49]).

Melatonin and Light Combination Treatment

Apart from the case of blind patients, patients generally receive exogenous melatonin or other melatonin receptor agonists while exposed to a light-dark cycle, which is, as noted earlier, the strongest circadian resetting agent.[1] In general, light has opposite phase shifting effects to melatonin, such that evening light phase delays and morning light phase advances.[1] Consequently, when administering melatonin or other melatonin receptor agonists, phase shifting effects can be altered depending on whether the concomitant light exposure is facilitating or opposing the melatonin agonist phase shift.[50–52] Thus, in the case of sighted patients, concomitant light exposure and/or light avoidance should also be included in the treatment plan.

EVALUATION OF OUTCOME

A continued limitation in the diagnosis and treatment of circadian rhythm sleep-wake disorders is the lack of an FDA-approved test of circadian timing. Although some progress has been made in this regard[53] since our last review,[1] clinicians should still use symptom improvement to gauge treatment response. This approach is similar to the treatment of most insomnias, in which the use of sleep diaries and rating scales can be useful. Wrist actigraphy offers a more objective measure, although, in clinical practice, the authors find it is more useful in determining the consistency of rest/activity and light/dark timing (discussed earlier).

SUMMARY

This article focuses on melatonin and other melatonin receptor agonists and summarizes their circadian phase shifting and sleep-enhancing properties, along with their associated possible safety concerns. The circadian system and circadian rhythm sleep-wake disorders are described, along with the latest AASM recommendations for the use of exogenous melatonin in treating them. In addition, the practical aspects of using exogenous melatonin obtainable over the counter in the United States, consideration of the effects of concomitant light exposure, and assessing treatment response are discussed.

ACKNOWLEDGMENTS

The authors thank Muneer Rizvydeen for his assistance in creating the figure. H.J. Burgess and J.S. Emens are supported by grants from the National Center for Complementary and Integrative Health (R34AT008347), National Heart, Lung, and Blood Institute (R01HL125893 and R01HL140577), National Institute of Nursing Research (R21NR014377), and National Institute on Alcohol Abuse and Alcoholism (R01AA023839). The content is solely the responsibility of the authors and does not necessarily represent the official views of the National Institutes of Health.

DISCLOSURE

H.J. Burgess is a consultant for Natrol, LLC. J.S. Emens has nothing to disclose.

REFERENCES

1. Emens J, Burgess HJ. Effect of light and melatonin and other melatonin receptor agonists on human circadian physiology. Sleep Med Clin 2015;10:435–53.
2. Auger RR, Burgess HJ, Emens JS, et al. Clinical practice guideline for the treatment of intrinsic circadian rhythm sleep-wake disorders: advanced sleep-wake phase disorder (ASWPD), delayed sleep-wake phase disorder (DSWPD), non-24-hour sleep-wake rhythm disorder (N24SWD), and irregular sleep-wake rhythm disorder (ISWRD). An update for 2015: an American Academy of Sleep Medicine clinical practice guideline. J Clin Sleep Med 2015;11(10):1199–236.
3. Buhr ED, Takahashi JS. Molecular components of the mammalian circadian clock. Handb Exp Phar Macol 2013;217:3–27.
4. Wright KP, Hull JT, Hughes RJ, et al. Sleep and wakefulness out of phase with internal biological time impairs learning in humans. J Cogn Neurosci 2006;18(4):508–21.
5. Scheer FA, Hilton MF, Mantzoros CS, et al. Adverse metabolic and cardiovascular consequences of circadian misalignment. Proc Natl Acad Sci U S A 2009;106(11):4453–8.
6. Levandovski R, Dantas G, Fernandes LC, et al. Depression scores associate with chronotype and social jetlag in a rural population. Chronobiol Int 2011;28(9):771–8.
7. Watson NF, Badr MS, Belenky G, et al. Recommended amount of sleep for a healthy adult: a joint consensus statement of the American Academy of Sleep Medicine and Sleep Research Society. Sleep 2015;38(6):843–4.
8. Reid KJ, Burgess HJ. Circadian rhythm sleep disorders. Prim Care 2005;32:449–73.
9. Redman J, Armstrong S, Ng KT. Free-running activity rhythms in the rat: entrainment by melatonin. Sci Ence 1983;219(4588):1089–91.
10. Arendt J, Bojkowski C, Folkard S, et al. Some effects of melatonin and the control of its secretion in hu mans. In: Evered D, Clark S, editors. Photoperiodism, melatonin, and the pineal. London: Pitman; 1985. p. 266–83.
11. Lewy AJ, Bauer VK, Ahmed S, et al. The human phase response curve (PRC) to melatonin is about

12 hours out of phase with the PRC to light. Chrono Biol Int 1998;15:71–83.
12. Burgess HJ, Revell VL, Molina TA, et al. Human phase response curves to three days of daily melatonin: 0.5 mg versus 3.0 mg. J Clin Endocrinol Metab 2010;95(7):3325–31.
13. Reppert SM, Weaver DR, Godson C. Melatonin receptors step into the light: cloning and classification of subtypes. Trends Pharmacol Sci 1996;17:100–2.
14. Dubocovich ML. Melatonin receptors: role on sleep and circadian rhythm regulation. Sleep Med 2007; 8(Suppl 3):34–42.
15. National Sleep Foundation. Sleep in America Poll. 2005. Available at: https://sleepfoundation.org/sleep-polls-data/sleep-in-america-poll/2005-adult-sleep-habits-and-styles. Accessed January 2, 2018.
16. Bliwise DL, Ansari FP. Insomnia associated with valerian and melatonin usage in the 2002 National Health Interview Survey. Sleep 2007;30(7):881–4.
17. Fourtillan JB, Brisson AM, Gobin P, et al. Bioavailability of melatonin in humans after day-time administration of D(7) melatonin. Biopharm Drug Dispos 2000;21(1):15–22.
18. Herxheimer A, Petrie KJ. Melatonin for the prevention and treatment of jet lag. Cochrane Database Syst Rev 2002;2:CD001520.
19. Kennaway DJ. Potential safety issues in the use of the hormone melatonin in paediatrics. J Paediatr Child Health 2015;51(6):584–9.
20. Andersen LP, Gogenur I, Rosenberg J, et al. The safety of melatonin in humans. Clin Drug Investig 2016;36(3):169–75.
21. Rubio-Sastre P, Scheer FA, Gomez-Abellan P, et al. Acute melatonin administration in humans impairs glucose tolerance in both the morning and evening. Sleep 2014;37(10):1715–9.
22. Garaulet M, Gomez-Abellan P, Rubio-Sastre P, et al. Common type 2 diabetes risk variant in MTNR1B worsens the deleterious effect of melatonin on glucose tolerance in humans. Metabolism 2015; 64(12):1650–7.
23. Lewy AJ, Cutler NL, Sack RL. The endogenous melatonin profile as a marker of circadian phase position. J Biol Rhythms 1999;14(3):227–36.
24. Klerman EB, Gershengorn HB, Duffy JF, et al. Comparisons of the variability of three markers of the human circadian pacemaker. J Biol Rhythms 2002; 17(2):181–93.
25. Burgess HJ, Wyatt JK, Park M, et al. Home circadian phase assessments with measures of compliance yield accurate dim light melatonin onsets. Sleep 2015;38(6):889–97.
26. Sack RL, Brandes RW, Kendall AR, et al. Entrainment of free-running circadian rhythms by melatonin in blind people. N Engl J Med 2000;343(15):1070–7.
27. Lewy AJ, Emens JS, Lefler BJ, et al. Melatonin en trains free-running blind people according to a physiological dose-response curve. Chronobiol Int 2005;22(6):1093–106.
28. Lewy AJ, Emens JS, Sack RL, et al. Low, but not high, doses of melatonin entrained a free-running blind person with long circadian period. Chronobiol Int 2002;19(3):649–58.
29. Dollins AB, Zhdanova IV, Wurtman RJ, et al. Effect of inducing nocturnal serum melatonin concentrations in daytime on sleep, mood, body temperature, and performance. Proc Natl Acad Sci USA 1994;91(5): 1824–8.
30. Burgess HJ. Using bright light and melatonin to reduce jet lag. In: Perlis M, Aloia M, Kuhn B, editors. Behavioral treatments for sleep disorders: a comprehensive primer of behavioral sleep medicine treatment protocols. Burlington (New Jersey): Elsevier; 2011. p. 151–7.
31. Burgess HJ. Using bright light and melatonin to adjust to night work. In: Perlis M, Aloia M, Kuhn B, editors. Behavioral treatments for sleep disorders: a comprehensive primer of behavioral sleep medicine treatment protocols. Burlington (New Jersey): Elsevier; 2011. p. 159–65.
32. Buscemi N, Vandermeer B, Hooton N, et al. The efficacy and safety of exogenous melatonin for primary sleep disorders. A meta-analysis. J Gen Int Med 2005;20:1151–8.
33. Ferracioli-Oda E, Qawasmi A, Bloch MH. Meta-analysis: melatonin for the treatment of primary sleep disorders. PLoS One 2013;8(5):e63773.
34. Auld F, Maschauer EL, Morrison I, et al. Evidence for the efficacy of melatonin in the treatment of primary adult sleep disorders. Sleep Med Rev 2017;34:10–22.
35. Wyatt JK, Dijk DJ, Ritz-de Cecco A, et al. Sleep-facilitating effect of exogenous melatonin in healthy young men and women is circadian-phase dependent. Sleep 2006;29(5):609–18.
36. Scheer FA, Morris CJ, Garcia JI, et al. Repeated melatonin supplementation improves sleep in hypertensive patients treated with beta-blockers: a randomized controlled trial. Sleep 2012;35(10): 1395–402.
37. Sateia MJ, Buysse DJ, Krystal AD, et al. Clinical practice guideline for the pharmacologic treatment of chronic insomnia in adults: an American Academy of Sleep Medicine clinical practice guideline. J Clin Sleep Med 2017;13(2):307–49.
38. Krauchi K, Cajochen C, Pache M, et al. Thermoregulatory effects of melatonin in relation to sleepiness. Chronobiol Int 2006;23:475–84.
39. Reppert SM, Weaver DR, Rivkees SA, et al. Putative melatonin receptors in a human biological clock. Science 1988;242:78–81.
40. Erland LA, Saxena PK. Melatonin natural health products and supplements: presence of serotonin and significant variability of melatonin content. J Clin Sleep Med 2017;13(2):275–81.

41. Hahm H, Kujawa J, Augsburger L. Comparison of melatonin products against USP's nutritional supplements standards and other criteria. J Am Pharm Assoc (Wash) 1999;39(1):27–31.
42. Available at: http://well.blogs.nytimes.com/2015/03/30/gnc-to-strengthen-supplement-quality-controls. Accessed January 2, 2018.
43. Available at: http://www.usp.org/verification-services/program-participants. Accessed January 2, 2018.
44. ConsumerLab.com. Product review: melatonin supplements. Available at: http://www.consumerlab.com/results/melatonin.asp. Accessed January 2, 2018.
45. Crowley SJ, Eastman CI. Melatonin in the afternoons of a gradually advancing sleep schedule enhances the circadian rhythm phase advance. Psychopharmacol (Berl) 2013;225(4):825–37.
46. Emens JS, Eastman CI. Diagnosis and treatment of non-24-h sleep-wake disorder in the blind. Drugs 2017;77:637–50.
47. Emens JS, Laurie AL, Songer JB, et al. Non-24-hour disorder in blind individuals revisited: variability and the influence of environmental time cues. Sleep 2013;36(07):1091–100.
48. Emens J, Lewy A, Yuhas K, et al. Melatonin entrains free-running blind individuals with circadian periods less than 24 hours. Sleep 2006;29(Suppl):A62.
49. Duffy JF, Cain SW, Chang AM, et al. Sex difference in the near-24-hour intrinsic period of the human circadian timing system. Proc Natl Acad Sci USA 2011;108(Suppl 3):15602–8.
50. Revell VL, Burgess HJ, Gazda CJ, et al. Advancing human circadian rhythms with afternoon melatonin and morning intermittent bright light. J Clin Endocr Metab 2006;91:54–9.
51. Paul MA, Gray GW, Lieberman HR, et al. Phase advance with separate and combined melatonin and light treatment. Psychopharmacology (Berl) 2011;214(2):515–23.
52. Burke TM, Markwald RR, Chinoy ED, et al. Combination of light and melatonin time cues for phase advancing the human circadian clock. Sleep 2013;36(11):1617–24.
53. Burgess HJ, Park M, Wyatt JK, et al. Home dim light melatonin onsets with measures of compliance in delayed sleep phase disorder. J Sleep Res 2016;25(3):314–7.
54. Wade A, Ford I, Crawford G, et al. Efficacy of pro longed release melatonin in insomnia patients aged 55-80 years: quality of sleep and next-day alertness outcomes. Curr Med Res Opin 2007;23(10):2597–605.
55. Available at: http://www.ema.europa.eu/docs/en_GB/document_library/EPAR_-_Summary_for_the_public/human/000695/WC500026805.pdf. Accessed January 2, 2018.
56. Lockley SW, Dressman MA, Licamele L, et al. Tasimelteon for non-24-hour sleep-wake disorder in totally blind people (SET and RESET): two multicentre, randomised, double-masked, placebo-controlled phase 3 trials. Lancet 2015;386:1754–64.
57. Rajaratnam SM, Polymeropoulos MH, Fisher DM, et al. Melatonin agonist tasimelteon (VEC-162) for transient insomnia after sleep-time shift: two randomised controlled multicentre trials. Lancet 2009;373(9662):482–91.
58. Available at: https://wayback.archive-it.org/7993/20170405224953/https://www.fda.gov/downloads/AdvisoryCommittees/CommitteesMeetingMaterials/Drugs/PeripheralandCentralNervousSystemDrugsAdvisoryCommittee/UCM374388.pdf. Accessed January 2, 2018.
59. Richardson GS, Zee PC, Wang-Weigand S, et al. Circadian phase-shifting effects of repeated ramelteon administration in healthy adults. J Clin Sleep Med 2008;4(5):456–61.
60. Kuriyama A, Honda M, Hayashino Y. Ramelteon for the treatment of insomnia in adults: a systematic re view and meta-analysis. Sleep Med 2014;15(4):385–92.
61. Krauchi K, Cajochen C, Mori D, et al. Early evening melatonin and S-20098 advance circadian phase and nocturnal regulation of core body temperature. Am J Phys 1997;272:R1178–88.
62. Leproult R, Onderbergen AV, L'Hermite-Baleriaux M, et al. Phase-shifts of 24-h rhythms of hormonal release and body temperature following early evening administration of the melatonin agonist agomelatine in healthy older men. Clin Endocrinol 2005;63:298–304.
63. Quera-Salva MA, Hajak G, Philip P, et al. Comparison of agomelatine and escitalopram on nighttime sleep and daytime condition and efficacy in major depressive disorder patients. Int Clin Psychopharmacol 2011;26(5):252–62.
64. Freiesleben SD, Furczyk K. A systematic review of agomelatine-induced liver injury. J Mol Psychiatry 2015;3(1):4.
65. Taylor D, Sparshatt A, Varma S, et al. Antidepressant efficacy of agomelatine: meta-analysis of published and unpublished studies. BMJ 2014;348:gi888.
66. Mundey K, Benloucif S, Harsanyi K, et al. Phase-dependent treatment of delayed sleep phase syndrome with melatonin. Sleep 2005;28:1271–8.
67. Kayumov L, Brown G, Jindal R, et al. A randomized, double-blind, placebo-controlled crossover study of the effect of exogenous melatonin on delayed sleep phase syndrome. Psychosom Med 2001;63:40–8.
68. Rahman SA, Kayumov L, Shapiro CM. Antidepressant action of melatonin in the treatment of delayed sleep phase syndrome. Sleep Med 2010;11(2):131–6.

69. van Geijlswijk IM, van der Heijden KB, Egberts AC, et al. Dose finding of melatonin for chronic idiopathic childhood sleep onset insomnia: an RCT. Psycho-Pharmacol (Berl) 2010;212(3):379–91.
70. Smits MG, Nagtegaal EE, van der Heijden J, et al. Melatonin for chronic sleep onset insomnia in children: a randomized placebo-controlled trial. J Child Neurol 2001;16(2):86–92.
71. Van der Heijden KB, Smits MG, Van Someren EJ, et al. Effect of melatonin on sleep, behavior, and cognition in ADHD and chronic sleep-onset insomnia. J Am Acad Child Adolesc Psychiatry 2007;46(2):233–41.
72. Serfaty M, Kennell-Webb S, Warner J, et al. Double blind randomised placebo controlled trial of low dose melatonin for sleep disorders in dementia. Int J Geriatr Psychiatry 2002;17(12):1120–7.
73. Wright B, Sims D, Smart S, et al. Melatonin versus placebo in children with autism spectrum conditions and severe sleep problems not amenable to behaviour management strategies: a randomised controlled crossover trial. J Autism Dev Disord 2011;41(2):175–84.
74. Hack LM, Lockley SW, Arendt J, et al. The effects of low-dose 0.5-mg melatonin on the free-running circadian rhythms of blind subjects. J Biol Rhythms 2003;18:420–9.
75. Lockley SW, Skene DJ, James K, et al. Melatonin administration can entrain the free-running circadian system of blind subjects. J Endocrinol 2000;164: R1–6.
76. Auger RR, Burgess HJ, Emens J, et al. Do evidence-based treatments for circadian rhythm sleep-wake disorders make the GRADE? Updated guidelines point to need for more clinical research. J Clin Sleep Med 2015;11(10):1079–80.

Chronic Opioid Use and Sleep Disorders

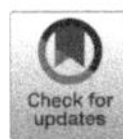

Shahrokh Javaheri, MD[a,b,*], Michelle Cao, DO[c,d]

KEYWORDS

• Opiates * poor sleep • Daytime sleepiness • Depression • Sleep-disordered breathing
• Central sleep apnea

KEY POINTS

- Chronic use of opioids has multitude negative effects on daytime function, including hypersomnolence, fatigue, depression, sleep architecture, and sleep-related breathing disorders, with resulting daytime consequences.
- Chronic opioid use is an established risk factor for sleep-disordered breathing, particularly for central sleep apnea (CSA).
- Patients on chronic opioid therapy may suffer from sleep-disordered breathing including CSA, obstructive sleep apnea (OSA), hypoventilation, all of which are not commonly unrecognized.
- For OSA, continuous positive airway pressure (CPAP) therapy is the treatment of choice; however, treatment-emergent CSA may occur when CPAP is used in patients on chronic opioids.
- New-generation servo ventilators are effective in treating both CSA and OSA; however, the algorithms are complex and require understanding and appropriate adjustments of settings for effective therapy.

INTRODUCTION

Opioid medications are considered a significant component in the multidisciplinary management of chronic pain. In the past two decades, the use of opioid medications has dramatically risen in part because of an increased awareness by health care providers to treat chronic pain more effectively. In addition, patients are encouraged to seek treatment. The release of a sentinel joint statement in 1997 by the American Academy of Pain Medicine and the American Pain Society in a national effort to increase awareness and support the treatment of chronic pain has undoubtedly contributed to the opioid crisis.[1] This effort and among others consequently led to an epidemic of opioid misuse (ie, without prescription or as directed by provider), abuse, and death related to overdose. One national large-scale survey reported that 91.8 million Americans used prescription opioids, 11.5 million misused them, and 1.9 million had opioid use disorder.[2] Cumulative data reported that increased use of opioids has resulted in increased morbidity and mortality, with more than 33,000 deaths because of opioid overdose in 2015,[3,4] with a staggering increase to approximately 70,0000 in 2020. Opioid-related deaths are most often from prescription opioid pain relievers and illicit use of synthetic compounds, including heroin and fentanyl.[4] With the support

Sleep Med Clin 13 (2018) 271-281 https://doi.org/10.1016/j.jsmc.2018.02.002. 1556-407X/18/© 2018 Elsevier Inc.

[a] Division of Pulmonary and Sleep Medicine, Bethesda North Hospital, 10535 Montgomery Road, Suite 200, Cincinnati, OH 45242, USA; [b] Division of Medicine, The Ohio State University, 181 Taylor Avenue, Columbus, OH 43203, USA; [c] Division of Pulmonary, Allergy, Critical Care Medicine, Stanford University School of Medicine, 300 Pasteur Drive, H3143, Stanford, CA 94305, USA; [d] Division of Sleep Medicine, Stanford University School of Medicine, 450 Broadway Street, Redwood City, CA 94063, USA
* Corresponding author. 10535 Montgomery Road, Suite 200, Cincinnati, OH 45242.
E-mail address: shahrokhjavaheri@icloud.com

Sleep Med Clin 17 (2022) 433–444
https://doi.org/10.1016/j.jsmc.2022.06.008
1556-407X/22/© 2022 Elsevier Inc.

of the Secretary of Health and Human Services, President Donald Trump declared the opioid crisis a national public health emergency.[4]

Opium contains alkaloids such as morphine and codeine that are ligands of the mu-opioid receptor and has been used for years for pain management. The antinociceptive effect of opioids is mediated by activation of mu-opioid receptors in the dorsal horn of the spinal cord and brainstem descending inhibitory pathways. The initial acceptance of opioid use for the relief of chronic pain more than 20 years ago is now being challenged on the efficacy and safety of these prescription practices. There is strong evidence to support the short-term use of opioids for chronic pain, but support for long-term opioid use is lacking.[3] There are no studies of opioid therapy versus placebo, or non-opioid therapy for chronic pain evaluating long-term (>1 year) outcomes related to pain, function, or quality of life. Most placebo-controlled randomized clinical trials were less than or equal to 6 weeks in duration.[5] Long-term use results in reduction or loss of analgesic efficacy because of pharmacologic tolerance or opioid-induced hyperalgesia (ie, worsening pain sensitivity). In the long run, among many other consequences, chronic use of opioids is associated with sleep dysfunction, leading to symptoms of excessive daytime sleepiness, daytime fatigue, depression, and notably, respiratory depression during sleep.

The diurnal adverse consequence of opioids, both while awake and in sleep, are well known. Daytime hypersomnolence, fatigue, depression, co-pharmacy with benzodiazepines and/or antidepressants, and consequently poor general health quality are common in chronic opioid users. There may be a bidirectional relationship between poor sleep quality, sleep-disordered breathing (SDB), and daytime function. Chronic use of opioids is associated with disrupted sleep architecture and SDB, which encompasses a spectrum of ventilatory derangements, including hypoventilation, hypoxemia, obstructive and central apneas, periodic breathing, and ataxic or irregular breathing. The authors believe that a complex relationship exists between chronic pain, chronic use of opioids, sleep disorders, and daytime symptoms (**Fig. 1**).

OPIOIDS AND DAYTIME FUNCTION

Opioids have adverse effects on sleep and daytime function—effects that could be bidirectional. These effects could be modulated by the presence of chronic pain when present. Excessive daytime sleepiness, fatigue, depression, neurocognitive dysfunction, and poor general health are common in patients using opioids chronically. On the other hand, disrupted sleep architecture and SDB are frequently observed during polysomnography, together interacting in a complex manner (see **Fig. 1**).

In an early pilot study from Australia, Teichtahl and colleagues[6] assessed the sleep and daytime function of 10 young patients (mean age 35 years) in a stable methadone maintenance program (MMP) with nine control patients matched for age, gender, and body mass index. The methadone dose ranged between 50 mg per day and 120 mg per day. All patients were assessed by a psychologist and a physician. Compared with the control group, patients in the MMP were significantly more depressed based on the Beck Depression Inventory (BDI) scale, had more daytime sleepiness based on the Epworth Sleepiness Scale (ESS) (mean score of 11 for MMP group vs 3 for control group), and, not surprisingly, had significantly lower scores on general health quality. All MMP patients smoked tobacco cigarettes and eight were admitted to regular cannabis use. Five MMP patients regularly used the benzodiazepine diazepam, with a daily dose of 20 mg to 30 mg.[6]

As discussed previously, poor sleep is common in patients on chronic opiates. Teichtahl and colleagues showed that polysomnograms on MMP patients showed significantly lower sleep efficiency, lower percentage of stage N3 and rapid eye movement (REM) sleep, and higher percentage of stage N2 sleep compared with controls. Six patients had a central apnea index (CAI) greater than five events per hour (normal <5), four had a CAI greater than 10 events per hour, and three of these showed periodic breathing patterns during sleep (**Fig. 2**). Not surprisingly, the control group did not have central sleep apnea (CSA) because it is a rare occurrence in the general population.

In a larger and more comprehensive study, the same investigators reported on 50 subjects on methadone chronically and 20 control subjects, matched for age and body mass index.[7] All subjects underwent polysomnography and blood toxicology. In addition, all subjects completed questionnaires, including the ESS, the Functional Outcome of Sleep Questionnaire (FOSQ), the BDI version 2 (BDI-II), and the Modified Mini-Mental State Examination (MMMSE). The FOSQ comprises five subscales evaluating general productivity, social outcome, activity level, vigilance, intimate relationship, and sexual activity.[8] BDI-II includes four items (agitation, worthlessness, concentration difficulty, and loss of energy) designed to assess for symptoms of depression. The MMMSE was designed to assess for

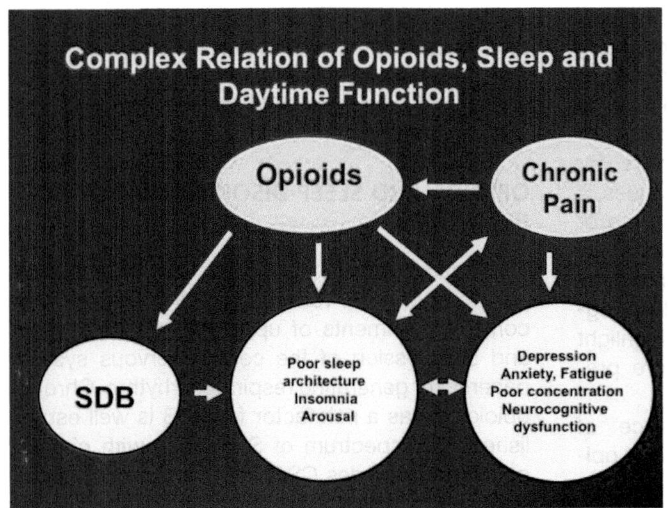

Fig. 1. Bidirectional relationship between opioids, chronic pain, and sleep.

neurocognitive impairment or organic mental disorders.[9] In this study, ESS, FOSQ, and BDI scores were significantly worse in patients on methadone compared with controls. The MMMSE showed a trend toward significance ($P = .09$).[7]

From these studies, it cannot be determined conclusively if chronic opioid use was the cause of depression. Emerging epidemiologic evidence suggests, however, that chronic use of opioids is associated with incident depression and changes in neuronal mechanisms impacting relevant neurologic pathways.[10] Similarly, patients with remitted depression seemed at increased risk of relapse after exposure to chronic opioid analgesics.[11] These findings highlight the "depressogenic" effect of opioids and the importance of a careful

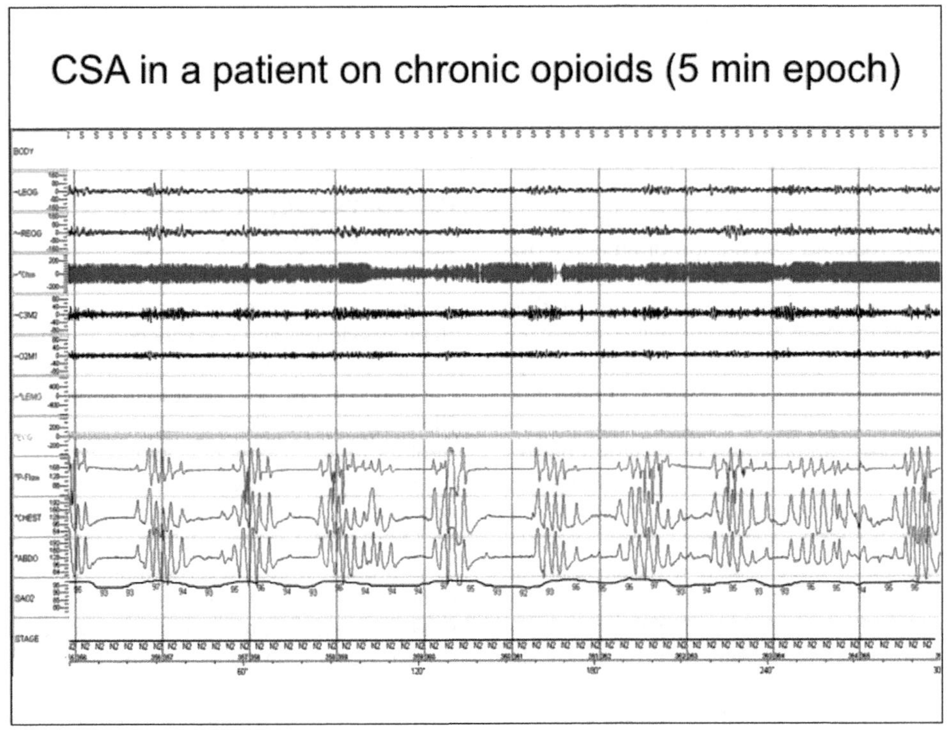

Fig. 2. An example of periodic breathing, central apneas, and ataxic breathing pattern in a patient on chronic opioids.

assessment of the past medical history of mood disturbances and depression as well as monitoring for the emergence of mood dysfunction before and during the administration of opioids. The studies suggest that higher doses of opioids[12] and chronicity[13] are potential risk factors for depression. In a study by Merrill and colleagues,[12] more than 60% of patients receiving 120 mg or higher daily equivalent of morphine were clinically depressed, a 2.6-fold higher risk (95% confidence interval, 1.5–4.4) than in patients on low-dose regimens (<20 mg daily). These data further highlight the importance of risk stratification before prescribing opioids for chronic use.

The daytime symptoms and presence of depression in association with chronic use of opioids are emphasized. In some of these studies, polysomnography was not performed, which might otherwise have discovered the presence of disrupted sleep architecture and SDB, both contributing to daytime impairment. Adverse effects of opioids on sleep and breathing are briefly reviewed.

OPIOIDS AND SLEEP

As depicted in **Fig. 1**, depression and anxiety may cause insomnia and poor sleep quantity and quality, and the latter could further contribute to a variety of daytime symptoms. Opioid use, although sedating, may interrupt sleep and impair sleep quality. To make matters more complicated, acute versus chronic opioid use (and withdrawal) have differing effects on sleep and daytime symptoms. Dimsdale and colleagues[14] evaluated the effects of one dose of sustained-release morphine versus methadone on sleep architecture in healthy subjects. The investigators reported that both drugs significantly reduced percentage of time in slow-wave sleep (stage N3) and increased percentage of time in sleep stage N2, whereas neither drug had an effect on sleep efficiency, wake after sleep onset, or total sleep time. The latter findings perhaps were not surprising because control individuals were enrolled. Xiao and colleagues[15] compared sleep architecture of healthy controls and methadone-treated patients. Patients treated with chronic methadone had lower sleep efficiency, shorter total sleep time, more arousals, and a lower percentage of slow-wave sleep (stage N3). Correspondingly, the Pittsburgh Sleep Quality Index and ESS scores were significantly higher than in control subjects. Although this study did not report a reduction in REM sleep, another study reported suppression of REM sleep with chronic opioid use.[6] Similar to SDB, the effects of opioids on sleep architecture seem dose dependent.[7,15]

The authors conclude that chronic use of opioids is associated with disturbed sleep architecture, low sleep efficiency, decreased slow-wave sleep and perhaps REM sleep, and daytime consequences.

OPIOIDS AND SLEEP-DISORDERED BREATHING

SDB associated with chronic opioid use is a complex form of sleep-related breathing disorder that combines elements of upper airway obstruction and suppression of the central nervous system pacemaker generating respiratory rhythm. Chronic opioid use as a risk factor for SDB is well established. The spectrum of SDB seen with chronic opioid use includes CSA, hypoventilation, hypoxemia, and ataxic or cluster breathing (see **Fig. 2**). Studies showed that 30% to 90% of patients on chronic opioids have some form of SDB.[16–18] A review of 560 patients with chronic opioid use reported an overall CSA prevalence of 24%.[19] A morphine equivalent daily dose of 200 mg or more was strongly associated with severity of SDB, specifically CSA.[20] A recent case-control study highlighted the risk of CSA specifically with chronic opioid therapy in combination with central nervous system active agents. In this study, the authors compared CSA prevalence in opioid users, nonopioid central nervous system active medications (CNSAM) users, combination users (opioids + nonopioid CNSAM), and controls. Opioid users had a twofold increase in CSA odds, and the combination group had a fivefold odd of CSA compared with controls, whereas the nonopioid group did not have CSA.[21]

Pathophysiology of Opioid-Induced Sleep-Disordered Breathing

Obstructive sleep apnea (OSA) and CSA induced by chronic use of opioid has been discussed in detail previously and is discussed briefly.[22] Experimental studies in neonatal rats have improved understanding of how respiration is controlled. Discovered in the 1990s, there are two distinct respiratory rhythm generators located in the ventrolateral medullary portion of the neonatal rat brainstem, the pre-Botzinger complex (pre-BotC) and the retrotrapezoid nucleus/parafacial respiratory group, which are normally coupled and generate normal respiratory rhythm.[23,24] In animal studies, the pre-BotC seems the dominant site for rhythm generation and contains the neurokinin-1 receptor (NK1R) and m-opioid receptor.[25] In neonatal rodents, stimulation with m-opioid agonists results in respiratory rate suppression.[26] Lesions in this area show apneas during sleep and an irregular breathing pattern during wakefulness and sleep.[27] A study in adult rats showed that accumulative loss of pre-BotC NK1R neurons led to progressive disturbances in sleep-related breathing initially in REM sleep, followed by Non-rapid eye movement (NREM) sleep, with greater than 80% of neuronal loss in wakefulness. The abnormal breathing events were characterized by central hypopneas and central apneas and, when most severe, they were characterized as ataxic breathing.[28] In human polysomnographic studies, however, central apneas occur primarily in non-REM sleep.

Chronic opioid use contributes to an increased incidence and severity of SDB for several reasons: enhanced relaxation of upper airway musculature, alterations in hypercapnic and hypoxic ventilatory responses, and depression of respiratory rhythm generation. During sleep, activity of the dilator muscles of the upper airway is reduced[29] and in those who are prone to airway collapse (eg, anatomically small upper airway), opioids may further decrease the activity of these muscles and increase the likelihood of upper airway obstruction. The authors postulate that opioid-induced SDB is secondary to a combined effect of upper airway obstruction and suppression of the pacemaker generating breathing rhythm. There are no human studies on the pathophysiology of opioid-induced SDB.

Although large, randomized studies have not been conducted, available data show that opioid-induced SDB may not respond to conventional positive airway pressure (PAP) devices and requires advanced PAP modes for effective treatment.[30–33]

MANAGEMENT GOALS

- Management of patients with opioid-related CSA is extremely challenging. The first and most important step is to assess the ongoing need for opioids and, when possible, reduce dosage of opioids. This discussion should be made together with provider and patient within the first 4 weeks of initiating therapy and every 3 months or more frequently as part of the treatment plan. In an effort to minimize opioid over-prescription and abuse, the Centers for Disease Control and Prevention recently published guidelines for prescribing opioids for chronic pain.[5] This guideline provides recommendations for clinicians who are prescribing opioids for chronic pain outside active cancer treatment, palliative care, and end-of-life care. The guideline addresses (1) when to initiate or continue opioids for chronic pain; (2) opioid selection, dosage, duration, follow-up, and discontinuation; and (3) assessing risk and addressing the harms of opioid use.[5] The state prescription drug monitoring program data should be used to determine whether patients are receiving opioid dosages or dangerous combinations that put them at high risk for overdose.
- Consider nonopioid pharmacologic therapies when possible.
- If an opioid is indicated, treatment should be initiated with immediate-release preparations rather than extended-release or long-acting preparations. The lowest effective dosage should be prescribed.
- Discontinue or taper opioid dosages if possible, as clinically appropriate.
- For patients with underlying risk for respiratory depression or those with symptoms suggestive of SDB, diagnostic testing and treatment are indicated.

PHARMACOLOGIC STRATEGIES

When possible, supervised taper or withdrawal of opioids is recommended, but this is difficult to achieve. Unfortunately, pharmacologic interventions for SDB are limited. Discontinuation of opioids is the best option and studies have shown the elimination of SDB by detoxification.[34,35] Importantly, these two studies[34,35] using polysomnography have unequivocally proved that opioids are a cause of SDB in humans.

Buprenorphine/Naloxone

Buprenorphine, a partial mu-opioid agonist, is widely used for the treatment of opioid dependency and chronic pain. Buprenorphine is a potent partial mu-agonist with a much higher receptor affinity than morphine and long dissociation half-life. The medication maintains an analgesic dose-response across all levels without an increase in respiratory depression. In 2002, the US Food and Drug Administration approved buprenorphine monotherapy and a combination product of buprenorphine/naloxone for opioid detoxification therapy. Prescriptions for buprenorphine have exponentially risen because of its supposedly attractive safety profile regarding respiratory suppression compared with other full m-agonists, such as methadone.

Farney and colleagues[36] reported that even at routine standard doses, buprenorphine showed significant respiratory impairment during sleep, with 63% showing evidence of mild SDB on polysomnography (an apnea-hypopnea index [AHI] >5 events/h), 17% of patients showing moderate-to-severe SDB (AHI >15 events/h), and 38% of patients had nocturnal hypoxemia (oxygen saturation as measured by pulse oximetry [SpO_2] <90% for 10% of total sleep time). The investigators concluded that clinically significant SDB occurred in many patients on buprenorphine/naloxone for opioid withdrawal therapy. Of significance, the respiratory disturbances consisted predominantly of central apneas and ataxic breathing, both of which are common respiratory events associated with opioids.

Acetazolamide

Opioids can cause continuous positive airway pressure (CPAP)-emergent CSA.[33] A case report described positive results with the use of acetazolamide, 250 mg, plus CPAP in the treatment of CSA secondary to chronic opioid use.[37] When the medication was discontinued after 5 months of treatment, central apneas reappeared while on CPAP.

Ampakines

Ampakines are a family of compounds that modulate the action of the excitatory neurotransmitter glutamate at the AMPA receptors by altering channel kinetics. Several studies using rat models showed that ampakines, acting through glutamate-mediated neurotransmission via AMPA receptors, alleviate opiate-induced respiratory depression of central respiratory rhythmogenesis, which is hypothesized to originate from the preBotC.[38,39] Studies using adult rats showed that CX717, a synthetic ampakine compound, alleviates fentanyl-induced respiratory depression without inhibiting analgesia or sedation.[40–42]

Preliminary findings suggest that ampakines may be beneficial in counteracting opiate-induced respiratory depression and maintain upper airway patency while preserving opioid's analgesic effect. In a study on 16 healthy human subjects, CX717 counteracted alfentanil-induced respiratory depression without affecting opiate-mediated analgesia.[43] Lorier and colleagues[43] showed that opiates induced upper airway obstruction by acting on the presynaptic inhibition of the hypoglossal (XII) motor neuron, affecting the tongue muscle involved in maintaining upper airway patency. Ampakines (CX 614 and CX717) successfully counteracted m-opioid receptor-mediated depression of hypoglossal (XII) motor-neuron inspiratory activity.[44] Dai and colleagues[45] showed the use of a synthetic ampakine compound XD-8-17C to reverse opioid-induced acute respiratory depression without having an impact on the antinociceptive efficacy of morphine in rat model. Treatment with XD-8-17C reversed respiratory depression with restoration of arterial blood gas and lung function parameters to normal range. These findings show promise in novel therapeutic agents that protect against opioid-induced respiratory impairment without loss of analgesia.

Oxygen Therapy

The role of oxygen therapy for SDB secondary to chronic opioid use has not been established. To date, there are no studies evaluating the role of oxygen therapy as a single agent for the treatment of SDB because of chronic opioid use. Supplemental oxygen in combination with PAP therapy, however, has been reported and is discussed later. Given the understanding of the hypoxic and hypercapnic ventilatory responses, adding oxygen to patients with an already reduced hypercapnic ventilatory response may further worsen hypercapnia. Oxygen therapy may prolong hypoxemia or the duration of central apneas. On the other hand, in patients with elevated hypercapnic or hypoxic ventilatory responses (high loop gain), oxygen may stabilize respiration and abolish central apneas by reducing ventilatory chemoresponsiveness.

Chowdhuri and colleagues[46] used a protocol consisting of CPAP followed by CPAP + oxygen, then bilevel PAP (BPAP) + oxygen, escalating in a stepwise titration to eliminate central apneas in veterans ($N = 162$) at an academic Veterans Affairs (VA) medical center; 47 patients were on opioid therapy for chronic pain, in whom CPAP, CPAP + oxygen, or BPAP + oxygen eliminated CSA in 54%, 28%, and 10% of the cases, respectively. The results showed that in individuals who fail initial CPAP therapy during a titration study, a majority of residual central apneas can be eliminated effectively by adding oxygen to PAP therapy. Obtaining oxygen using this protocol, however, may not be feasible in a non-VA setting given the current stringent oxygen criteria set forth by the Centers for Medicare and Medicaid Services.

POSITIVE AIRWAY PRESSURE THERAPY

See **Table 1** on studies using PAP therapy.

Continuous Positive Airway Pressure

Treatment of SDB secondary to chronic opioid use is challenging due to the presence of both OSA and CSA. In patients with OSA, the first treatment option is treatment with CPAP. As discussed later, however, treatment-emergent CSA may emerge. CPAP does not treat central apneas associated

Table 1
Studies using positive airway pressure therapies for opioid-induced central sleep apnea

Study	Design	Intervention	Outcomes
Shapiro et al.[52] 2015	Prospective, randomized, crossover $N = 34$ First-night titration then followed for 3 mo on ASV in the home setting	All subjects underwent CPAP, ASV without mandatory PS, ASV manual (PS min 6 cm H_2O) titration— then sent home with ASV with or without mandatory PS.	Significant reduction in AHI and CAI with ASV on initial titration, and at 3 mo compared with baseline diagnostic PSG and CPAP titration
Javaheri et al.,[53] 2014	Prospective trial $N = 20$ acute 17 followed for a minimum of 9 mo up to 6 y	All subjects underwent CPAP titration with persistent CSA; 9 subjects underwent second CPAP titration with persistent CSA; all subjects underwent ASV titration.	Significant reductions in AHI and CAI and improvement in oxyhemoglobin saturation on ASV compared with/diagnostic PSG and CPAP titration Mean adherence = 5.1 h ± 2.5 h
Cao et al.,[51] 2014	Prospective, randomized crossover $N = 18$	All subjects underwent 1 night with bilevel ST titration, then crossover to 1 night with ASV titration.	ASV normalized AHI and CAI compared with bilevel ST (83.3% vs 33.3%, respectively)
Chowdhuri et al.,[46] 2012	Retrospective, using the protocol at a VA medical center $N = 47$ (opioid-induced CSA)	All subjects underwent a routine protocol, which consisted of CPAP titration, then CPAP + O_2, then bilevel + O_2 for persistent central apneas.	CPAP, CPAP + O_2, or BPAP + O_2 eliminated CSA in 54%, 28%, and 10% of cases, respectively. Using a protocol resulted in a significant decline in AHI, CAI and an increase in SpO_2.
Ramar et al.,[55] 2012	Retrospective $N = 47$	Comparative review on ASV titration for CSA because of opioids vs systolic heart failure	ASV was successful in 59.6% (28 of 47) in the c opioid group (AHI <10 events/h).
Guilleminault et al.,[30] 2010	Retrospective $N = 44$	All subjects underwent systematic protocol consisting of CPAP, bilevel S, and bilevel ST titration for persistent CSA.	Bilevel ST significantly reduced CAI (1.70 ± 0.58 events/h) compared with CPAP (13.81 ± 2.77 events/h) and bilevel S (11.52 ± 2.12 events/h).
Alattar and Scharf,[48] 2009	Retrospective case series $N = 5$	All 5 subjects underwent diagnostic PSG, then CPAP, then bilevel ST titration (4 subjects).	Three patients responded to bilevel ST with reduction of AHI from severe to mild.
Javaheri et al.,[32] 2008	Retrospective case series $N = 5$	All underwent diagnostic PSG, followed by CPAP titration, then ASV titration due to an increase in central apneas on CPAP	CPAP titration resulted in increased CAI from 26 to 27 events/h. Mean CAI was 0 events/h on ASV compared with 37 events/h on CPAP.

(*continued on next page*)

Table 1
(*continued*)

Study	Design	Intervention	Outcomes
Farney et al.,[31] 2008	Retrospective $N = 22$	All underwent diagnostic PSG, followed by CPAP titration, then ASV titration due to an increase in central apneas on CPAP.	ASV improved CAI compared with CPAP but did not reach significance, presumably due to an increase in obstructive events. Mean AHI was 66 events/h at baseline, 70 events/h on CPAP, and 54 events/h on ASV. Hypopnea index increased from 14.5 events/h to 35.7 events/h on ASV.
Allam et al.,[33] 2007	Retrospective $N = 100$ (category of CSA included CompSA, idiopathic CSA, and CSA/CSR) 13 subjects used opioids chronically (within CompSA and CSA category).	All subjects underwent diagnostic PSG, followed by CPAP, bilevel S, bilevel ST, and ASV titration for persistently elevated CAI.	ASV significantly improved AHI to a mean of 5 events/h vs diagnostic PSG and CPAP titration night. Sixty-four patients responded to ASV with a mean AHI <10 events/h[a]

Abbreviations: CompSA, complex sleep apnea; CSR, Cheyne–Stokes respiration; PS, pressure support; PSG, polysomnogram.

[a] No specific data on those using opioids (lumped into complex sleep apnea and CSA success category).

with opioid use but rather increases the frequency of central apnea events.[30–32] Farney and colleagues[47] reported one of the earliest cases, of three patients who developed opioid-induced CSA that was unresponsive to CPAP. Allam and colleagues[33] undertook a retrospective study of 100 patients who failed conventional CPAP therapy for various types of CSA, including those due to opioids. These patients were successfully treated with an adaptive servo ventilator (ASV). In an early study,[31] Javaheri and colleagues[32] reported five patients with severe sleep apnea (overall AHI 70 ± 19, CAI 26 ± 27 events/h) who failed CPAP therapy (central apnea events increased on CPAP, CAI 37 ± 21 events/h). Farney and colleagues[31] performed a retrospective analysis of 22 patients with severe sleep apnea (AHI 66 ± 37 events/h), of whom 18 of 22 failed CPAP therapy (AHI on CPAP 70 ± 33 events/h). Guilleminault and colleagues[30] performed a case-control study evaluating 44 patients with severe OSA on chronic opioid therapy and observed CPAP-emergent CSA (diagnostic CAI = 0.6 ± 1 events/h, CPAP CAI = 14 ± 3 events/h).

Bilevel Positive Airway Pressure

Alattar and Scharf[48] reported four patients with opioid-induced CSA who failed CPAP and bilevel therapy; three of the four bilevel patients required supplemental oxygen due to persistent nocturnal hypoxemia.[48] Guilleminault and colleagues[30] attempted BPAP therapy on 44 patients with comorbid OSA and CPAP-emergent CSA secondary to opioids. Although BPAP effectively treated obstructive respiratory events, central apneas present on CPAP persisted (bilevel CAI = 12 ± 2 events/h). Patients continued to complain of nocturnal awakenings and daytime hypersomnolence on CPAP and BPAP.[30]

Bilevel Spontaneous Timed

BPAP with the backup respiratory rate (ie, bilevel spontaneous timed [ST]) has shown some success in treating CSA associated with chronic opioid use. Alattar and Scharf[48] reported five patients on methadone maintenance with central apneas (AHI ranged 28–106 events/h with >50% central apneas) that improved on BPAP therapy with backup respiratory rate. A case-control study by Guilleminault and colleagues[30] in 44 chronic opioid users with OSA (mean AHI 44 ± 1 events/h) reported a high rate of central apneas on treatment with CPAP (CAI 14 ± 3 events/h) and BPAP (CAI 12 ± 2 events/h). Bilevel ST, however, effectively eliminated central apneas (CA11.7 ± 0.6 events/h) and OSAs and improved nocturnal oxyhemoglobin saturation and daytime hypersomnolence.

Adaptive Servo Ventilator

More recent literature supports the use of ASV over other modes of PAP therapy. New-generation pressure support (PS) servo ventilators use a breath-by-breath algorithm to analyze a patient's ventilatory status with real-time corresponding adjustments.[49] With this platform, dynamic anticyclic PS is applied during the "undershoot period" and a sloughing off of PS during the "overshoot period." This platform has been used with increasing popularity for other types of SDB, including treatment-emergent central apneas and complex sleep apneas, idiopathic CSAs, periodic breathing, and most recently, CSAs associated with chronic opioid use.[50] It has been shown to improve respiratory disturbances in patients with complex sleep apnea and mixed sleep apnea and is more effective than both CPAP and bilevel therapy.

Initial studies on ASV for CSA secondary to chronic opioid use were carried out by Farney and colleagues[31] and Javaheri and colleagues.[32] Farney and colleagues[31] conducted a retrospective study with ASV to treat comorbid OSA and CSA in chronic opioid users with somewhat disappointing results; 22 chronic opioid using patients referred for suspected SDB did not respond to CPAP and were subsequently placed on ASV. In this study, the end-expiratory pressure (EEP) was fixed at 5 cm H_2O (not titrated up for obstructive events), whereas the backup respiratory rate was set at 15 breaths per minute. With EEP set at 5 cm H_2O, it is likely below the pressure required to maintain upper airway patency; therefore, obstructive events persisted. Around the same time, Javaheri and colleagues[32] evaluated five consecutive patients with SDB on chronic opioid therapy and found that the ASV effectively eliminated central apneas (AHI decreased from 70 events/h to 20 events/h, with a CAI of 0 events/h). In contrast to the study by Farney and colleagues,[31] the EEP was titrated to effectively eliminate obstructive events. EEP titration with appropriate adjustment of both inspiratory and expiratory pressures is critical in treating comorbid OSA and CSA.

Cao and colleagues[51] randomized patients to bilevel ST versus new-generation ASV with a one-night crossover design study. ASV with auto-titrating expiratory PAP was superior to bilevel ST in normalizing respiratory events, including central apneas (83.3% vs 33.3% respectively). Two studies evaluated extended ASV use in the home setting. Shapiro and colleagues[52] performed a prospective interventional study comparing CPAP versus ASV on patients with CSA secondary to opioid use on initial titration study, then followed patients in the home setting for 3 months. All patients were using opioids prescribed at greater than 100 mg morphine equivalent. At 3 months of home ASV use, the AHI and CAI were significantly reduced compared with baseline diagnostic levels and CPAP treatment. Javaheri and colleagues[53] conducted a stepwise titration protocol on 20 patients with CSA secondary to chronic opioid therapy. CPAP titration was ineffective in reducing central apneas at initial titration and again 4 weeks later. The mean CAI was 32 events per hour at baseline, which was reduced to 0 events per hour with ASV. Seventeen patients were followed for a period of 9 months up to 6 years, with persistently low CAI and a mean adherence of 5.1 $\pm$ 2.5 hours per night.[53]

A recent systematic review on current PAP therapies for opioid-induced CSA (n = 127 patients) showed conflicting results.[54] Opioid dosages ranged from 10 mg to 450 mg daily of morphine equivalent dose. CPAP was ineffective in reducing central apneic events. BPAP with and without supplemental oxygen achieved elimination of central apneas in 62% of patients. ASV yielded conflicting results with only 58% of participants achieving a CAI less than 10 events per hour. The investigators also found that the presence of ataxic breathing predicted a poor response to PAP therapy. Ramar and colleagues[55] also found a variable response to ASV. These data contrast with another study reporting good response, both acutely and chronically to ASV.[53] It must be emphasized that the complex algorithms of ASV devices and successful treatment of complex SDB require in-depth knowledge of these algorithms and the choice of appropriate pressure settings detailed elsewhere.[56,57]

SUMMARY

Chronic opioid use is an established risk factor for impaired sleep architecture and SDB, especially CSA. These sleep-related consequences result in daytime impairment, including daytime hypersomnolence, fatigue, depression, and neurocognitive impairment. A careful medical history assessment and close follow-up are essential in patients using chronic opioids. Meanwhile, a large number of patients on opioids are found dead in bed, and postmortem, no cause is found, except presence of opioids and other drugs in the blood. We speculate that either a terminal apnea, or an arrhythmia could be a potential cause. In regard to arrhythmia and opioids, an association between methadone and torsade de pointes was first described in 2002 and subsequently found to be mediated by a blockade of the human ion channel responsible for the delayed rectifier potassium current.[58] A boxed warning was added to Food and Drug Administration (FDA) labeling for methadone in 2006 about arrhythmia risk followed by a clinical practice guideline in 2009 recommending corrected QT interval screening.

SDB associated with chronic opioid use is a diagnostic challenge. When diagnosed, opiates should be tapered or discontinued. Optimal treatment modalities have not been extensively studied in long-term randomized trials as reflected by a paucity of the available literature. Although studies are limited, new-generation ASVs deserve further research and should be attempted in patients with SDB, including CSA induced by chronic opioid use, especially in those who do not respond to conventional modes of therapy, such as CPAP or BPAP. It is important to screen for sleep related or daytime hypoventilation, and if present, consider BPAP with backup respiratory rate over ASV. The overall impact of ASV on SDB induced by chronic opioid use on long-term morbidity and mortality is unknown.

REFERENCES

1. American Academy of Pain Medicine and the American Pain Society. The use of opioids for the treatment of chronic pain. A consensus statement from the American Academy of Pain Medicine and the American Pain Society. Clin J Pain 1997;13(1):6–8.
2. Han B, Compton WM, Blanco C, et al. Prescription opioid use, misuse, and use disorders in U.S. Adults: 2015 national survey on drug use and health. Ann Intern Med 2017;167:293–301.
3. Ballantyne JC. Opioid for the treatment of chronic pain: mistakes made, lessons learned, and future directions. Anesth Analg 2017;125:1769–78.
4. Rutkow J, Vernick JS. Emergency legal authority and the opioid crisis. N Engl J Med 2017;377(26): 2512–4.
5. Dowell D, Haegerich T, Chou R, et al. CDC guideline for prescribing opioids for chronic pain - United States, 2016. MMWR Recomm Rep 2016;65(1): 1–49.
6. Teichtahl H, Prodromidis A, Miller B, et al. Sleep disordered breathing in stable methadone programme patients: a pilot study. Addiction 2001;96: 395–403.
7. Wang D, Teichtahl M, Drummer O, et al. Central sleep apnea in stable methadone maintenance treatment patients. Chest 2005;128:1348–56.
8. Weaver TE, Laizner AM, Evans LK, et al. An instrument to measure functional status outcomes for disorders of excessive sleepiness. Sleep 1997;20: 835–43.
9. Patten SB, Fick GH. Clinical interpretation of the mini-mental state. Gen Hosp Psychiatry 1993;15:254–9.
10. Fischer B, Murphy Y, Kurdyak P, et al. Depression - a major but neglected consequence contributing to the health toll from prescription opioids? Psychiatry Res 2016;243:331–4.
11. Scherrer JF, Salas J, Copeland LA, et al. Increased risk of depression recurrence after initiation of prescription opioids in non-cancer pain patients. J Pain 2016;17(4):473–82.
12. Merrill JO, Von Korff M, Banta-Green CJ, et al. Prescribed opioid difficulties, depression and opioid dose among chronic opioid therapy patients. Gen Hosp Psychiatry 2012;34(6):581–7.
13. Scherrer JF, Svrakic DM, Freedland KE, et al. Prescription opioid analgesics increase the risk of depression. J Gen Intern Med 2014;29(3):491–9.
14. Dimsdale JE, Norman D, DeJardin D, et al. The effect of opioids on sleep architecture. J Clin Sleep Med 2007;3(1):33–6.
15. Xiao L, Tang Y, Smith AK, et al. Nocturnal sleep architecture disturbances in early methadone treatment patients. Psychiatry Res 2010;179:91–5.
16. Mogri M, Desai H, Webster L, et al. Hypoxemia in patients on chronic opiate therapy with and without sleep apnea. Sleep Breath 2009;13(1):49–57.
17. Webster LR, Choi Y, Desai H, et al. Sleep-disordered breathing and chronic opioid therapy. Pain Med 2008;9(4):425–32.
18. Sharkey KM, Kurth ME, Anderson BJ, et al. Obstructive sleep apnea is more common than central sleep apnea in methadone maintenance patients with subjective sleep complaints. Drug Alcohol Depend 2010;108(1–2):77–83.
19. Correa D, Farney RJ, Chung F, et al. Chronic opioid use and central sleep apnea: a review of the prevalence, mechanisms, and perioperative considerations. Anesth Analg 2015;120:1273–85.
20. Walker JM, Farney RJ, Rhondeau SM, et al. Chronic opioid use is a risk factor for the development of central sleep apnea and ataxic breathing. J Clin Sleep Med 2007;3(5):455–61.
21. Gavidia R, Emenike A, Meng A, et al. The influence of opioids and nonopioid central nervous system active medications on central sleep apnea: a case-control study. J Clin Sleep Med 2021;17(1):55–60.
22. Chowdhuri S, Javaheri S. Sleep disordered breathing caused by chronic opioid use: diverse manifestations and their management. Sleep Med Clin 2017; 12(4):573–86.
23. Smith JC, Ellenberger HH, Ballanyi K, et al. Pre-Botzinger complex: a brainstem region that may generate respiratory rhythm in mammals. Science 1991;254(5032):726–9.
24. Feldman JL, Del Negro CA. Looking for inspiration: new perspectives on respiratory rhythm. Nat Rev Neurosci 2006;7(3):232–42.

25. Gray PA, Janczewski WA, Mellen N, et al. Normal breathing requires preBotzinger complex neurokinin-1 receptor-expressing neurons. Nat Neurosci 2001;4(9):927–30.
26. Gray PA, Rekling JC, Bocchiaro CM, et al. Modulation of respiratory frequency by peptidergic input to rhythmogenic neurons in the preBotzinger complex. Science 1999;286(5444):1566–8.
27. McKay LC, Janczewski WA, Feldman JL. Sleep-disordered breathing after targeted ablation of preBotzinger complex neurons. Nat Neurosci 2005;8(9):1142–4.
28. McKay LC, Feldman JL. Unilateral ablation of preBotzinger complex disrupts breathing during sleep but not wakefulness. Am J Respir Crit Care Med 2008;178(1):89–95.
29. Edwards BA, White DP. Control of the pharyngeal musculature during wakefulness and sleep: implications in normal controls and sleep apnea. Head Neck 2011;33(Suppl 1):S37–45.
30. Guilleminault C, Cao M, Yue HJ, et al. Obstructive sleep apnea and chronic opioid use. Lung 2010;188(6):459–68.
31. Farney RJ, Walker JM, Boyle KM, et al. Adaptive servoventilation (ASV) in patients with sleep disordered breathing associated with chronic opioid medica tions for non-malignant pain. J Clin Sleep Med 2008;4(4):311–9.
32. Javaheri S, Malik A, Smith J, et al. Adaptive pressure support servoventilation: a novel treatment for sleep apnea associated with use of opioids. J Clin Sleep Med 2008;4(4):305–10.
33. Allam JS, Olson EJ, Gay PC, et al. Efficacy of adaptive servoventilation in treatment of complex and central sleep apnea syndromes. Chest 2007;132(6):1839–46.
34. Javaheri S, Patel S. Opioids cause central and complex sleep apnea in humans and reversal with discontinuation: a plea for detoxification. J Clin Sleep Med 2017;13(6):829–33.
35. Davis MJ, Livingston M, Scharf SM. Reversal of central sleep apnea following discontinuation of opioids. J Clin Sleep Med 2012;8(5):579–80.
36. Farney RJ, McDonald AM, Boyle KM, et al. Sleep disordered breathing in patients receiving therapy with buprenorphine/naloxone. Eur Respir J 2013;42:394–403.
37. Glidewell RN, Orr WC, Imes N. Acetazolamide as an adjunct to CPAP treatment: a case of complex sleep apnea in a patient on long-acting opioid therapy. J Clin Sleep Med 2009;5(1):63–4.
38. Ren J, Poon BY, Tang Y, et al. Ampakines alleviate respiratory depression in rats. Am J Respir Crit Care Med 2006;174(12):1384–91.
39. Ren J, Greer JJ. Modulation of perinatal respiratory rhythm by GABA(A)-and glycine receptor- mediated chloride conductances. Adv Exp Med Biol 2008;605:149–53.
40. Greer JJ, Ren J. Ampakine therapy to counter fentanyl-induced respiratory depression. Respir Physiol Neurobiol 2009;168(1–2):153–7.
41. Ren J, Ding X, Funk GD, et al. Ampakine CX717 protects against fentanyl-induced respiratory depression and lethal apnea in rats. Anesthesiology 2009;110(6):1364–70.
42. Ren J, Lenal F, Yang M, et al. Coadministration of the AMPAKINE CX717 with propofol reduces respiratory depression and fatal apneas. Anesthesiology 2013;118(6):1437–45.
43. Oertel BG, Felden L, Tran PV, et al. Selective antagonism of opioid-induced ventilatory depression by an ampakine molecule in humans without loss of opioid analgesia. Clin Pharmacol Ther 2010;87(2):204–11.
44. Lorier AR, Funk GD, Greer JJ. Opiate-induced suppression of rat hypoglossal motoneuron activity and its reversal by ampakine therapy. PLoS One 2010;5(1):e8766.
45. Dai W, Xiao D, Gao X, et al. A brain-targeted ampakine compound protects against opioid-induced respiratory depression. Eur J Pharmacol 2017;809:122–9.
46. Chowdhuri S, Ghabsha A, Sinha P, et al. Treatment of central sleep apnea in US veterans. J Clin Sleep Med 2012;8(5):555–63.
47. Farney RJ, Walker JM, Cloward TV, et al. Sleep-disordered breathing associated with long-term opioid therapy. Chest 2003;123(2):632–9.
48. Alattar MA, Scharf SM. Opioid-associated central sleep apnea: a case series. Sleep Breath 2009;13(1):201–6.
49. Javaheri S, Goetting MG, Khayat R, et al. The performance of two automatic servo-ventilation devices in the treatment of central sleep apnea. Sleep 2011;34(12):1693–8.
50. Javaheri S. Positive airway pressure treatment of central sleep apnea with emphasis on heart failure, opioids, and complex sleep apnea. In: Berry RB, editor. Sleep medicine clinics. Philadelphia: WB Saunders; 2010. p. 407–17.
51. Cao M, Cardell C, Willes L, et al. A novel adaptive servoventilation (ASVauto) for the treatment of central sleep apnea associated with chronic use of opioids. J Clin Sleep Med 2014;10(8):855–61.
52. Shapiro CM, Chung SA, Wylie PE, et al. Home-use of servo-ventilation therapy in chronic pain patients with central sleep apnea: initial and 3-month follow up. Sleep Breath 2015;19:1285–92.
53. Javaheri S, Harris N, Howard J, et al. Adaptive servoventilation for treatment of opioid-associated central sleep apnea. J Clin Sleep Med 2014;10(6):637–43.

54. Reddy R, Adamo D, Kufel T, et al. Treatment of opioid-related central sleep apnea with positive airway pressure: a systematic review. J Opioid Manag 2014;10(1):57–62.
55. Ramar K, Ramar P, Morgenthaler T. Adaptive servo-ventilation in patients with central or complex sleep apnea related to chronic opioid use and congestive heart failure. J Clin Sleep Med 2012;8(5):569–76.
56. Javaheri S, Brown L, Randerath W. Positive airway pressure therapy with adaptive servo-ventilation (Part 1: operational algorithms). Chest 2014;146:514–23.
57. Javaheri S, Brown L, Randerath W. Positive airway pressure therapy with adaptive servo-ventilation (Part II: clinical Applications). Chest 2014;146:855–68.
58. Katchman AN, McGroary KA, Kilborn MJ, et al. Influence of opioid agonists on cardiac human ether-a-go-go related gene K(+) currents. J Pharmacol Exp Ther 2002;303:688–94.

Pharmacologic Treatment of Sleep Disorders in Pregnancy

Laura P. McLafferty, MD[a,*], Meredith Spada, MD[b], Priya Gopalan, MD[b]

KEYWORDS

• Pregnancy • Sleep disorders • Sleep aids • Insomnia • Restless legs syndrome • Narcolepsy

KEY POINTS

- Sleep disorders during pregnancy have adverse effects on both mother and fetus that may necessitate pharmacologic treatment.
- In addition to general side effects, sleep medications in pregnancy may affect fetal development, timing and duration of delivery, and postnatal outcomes.
- Pharmacologic treatment of sleep disorders in pregnancy must include an individualized assessment of benefit and risk for both the patient and her unborn child.

INTRODUCTION

Pregnancy is a unique physiologic state whose characteristics often predispose women to new-onset sleep disturbances or exacerbations of pre-existing sleep disorders. Pregnancy-related factors that can disrupt sleep include heartburn, nocturnal oxytocin secretion, nocturia, and fetal movement. Sleep disorders in pregnancy include insomnia (primary and secondary), restless legs syndrome (RLS), and narcolepsy.[1]

Primary and Secondary Insomnia

Sleep duration decreases during the later phases of pregnancy.[2] Factors associated with shorter sleep duration include nulliparity, younger maternal age, advanced gestational age, and elevated blood pressure.[3] Excessive sleep disruption places pregnant and postpartum women at risk of new-onset and recurrent mood disturbance,[4] and is associated with increased risk of longer labor duration and need for caesarean delivery in nulliparous women,[5] as well as risk of preterm birth.[6] For primary insomnia, treatment strategies include cognitive behavioral and pharmacologic therapies.[1] For secondary insomnia, therapeutic management should include treatment of the underlying psychiatric and/or medical disorder.

Restless Legs Syndrome

Patients with RLS describe an unpleasant sensation that causes an overwhelming urge to move their legs. This sensation tends to worsen at night and during periods of rest. RLS is found in more than one-fourth of pregnant women[7,8] and almost two-thirds have no symptoms before pregnancy.[9] For most women, symptoms resolve postdelivery.[10] RLS is linked to dopamine metabolism dysfunction in the central nervous system,[1] which, in pregnancy, may be linked to serum iron deficiency due to increased iron requirements,[8] folate deficiency,[11] and hormones such as estradiol.[12] Management strategies include pharmacologic therapy and reducing exposure to known triggers such as caffeine, smoking, and certain drugs.[1]

Sleep Med Clin 13 (2018) 243-250 https://doi.org/10.1016/j.jsmc.2018.02.004 1556-407X/18/© 2018 Elsevier Inc.

[a] Department of Psychiatry and Human Behavior, Thomas Jefferson University, Thompson Building, Suite 1652, 1020 Sansom Street, Philadelphia, PA 19107, USA; [b] Department of Psychiatry, Western Psychiatric Institute and Clinic, University of Pittsburgh Medical Center, 3811 O'Hara Street, Pittsburgh, PA 15213, USA
* Corresponding author.
E-mail address: laura.mclafferty@jefferson.edu

Sleep Med Clin 17 (2022) 445–452
https://doi.org/10.1016/j.jsmc.2022.06.009
1556-407X/22/

Narcolepsy

It is a clinical syndrome of daytime sleepiness caused by dysfunctional transition between sleep stages and is often accompanied by cataplexy, hypnagogic hallucinations, and sleep paralysis.[13] Given the peak incidence of narcolepsy from adolescence to early in the third decade of life, afflicted women are likely to have a pregnancy affected by the condition, and 40% report worsening symptoms in pregnancy.[1,14] Pregnant women with narcolepsy have higher rates of anemia and glucose intolerance, although there is no significant difference in mean weight and gestational age at birth.[14] Labor may be a trigger for cataplexy.[1]

SLEEP MEDICATIONS IN PREGNANCY

The goals of treating sleep disorders in pregnancy include the promotion of restorative sleep and the benefits it brings to both mother and fetus. Pregnancy is unique, however, in the presence of a fetus, who is also affected by any medication the patient takes. The prescribing of any sleep aid in pregnancy must include consideration of the risks and benefits of that medication for both mother and fetus.[15] The following pharmacologic agents and their perinatal effects are organized according to the sleep disorders they are intended to treat.

Primary and Secondary Insomnia

Benzodiazepines

Benzodiazepines function at the limbic, thalamic, and hypothalamic levels of the central nervous system to enhance neurotransmission of gamma-aminobutyric acid (GABA). They work via a modulatory site on the $GABA_A$ receptor complex to produce their sedative, anxiolytic, and antiepileptic effects are, used for the treatment of insomnia, anxiety, and seizures.[16,17] Although better suited for the short-term treatment of insomnia and anxiety, long-term use for these purposes is common and is associated with significant morbidity, including dependence and withdrawal, drowsiness and cognitive dulling, falls, and fractures.[18,19] They are commonly prescribed for the treatment of perinatal insomnia[16] and, because half of pregnancies are unplanned, there is the potential for accidental early fetal exposure.[20]

Benzodiazepines readily cross the placenta. However, despite access to fetal tissues because of placental transfer, studies indicate that benzodiazepines are not teratogenic.[21,22] Although early case-control investigations reported increased incidence of cleft lip or palate with benzodiazepines,[23,24] these findings have not been replicated in subsequent research.[21,25–27] Evidence does suggest, however, that benzodiazepines may contribute to increased rates of preterm birth and low birthweight.[28]

Hypnotic benzodiazepine receptor agonists

Medications in the hypnotic benzodiazepine receptor agonist (HBRA) class, also known as Z-drugs, include the imidazopyridine zolpidem; the pyrazolopyrimidine zaleplon; and the cyclopyrrolone, zopiclone (not commercially available on the market in the United States), and eszopiclone (the active enantiomer of zopiclone). HBRAs are now the most commonly prescribed hypnotics worldwide, including among pregnant women. Although not chemically related to benzodiazepines, they are agonists at the $GABA_A$ receptor, reducing sleep latency and improving sleep quality,[29,30] and they are thought to have minimal disruption of sleep architecture. Many potential adverse reactions have been noted, including memory loss, daytime fatigue, hallucinations, and tolerance or physiologic dependence.[31,32] HBRAs, such as benzodiazepines, cross the human placenta and rapidly clear the fetal circulation.[33,34] HBRAs do not seem to increase the risk for congenital malformations at usual clinical doses.[28,34–37] There is a case report, however, of neural tube defects occurring with high-dose exposure to zolpidem in the first trimester of pregnancy.[38] HBRAs may increase rates of preterm birth, low birthweight, and/or small-for-gestational-age infants[34,39]; however, studies were small and results showed statistical but likely no clinical significance.

Antidepressants

Regardless of class, all currently available antidepressants are thought to work through the modulation of the monoamine neurotransmitters, serotonin, norepinephrine, and dopamine, for the treatment of depression and anxiety. Given the sedating nature of some antidepressants, including tricyclic antidepressants (TCAs), the piperazinoazepine agent mirtazapine, and the serotonin-2 receptor antagonist and serotonin reuptake inhibitor, trazodone, it comes as no surprise that these medications are sometimes used off-label for the treatment of perinatal insomnia.[40] Doxepin and amitriptyline are TCAs that are often used as sleep aids at low doses. Their hypnotic effects are thought to be related to their antihistaminergic properties. TCAs carry the risk of significant morbidity given their action at multiple receptor sites; side effects include confusion, constipation, blurred vision, weight gain, tachycardia, cardiac arrhythmias, and death in overdose. Low-dose doxepin for insomnia seems to be relatively well tolerated in the general adult population.[41] Treatment providers often take advantage of the main side effects of mirtazapine, namely drowsiness, increased appetite, and weight gain, for the treatment of depression with concomitant insomnia and poor appetite.[42] Originally developed as an antidepressant, trazodone is now almost exclusively used for the treatment of insomnia,[43] is generally well tolerated, and has been shown to improve sleep efficacy and shorten sleep onset latency.[44]

In contemporary studies, antidepressant use in the perinatal period does not seem to confer an increased risk for congenital malformations.[45,46] Studies do seem to support a small but increased risk for low birthweight and preterm birth,[46,47] although this is significantly confounded by underlying illness state. When used in late pregnancy, studies show a small but an increased risk for respiratory symptoms, including persistent pulmonary hypertension of the newborn. However, the absolute risk is extremely low.[46,48] A systematic review of mirtazapine use in pregnant women found a possible increased risk of spontaneous abortion. However, this may have been related to underlying psychiatric disease. No association was found between prenatal mirtazapine use and congenital malformations.[49] The only study evaluating the effects of trazodone on the neonate was by Khazaie and colleagues,[50] which compared trazodone with other treatments of perinatal insomnia.

Antidepressant use in pregnancy has been associated with a constellation of adverse neurobehavioral effects in newborns (irritability, tremors, jitteriness, and sleep disturbances), known as neonatal adaptation syndrome, although these symptoms are generally transient and short-lived.[51,52] Additional neurologic effects noted in the neonate include abnormal general movements.[51] However, these results must be interpreted carefully because untreated depression has been implicated in many of the same processes.[53]

Antipsychotics

Antipsychotic medications work primarily as antagonists at dopamine receptors, although there is considerable variability in their receptor profiles. Although the first-generation antipsychotics are largely uniform in their D2 receptor antagonism (though to varying potencies), the second-generation antipsychotics do not uniformly have this effect and are largely known for serotonin antagonism. Although the off-label use of these medications for insomnia has become a widespread practice, their side-effect profile should preclude their use in pregnancy for the primary indication of insomnia. However, the sedating effects of many of the antipsychotics may be helpful in the treatment of psychosis and mood disorders. Sedating second-generation antipsychotics include clozapine, olanzapine, quetiapine, and risperidone, the last 3 having the largest number of studies. Of these, olanzapine and clozapine cross the placenta at higher rates than quetiapine and risperidone due to the level of protein binding. In vivo studies of antipsychotic levels during pregnancy suggest a decrease in maternal serum levels during the third trimester, consistent with other classes of medications and in line with the pharmacokinetic changes that occur during pregnancy.[54]

Second-generation antipsychotics have an emerging body of research that validates their safety profile during the perinatal period. Recent studies have found no association with congenital malformations[55,56] or gestational diabetes.[57] Sorensen and colleagues[58] found no difference in spontaneous abortion rates between pregnant women who stayed on their antipsychotic medications versus those who discontinued them; however, they did find a 2-fold increase in the risk of stillbirth, with an absolute risk difference of 1.2% versus 0.6%. Both medication-exposed groups had higher rates of stillbirths and spontaneous abortions compared with unexposed women but absolute numbers remained low in all groups.[58] The US Federal Drug Administration issued a class warning in 2011 for withdrawal symptoms and extrapyramidal symptoms in neonates born to mothers on antipsychotics.[59]

Melatonin and melatonin receptor agonists

Melatonin is a naturally produced neurotransmitter that modulates circadian rhythms in all mammals. It is known to have effects on sexual maturation and elevated secretion of endogenous melatonin during pregnancy.[60] Endogenous melatonin is also produced in the placenta, and protects against molecular damage and cellular dysfunction arising from oxidative stress.[61] However, only limited data are available for the use of exogenous melatonin in pregnancy. Studies investigating the neonatal effects of melatonin are primarily in mice. They show conflicted results, with some showing evidence of neuroprotection in the setting of toxin exposure,[62] whereas others have shown disruption to reproductive hormone development[63] and postpartum circadian rhythm.[64]

Antihistamines

Diphenhydramine and hydroxyzine are widely accepted for use during pregnancy, yet there are few studies in humans to confirm their safety profiles. Khazaie and colleagues[50] evaluated the effect of insomnia treatment during the third trimester of pregnancy on postpartum depression symptoms in 54 pregnant women who were randomly assigned to trazodone 50 mg per day, diphenhydramine 25 mg per day, or placebo treatment. Trazodone and diphenhydramine significantly improved sleep duration and sleep efficiency compared with placebo at 2 and 6 weeks of treatment ($P < .0001$), and both medications improved depressive symptoms. Doxylamine is present in numerous over-the-counter sleep aids and has been investigated almost exclusively in the context of treatment of nausea and vomiting.

Einarson and colleagues[65] prospectively compared 53 pregnant women on hydroxyzine with 23 women on cetirizine and a control group, and found no differences in rates of livebirths, spontaneous or therapeutic abortion, or stillbirth. A case report of a neonatal withdrawal syndrome with 150 mg (mg) of hydroxyzine was reported in 2005.[66] The Israel Teratogen Information Service followed 37 pregnancies with exposure to hydroxyzine and found no increased risk of congenital malformations.[67] A study by Li and colleagues[68] showed no significant associations between diphenhydramine and doxylamine and congenital malformations. Diphenhydramine was investigated in the setting of hyperemesis gravidarum and showed no effects on perinatal outcomes.[69] Another study found a possible association between diphenhydramine, doxylamine, and birth defects but was significantly confounded by recall bias and limited by relatively small numbers.[70]

Restless Legs Syndrome

Dopamine agonists

The nonergot dopamine agonists, including pramipexole, ropinirole, and rotigotine, are considered first-line medications for the treatment of RLS in nonpregnant adults. Additionally, carbidopa-levodopa can be used for RLS symptoms that occur intermittently in the evening, at bedtime, on waking during the night, or for symptoms associated with specific activities, such as long car rides.[71] Ergot agonists, such as bromocriptine and cabergoline, as well as pergolide, should be avoided for the treatment of RLS because they have been associated with cardiac valvular fibrosis and other fibrotic reactions.[72,73] Minor potential side effects of the nonergot dopamine agonists include nausea and lightheadedness (which generally resolve within 10–14 days), and less common adverse reactions include nasal stuffiness, constipation, insomnia, and leg edema (which are reversible with discontinuation of treatment). At higher doses, hypersomnia may occur.[71] Treatment-limiting adverse reactions include the development of augmentation (ie, a worsening of RLS symptoms earlier in the day after an evening dose of medication) and impulse control disorders.[74,75]

The literature regarding the pharmacologic treatment of RLS in pregnancy is scarce. As such, a task force of 9 experts was chosen by the International RLS Study Group (IRLSSG) to develop guidelines for the diagnosis and treatment of RLS during pregnancy and lactation.[76] In 2015, the IRLSSG task force outlined nonpharmacologic treatment approaches, a rationale for iron supplementation, and, finally, pharmacologic treatment approaches for perinatal RLS. As with other medications, the task force called for a risk-benefit approach regarding the use of dopamine agonists for the treatment of RLS in pregnancy.[76]

Although there is more evidence for the effectiveness of the nonergot dopamine agonists for the treatment of RLS compared with carbidopa-levodopa, there are more safety data for carbidopa-levodopa in pregnancy.[76] Carbidopa-levodopa use during pregnancy has been reported in 38 cases of RLS in pregnancy without evidence for major malformations or other adverse outcomes.[77] However, the combination of levodopa with benserazide should be avoided owing to a possible adverse effect on bone development.[76] Due to limited data regarding the safety of nonergot dopamine agonists in pregnancy, the IRLSSG task force rated these medications as "insufficient evidence to reach consensus" for use in the treatment of RLS during pregnancy.[76] Task force recommendations include avoiding the ergot dopamine agonists for the treatment of RLS in pregnancy, given their potential for fibrotic reactions.[76,78]

Narcolepsy

Stimulants

Although stimulant use for the treatment of perinatal sleep disorders has not been systematically researched, clinical outcomes from studies on the treatment of attention-deficit hyperactivity disorder (ADHD) may guide the risk-benefit discussion of stimulant use for the management of narcolepsy in patients who require these medications. Animal studies on the use of stimulants in pregnancy have suggested structural and behavioral teratogenicity.[79,80] A Danish case-control study of 480 women taking methylphenidate, modafinil, or atomoxetine during pregnancy found a 2-fold increase in the risk of induced abortion and miscarriage in pregnancies exposed to these medications. However, in a case-crossover subanalysis of pregnant women with ADHD with and without medication exposure, the relative risk decreased, suggesting confounding by indication.[81] A multicenter prospective study comparing 382 women exposed to methylphenidate during pregnancy with a matched unexposed sample found a similar increased adjusted hazard ratio of 1.35, also confounded by indication.[82] The investigators did not find any associations with congenital or cardiovascular defects with perinatal use of methylphenidate.[82] A case-control study by Newport and colleagues[83] looking at the relationship between stimulants and hypertensive disorders of pregnancy is limited by a sample size (n = 12) that is too small to draw any meaningful conclusions.

Wake-promoting agents

In a retrospective case-control study of 25 women with narcolepsy with cataplexy, 6 pregnancies were determined to have occurred in which modafinil and methylphenidate were prescribed, and pregnancy outcomes were similar to controls.[84,85] There are no studies of armodafinil in pregnancy.

Sodium oxybate, gamma hydroxybutyrate, and other medications

There are no human studies on the use of sodium oxybate or gamma hydroxybutyrate during pregnancy. The management of narcolepsy in nonpregnant patients reports use of such medications as opioids, carbamazepine, valproic acid, clonidine, gabapentin, pregabalin, bromocriptine, and cabergoline.[1] Of these, opioids are not a first-line treatment and should not be used in this setting. Valproic acid and carbamazepine should not be used during pregnancy owing to known teratogenicity. Studies on gabapentin and pregabalin are limited to seizure indication and not studied for a narcolepsy indication. Bromocriptine and cabergoline are not recommended for use in pregnancy.[1]

SUMMARY

Sleep disorders, such as primary and secondary insomnia and RLS, have increased prevalence in pregnancy, whereas others, such as narcolepsy, have unique relationships with certain aspects of pregnancy, including delivery.[1] The roles of both mother and fetus in pregnancy affect provider consideration of sleep disorder outcome as well as treatment choice. Providers must keep in mind that literature on the use of sleep medications in pregnancy is often sparse or nonexistent.[15] Therefore, pharmacologic treatment of sleep disorders in pregnancy must include an individualized assessment of the potential risk of untreated disease for both mother and infant compared with the risks and benefits of maternal and fetal pharmacologic exposure.

CLINICS CARE POINTS

- Weigh the risks and benefits of any medication for both mother and fetus before prescribing any sleep aid during pregnancy.
- Consider pregnancy-related factors as well as primary sleep disorders, when managing new onset sleep disturbances or exacerbations of pre-existing sleep disorders during pregnancy.

DISCLOSURE

None of the authors has any relationship with a commercial company that has a direct financial interest in subject matter or materials discussed in the article or with a company making a competing product.

REFERENCES

1. Oyiengo D, Louis M, Hott B, et al. Sleep disorders in pregnancy. Clin Chest Med 2014;35:571–87.
2. Hertz G, Fast A, Feinsilver SH, et al. Sleep in normal late pregnancy. Sleep 1992;14:246–51.
3. Fernandez-Alonso AM, Trabalon-Pastor M, Chedraui P, et al. Factors related to insomnia and sleepiness in the late third trimester of pregnancy. Arch Gynecol Obstet 2012;286:55–61.
4. Okun ML, Hanusa BJ, Hall M, et al. Sleep complaints in late pregnancy and the recurrence of postpartum depression. Behav Sleep Med 2009;7:106–17.
5. Lee KA, Gay CL. Sleep in late pregnancy predicts length of labor and type of delivery. Am J Obstet Gynecol 2004;191:2041–6.
6. Okun ML, Schetter CD, Glynn LM. Poor sleep quality is associated with preterm birth. Sleep 2011;34: 1493–8.
7. Chen PH, Liou KC, Chen CP, et al. Risk factors and prevalence rate of restless legs syndrome among pregnant women in Taiwan. Sleep Med 2012;13: 1153–7.
8. Manconi M, Govoni V, De Vito A, et al. Pregnancy as a risk factor for restless legs syndrome. Sleep Med 2004;5:305–8.
9. Manconi M, Govoni V, De Vito A, et al. Restless legs syndrome in pregnancy. Neurology 2004;63:1065–9.

10. Uglane MT, Westad S, Backe B. Restless legs syndrome in pregnancy is a frequent disorder with a good prognosis. Acta Obstet Gynecol Scand 2011;90(9):1046–8.
11. Lee KA, Zaffke ME, Baratte-Beebe K. Restless legs syndrome and sleep disturbance during pregnancy: the role of folate and iron. J Womens Health Gend Based Med 2001;10:335–41.
12. Djaza A, Wehrle R, Lancel M, et al. Elevated estradiol plasma levels in women with restless legs during pregnancy. Sleep 2009;32:169–74.
13. Scammell TE. The neurobiology, diagnosis, and treatment of narcolepsy. Ann Neurol 2003;53: 154–66.
14. Maurovat-Horvich E, Kemlink D, Hogl B, et al. Narcolepsy and pregnancy: a retrospective European evaluation of 249 pregnancies. J Sleep Res 2013; 22:496–512.
15. McAllister-Williams RH, Baldwin DS, Cantwell R, et al. British Association for Psychopharmacology consensus guidance on the use of psychotropic medication preconception, in pregnancy and postpartum 2017. J Psychopharmacol 2017;31(5): 519–52.
16. Iqbal MM, Sobhan T, Ryals T. Effects of commonly used benzodiazepines on the fetus, the neonate, and the nursing infant. Psychiatr Serv 2002;53(1): 39–49.
17. Hood SD, Norman A, Hince DA, et al. Benzodiazepine dependence and its treatment with low dose flumazenil. Br J Clin Pharmacol 2014;77(2):285–94.
18. Ballinger BR. New drugs. Hypnotics and anxiolytics. BMJ 1990;300(6722):456–8.
19. Pollmann AS, Murphy AL, Bergman JC, et al. Deprescribing benzodiazepines and Z-drugs in community-dwelling adults: a scoping review. BMC Pharmacol Toxicol 2015;16:19.
20. Koren G, Pastuszak A, Ito S. Drugs in pregnancy. N Engl J Med 1998;338:1128–37.
21. Ban L, West J, Gibson JE, et al. First trimester expo sure to anxiolytic and hypnotic drugs and the risks of major congenital anomalies: a United Kingdom population-based cohort study. PLoS One 2014; 9(6):e100996.
22. Enato E, Moretti M, Koren G. The fetal safety of benzodiazepines: an updated meta-analysis. J Obstet Gynaecol Can 2011;33(1):46–8.
23. Saxen I. Associations between oral clefts and drugs taken during pregnancy. Int J Epidemiol 1975;4(1): 37–44.
24. Safra MJ, Oakley GP. Association between cleft lip with or without cleft palate and prenatal exposure to diazepam. Lancet 1975;2(7933):478–80.
25. Cates C. Benzodiazepine use in pregnancy and ma jor malformations or oral clefts. Pooled results are sensitive to zero transformation used. BMJ 1999; 319(7214):918–9.
26. Czeizel A. Lack of evidence of teratogenicity of benzodiazepine drugs in Hungary. Reprod Toxicol 1987;1(3):183–8.
27. Rosenberg L, Mitchell AA, Parsells JL, et al. Lack of relation of oral clefts to diazepam use during preg nancy. N Engl J Med 1983;309(21):1282–5.
28. Wikner BN, Kallen B. Are hypnotic benzodiazepine receptor agonists teratogenic in humans? J Clin Psychopharmacol 2011;31(3):356–9.
29. Sullivan SS, Guilleminault C. Emerging drugs for insomnia: new frontiers for old and novel targets. Expert Opin Emerg Drugs 2009;14(3):411–22.
30. Gunja N. The clinical and forensic toxicology of Z-drugs. J Med Toxicol 2013;9(2):155–62.
31. Siriwardena AN, Qureshi MZ, Dyas JV, et al. Magic bullets for insomnia? Patients' use and experiences of newer (Z drugs) versus older (benzodiazepine) hypnotics for sleep problems in primary care. Br J Gen Pract 2008;58(551):417–22.
32. Huedo-medina TB, Kirsch I, Middlemass J, et al. Effectiveness of non-benzodiazepine hypnotics in treatment of adult insomnia: meta-analysis of data submitted to the Food and Drug Administration. BMJ 2012;345:e8343.
33. Askew JP. Zolpidem addiction in a pregnant woman with a history of second-trimester bleeding. Pharmacotherapy 2007;27(2):306–8.
34. Juric S, Newport DJ, Ritchie JC, et al. Zolpidem (Ambien) in pregnancy: placental passage and outcome. Arch Womens Ment Health 2009;12(6): 441–6.
35. Diav-citrin O, Okotore B, Lucarelli K, et al. Pregnancy outcome following first-trimester exposure to zopiclone: a prospective controlled cohort study. Am J Perinatol 1999;16(4):157–60.
36. Wilton LV, Pearce GL, Martin RM, et al. The outcomes of pregnancy in women exposed to newly marketed drugs in general practice in England. Br J Obstet Gynaecol 1998;105(8):882–9.
37. Wikner BN, Stiller CO, Bergman U, et al. Use of ben zodiazepines and benzodiazepine receptor ago nists during pregnancy: neonatal outcome and congenital malformations. Pharmacoepidemiol Drug Saf 2007;16(11):1203–10.
38. Sharma A, Sayeed N, Khees CR, et al. High dose zolpidem induced fetal neural tube defects. Curr Drug Saf 2011;6(2):128–9.
39. Wang LH, Lin HC, Lin CC, et al. Increased risk of adverse pregnancy outcomes in women receiving zolpidem during pregnancy. Clin Pharmacol Ther 2010;88(3):369–74.
40. Winokur A, Gary KA, Rodner S, et al. Depression, sleep physiology, and antidepressant drugs. Depress Anxiety 2001;14(1):19–28.
41. Wilt TJ, Macdonald R, Brasure M, et al. Pharmacologic treatment of insomnia disorder: an evidence report for a clinical practice guideline by the Amer-

ican College of Physicians. Ann Intern Med 2016; 165(2):103–12.
42. Djulus J, Koren G, Einarson TR, et al. Exposure to mirtazapine during pregnancy: a prospective, comparative study of birth outcomes. J Clin Psychiatry 2006;67(8):1280–4.
43. Wong J, Motulsky A, Abrahamowicz M, et al. Off-label indications for antidepressants in primary care: descriptive study of prescriptions from an indication based electronic prescribing system. BMJ 2017; 356:j603.
44. Mashiko H, Niwa S, Kumashiro H, et al. Effect of trazodone in a single dose before bedtime for sleep disorders accompanied by a depressive state: dose-finding study with no concomitant use of hypnotic agent. Psychiatry Clin Neurosci. 1999 Apr;53(2): 193–4.
45. Einarson TR, Einarson A. Newer antidepressants in pregnancy and rates of major malformations: a meta-analysis of prospective comparative studies. Pharmacoepidemiol Drug Saf 2005;14(12):823–7.
46. Tak CR, Job KM, Schoen-gentry K, et al. The impact of exposure to antidepressant medications during pregnancy on neonatal outcomes: a review of retro spective database cohort studies. Eur J Clin Pharmacol 2017;73(9):1055–69.
47. Huang H, Coleman S, Bridge JA, et al. A meta-analysis of the relationship between antidepressant use in pregnancy and the risk of preterm birth and low birth weight. Gen Hosp Psychiatry 2014;36(1):13–8.
48. Huybrechts KF, Bateman BT, Palmsten K, et al. Antidepressant use late in pregnancy and risk of persistent pulmonary hypertension of the newborn. JAMA 2015;313(21):2142–51.
49. Smit M, Dolman KM, Honig A. Mirtazapine in preg nancy and lactation - a systematic review. Eur Neuropsychopharmacol 2016;26(1):126–35.
50. Khazaie H, Ghadami MR, Knight DC, et al. Insomnia treatment in the third trimester of pregnancy reduces postpartum depression symptoms: a randomized clinical trial. Psychiatry Res 2013;210(3):901–5.
51. De vries NK, Van der veere CN, Reijneveld SA, et al. Early neurological outcome of young infants exposed to selective serotonin reuptake inhibitors during pregnancy: results from the observational SMOK study. PLoS One 2013;8(5):e64654.
52. Grigoriadis S, Vonderporten EH, Mamisashvili L, et al. The effect of prenatal antidepressant exposure on neonatal adaptation: a systematic review and meta-analysis. J Clin Psychiatry 2013;74(4): e309–20.
53. Wisner KL, Sit DK, Hanusa BH, et al. Major depression and antidepressant treatment: impact on pregnancy and neonatal outcomes. Am J Psychiatry 2009;166(5):557–66.
54. Westin AA, Brekke M, Molden E, et al. Treatment with antipsychotics in pregnancy: changes in drug disposition. Clin Pharmacol Ther 2018;103(3): 477–84.
55. Huybrechts KF, Hernández-Díaz S, Patorno E. Antipsychotic use in pregnancy and the risk for congenital malformations. JAMA Psychiatry 2016;73(9): 938–46.
56. Cohen LS, Viguera AC, McInerney KA. Reproductive safety of second-generation antipsychotics: current data from the Massachusetts General Hospital Na tional Pregnancy registry for atypical antipsychotics. Am J Psychiatry 2016;173(3):263–70.
57. Panchaud A, Hernandez-Diaz S, Freeman MP, et al. Use of atypical antipsychotics in pregnancy and maternal gestational diabetes. J Psychiatr Res 2017;95:84–90.
58. Sørensen MJ, Kjaersgaard MI, Pedersen HS, et al. Risk of fetal death after treatment with antipsychotic medications during pregnancy. PLoS One 2015 Jul 10;10(7):e0132280.
59. FDA. FDA drug safety communication: antipsychotic drug labels updated on use during pregnancy and risk of abnormal muscle movements and withdrawal symptoms in newborns. In: FDA drug safety and availability. Available at: http://www.fda.gov/Drugs/DrugSafety/ucm243903.htm. Accessed October 1, 2017.
60. Tamura H, Takasaki A, Taketani T, et al. Melatonin and female reproduction. J Obstet Gynaecol Res 2014;40(1):1–11.
61. Soliman A, Lacasse AA, Lanoix D, et al. Placental melatonin system is present throughout pregnancy and regulates villous trophoblast differentiation. J Pineal Res 2015;59(1):38–46.
62. Dubovicky M, Ujhazy E, Kovacovsky P, et al. Effect of melatonin on neurobehavioral dysfunctions induced by intrauterine hypoxia in rats. Cent Eur J Public Health 2004;12(Suppl):S23–5.
63. Dominguez Rubio AP, Correa F, Aisemberg J, et al. Maternal administration of melatonin exerts short- and long-term neuroprotective effects on the offspring from lipopolysaccharide-treated mice. J Pineal Res 2017. https://doi.org/10.1111/jpi.12439.
64. Davis FC. Melatonin: role in development. J Biol Rhythms 1997;12(6):498–508.
65. Einarson A, Bailey B, Jung G, et al. Prospective controlled study of hydroxyzine and cetirizine in pregnancy. Ann Allergy Asthma Immunol 1997; 78(2):183–6.
66. Serreau R, Komiha M, Blanc F, et al. Neonatal seizures associated with maternal hydroxyzine hydrochloride in late pregnancy. Reprod Toxicol 2005; 20(4):573–4.
67. Diav-Citrin O, Shechtman S, Aharonovich A. Pregnancy outcome after gestational exposure to loratadine or antihistamines: a prospective controlled cohort study. J Allergy Clin Immunol 2003;111(6): 1239–43.

68. Li Q, Mitchell AA, Werler MM, et al. Assessment of antihistamine use in early pregnancy and birth defects. J Allergy Clin Immunol Pract 2013;1(6): 666–74.
69. Nageotte MP, Briggs GG, Towers CV, et al. Droperidol and diphenhydramine in the management of hyperemesis gravidarum. Am J Obstet Gynecol 1996; 174(6):1801–5.
70. Gilboa SM, Strickland MJ, Olshan AF, et al. Use of antihistamine medications during early preg- nancy and isolated major malformations. Birth Defects Res A Clin Mol Teratol 2009;85(2):137–50.
71. Silber MH, Becker PM, Earley C, et al. Willis-Ekbom Disease Foundation revised consensus statement on the management of restless legs syndrome. Mayo Clin Proc 2013;88(9):977–86.
72. Andersohn F, Garbe E. Cardiac and noncardiac fibrotic reactions caused by ergot-and nonergot-derived dopamine agonists. Mov Disord 2009; 24(1):129–33.
73. Garcia-Borreguero D, Ferini-strambi L, Kohnen R, et al. European guidelines on management of rest less legs syndrome: report of a joint task force by the European Federation of Neurological Societies, the European Neurological Society and the Euro pean Sleep Research Society. Eur J Neurol 2012; 19(11):1385–96.
74. Lipford MC, Silber MH. Long-term use of pramipexole in the management of restless legs syndrome. Sleep Med 2012;13(10):1280–5.
75. Cornelius JR, Tippmann-Peikert M, Slocumb NL, et al. Impulse control disorders with the use of dopa- minergic agents in restless legs syndrome: a case- control study. Sleep 2010;33(1):81–7.
76. Picchietti DL, Hensley JG, Bainbridge JL, et al. Consensus clinical practice guidelines for the diag- nosis and treatment of restless legs syndrome/Willis- Ekbom disease during pregnancy and lactation. Sleep Med Rev 2015;22:64–77.
77. Dostal M, Weber-schoendorfer C, Sobesky J, et al. Pregnancy outcome following use of levodopa, pra- mipexole, ropinirole, and rotigotine for restless legs syndrome during pregnancy: a case series. Eur J Neurol 2013;20(9):1241–6.
78. Araujo B, Belo S, Carvalho D. Pregnancy and tumor outcomes in women with prolactinoma. Exp Clin Endocrinol Diabetes 2017;125(10):642–8.
79. Costa Gdr A, Galvao TC, Bacchi AD, et al. Inves tigation of possible teratogenic effects in the offspring of mice exposed to methylphenidate dur ing pregnancy. Reprod Biomed Online 2016;32(2):170–7.
80. Peters HT, Strange LG, Brown SSD, et al. The phar macokinetic profile of methylphenidate use in preg nancy: a study in mice. Neurotoxicol Teratol 2016; 54:1–4.
81. Haervig KB, Mortensen LH, Hansen AV, et al. Use of ADHD medication during pregnancy from 1999 to 2010: a Danish register-based study. Pharmacoepidemiol Drug Saf 2014;23(5):526–33.
82. Diav-Citrin O, Shechtman S, Arnon J, et al. Methylphenidate in pregnancy: a multicenter, prospective, comparative, observational Study. J Clin Psychiatry 2016;77(9):1176–81.
83. Newport DJ, Hostetter AL, Juul SH, et al. Prenatal psychostimulant and antidepressant exposure and risk of hypertensive disorders of pregnancy. J Clin Psychiatry 2016;77(11):1538–45.
84. Calvo-Ferrandiz E, Peraita-Adrados R. Narcolepsy with cataplexy and pregnancy: a case-control study. J Sleep Res 2017. https://doi.org/10.1111/jsr.12567.
85. Kuczkowski KM. Liquid ecstasy during pregnancy. Anaesthesia 2004;59(9):926.

Turning Over a New Leaf—Pharmacologic Therapy in Obstructive Sleep Apnea

Jan Hedner, MD, PhD, FERS, Ding Zou, MD, PhD*

KEYWORDS

- Comorbidity • Drug • Endotype • Non-positive airway pressure treatment
- Patient-reported outcomes • Precision medicine • Randomized controlled trial
- Sleep-disordered breathing

KEY POINTS

- Current therapies in obstructive sleep apnea (OSA) are hampered by limited compliance (positive airway pressure treatment) or efficacy (oral appliance therapy).
- Relevant experimental models of OSA are lacking. Recognition of pathophysiological endotypic traits in OSA has provided novel insights for tailored drug therapy.
- Multiple aspects (eg, comorbid conditions, patient-reported outcomes) should be considered in addition to apnea hypopnea index reduction when assessing outcome of drug treatment in OSA.
- There is currently no labeled pharmacologic treatment available in OSA. However, new candidates (eg, carbonic anhydrase inhibitors, norepinephrine reuptake inhibitor/antimuscarinic drug combinations) that address selective mechanisms are targeted in ongoing trials.

OVERVIEW

Obstructive sleep apnea (OSA) is a common condition that has turned out to provide a challenge for physicians and the health-care systems.[1] This particular form of sleep-disordered breathing is characterized by recurrent episodes of complete or partial obstruction of the upper airway, which causes periodic hypoxia and hypercapnia during sleep.[2] OSA leads to not only transient cortical arousals and sleep fragmentation but also to increased oxidative stress, autonomic dysregulation, and hemodynamic changes during sleep.[3] These consequences have been linked to daytime sleepiness as well as increased prevalence of cardiovascular/metabolic morbidities in terms of arterial hypertension, coronary heart disease, stroke, type 2 diabetes, and mortality in patients with OSA.[4]

Despite a high prevalence, treatment options for OSA are limited. So far, there is no generally effective drug available.[5] Several drug candidates have been proposed, and there are steps taken toward more strategic development programs in OSA. Previous attempts to generate a drug therapy were more or less serendipity driven, and the literature in the area is characterized by small-scale explorative studies. These studies have been reviewed in several publications in the area as well as in a Cochrane review.[6–8] There are now better-designed trials, which adequately address many of the potential pitfalls encountered in previous studies, under way. There are also considerable literatures on interventional strategies that address physiologic mechanisms involved in upper airway collapse during sleep.[9,10]

This article addresses some major methodologic problems encountered when designing clinical drug trials in OSA. In addition, we describe the conventional outcomes addressed in previous and ongoing drug studies. Finally, we address drugs with a potential effect on the various

Sleep Med Clin 13 (2018) 203-217 https://doi.org/10.1016/j.jsmc.2018.03.004
Center for Sleep and Vigilance Disorders, Department of Internal Medicine and Clinical Nutrition, Sahlgrenska Academy, University of Gothenburg, Medicinaregatan 8B, Box 421, Gothenburg SE-40530, Sweden
* Corresponding author.
E-mail address: Zou.ding@lungall.gu.se

Sleep Med Clin 17 (2022) 453–469
https://doi.org/10.1016/j.jsmc.2022.06.010
1556-407X/22/

pathophysiologic mechanisms that have been associated with OSA and associated conditions (eg, sleepiness, obesity, arterial hypertension, and gastroesophageal reflux).

Current Treatment Options

OSA is known to, pathophysiologically, involve anatomic predisposition for airway collapse, reduced compensatory neuromuscular control of the upper airway, and labile central neurochemical ventilatory control during sleep.[2] Continuous positive airway pressure (CPAP) is a highly efficacious treatment in OSA, which acts to splint the upper airway. However, CPAP does not seem to modulate the fundamental underlying mechanisms. Moreover, although the clinical utility of CPAP has been extremely well established for many years, the therapy is limited by poor compliance[11] and modest effect on long-term cardiovascular outcomes.[12] Not only do several patients reject this form of therapy completely, there are also many who use CPAP only during part of the night. Partial use of the device will frequently leave several hours of residual sleep apnea every night and thereby tentatively only provide partial therapy for the sleep and breathing disorder.[13] Most outcome studies in the area have considered a cutoff threshold of 4 hours per night for at least 70% of the nights as CPAP adherent, and there is evidence that this amount of use represents a minimum for long-term efficacious therapy.[14] However, susceptibility to the untoward effects of OSA is subject to considerable interindividual variation. Although 4 hours of unobstructed breathing may be adequate in some patients, it may only cover a fraction of a relevant sleep period in others.

With these limitations in mind, there is certainly an incentive to identify pharmacologic remedies in OSA. In fact, in a comparative sense, it may be argued that a drug therapy with only partial efficacy, for example, 50% reduction of OSA but present during 8 hours of sleep (alleviation of 50% of OSA), may result in a better therapeutic response than a mechanical device that induces a 100% reduction of OSA but only during 2 hours (alleviation of 25% of OSA) in an 8 hour sleeper. Clearly, future trials of pharmacologic therapies in OSA should introduce the component habitual sleep length in order to adequately compute effectiveness and the influence of therapy on various outcomes.[15] Incomplete compliance is also relevant for other mechanical therapies, such as oral appliance therapy,[16] whereby the possibility to monitor and quantify use is even more restricted compared with in CPAP therapy.

Obstructive Sleep Apnea as a Target in Clinical Trials

There are no established regulatory guidelines related to the design of clinical trial programs in sleep-disordered breathing. There is also uncertainty about appropriate clinical endpoints in trials and whether these should be focused on frequency markers, such as the apnea hypopnea index (AHI). However, the general trend is to go beyond the AHI[17–19] toward outcomes reflecting hypoxic exposure,[20,21] excessive daytime sleepiness,[22] and comorbidities such as hypertension or metabolic disease in OSA.

Multicenter trials need to observe the risk of interscorer variability in studies using polysomnography and potentially apply centralized scoring functions. The choice of the recording technique applied, for instance, use of thermistor or pressure cannula in protocols, may markedly influence the results (eg, apnea index). Other challenges in clinical trials in OSA include night-to-night variability resulting from the influence of body position change, variability related to differences between nights in sleep stage distribution (particularly in those with sleep stage-dependent OSA) or life-style related factors such as alcohol intake. Although there are guidelines addressing scoring rules of sleep and breathing events, there is a need to better define general standards to be applied in large-scale clinical trials.[23] Finally, as discussed later in this article, there is emerging evidence for distinct subendotypes of OSA. This finding implies that a certain pharmacologic remedy may be particularly useful in some patients but ineffective in others. Hence, insights gained in clinical trials may help us to subselect and better define such specific groups of patients (endotypes). The stricter, with respect to subendotype, our protocols are designed, the better the efficacy of the intervention is likely to be.

Another problematic dimension related to drug development in OSA is the choice of appropriate outcome variables in clinical trials. Most previous trials have used the AHI as a primary measure of efficacy. However, it should be recognized that a drug used for treatment of sleep apnea might also be designed to address comorbid conditions, such as cardiovascular or metabolic disease, cognitive function impairment, or daytime sleepiness; this could represent a useful end point in clinical trials (**Table 1**). This possibility has rarely been systematically explored in currently published studies. Future interventional trials in this area should benefit from a global evaluation that includes breathing events during sleep, daytime symptoms, target organ damage, and disease-specific outcome measurements of quality of life.[24]

Table 1
Challenges in clinical trials in obstructive sleep apnea

Specific to recordings or measurements	Interscorer variability in polysomnography; Inconsistent use or choice of sensors; Incomplete sleep classification in polygraphy studies;
Specific to the OSA disorder	Variation due to sex, age, race, disease onset; Night-to-night variability of the breathing disorder; Position-dependent OSA; Sleep stage-dependent OSA;
Specific to OSA endotypes	Anatomic predisposition for airway collapse; Poor compensatory neuromuscular control of the upper airway; Unstable central neurochemical ventilatory control (eg, high loop gain); Low arousal threshold; Systemic volume influence;
Specific to end-points	Efficacy OSA variable (eg, AHI (3% desaturation/ arousal hypopnea criterion), AHI (4% desaturation hypopnea criterion), hypoxic burden); Efficacy variable related to comorbidity (eg, obesity, arterial hypertension, type 2 diabetes, hyperlipidemia); Efficacy variable related to daytime sleepiness, cognitive function, quality of life;

The Endotype Approach

At least 4 physiologic traits that may result in OSA have been described.[25] These traits differ in several fundamental aspects and may pave the way for specific therapeutic approaches in OSA (**Fig. 1**).[26] A small or narrow upper airway provides an anatomic predisposition to airway collapse during sleep. Factors, such as local fat deposition, hypertrophied tonsils, or adenoids, may contribute in this dominating trait in OSA. A patient with a stronger dominance of this trait would be less likely to be responsive to a drug therapy addressing a dynamic intervention. However, therapies such as pharmacologically induced weight loss may certainly provide a therapeutic potential at least in a subgroup of these patients.[27]

A second trait is that of ineffective upper airway muscle responsiveness during sleep. The state of sleep per se is known to induce a reduction of dilatory muscle activity, which increases the risk of airway collapse. This effect is counteracted by arousing phenomena and increased central respiratory drive induced by, for example, mild hypercapnia. The net effect of such activation is increased pharyngeal upper airway dilating muscle activity. Reduced activity seems to compromise apnea in at least one-third of patients with clinical OSA.[25] Several drugs that might increase this activity have been explored in OSA, and this approach certainly provides a promising target in drug development.[28–30]

The third mechanism relates to the threshold for arousal from sleep. This important mechanism tends to stabilize respiration by providing a constant input to upper airway dilator muscles.[31] A modified arousal threshold may cause a mismatch between increased respiratory drive (as a consequence of a respiratory event) and upper airway muscle recruitment, which would likely induce a breathing instability. A particular clinical focus has been directed toward hypnotic drugs to increase the arousal threshold and provide a mechanism that improves airway patency in OSA.[32–35]

Finally, OSA was found to be associated with instability of the respiratory control system (high loop gain).[36] The oscillation of the ventilatory drive may periodically diminish pharyngeal dilatory muscle activity and contribute to pathogenesis of OSA. Loop gain can be pharmacologically modified and the mechanism has therefore been studied quite extensively in this condition.[37]

It should be emphasized that OSA reflects a combination of several these endotypic traits most likely in a nondelineated fashion. With a similar degree of deficiency, the dominant mechanism for OSA pathogenesis may vary between individual patients.

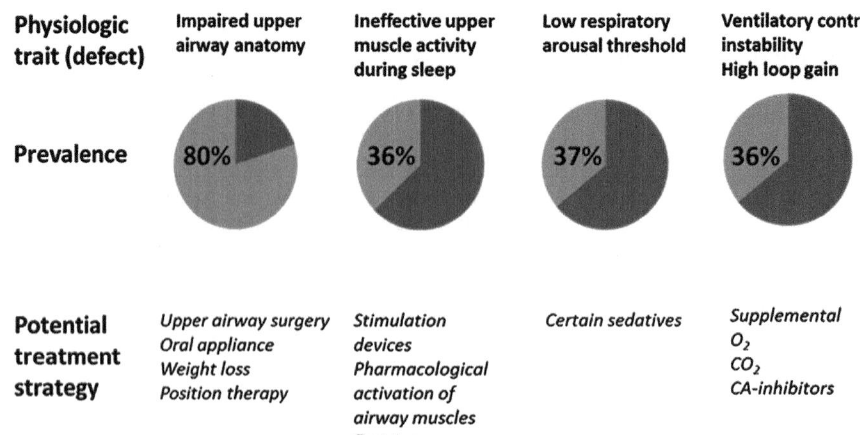

Physiologic trait (defect)
Impaired upper airway anatomy
Ineffective upper muscle activity during sleep
Low respiratory arousal threshold
Ventilatory control instability High loop gain
Prevalence
80%
36%
37%
36%
Potential treatment strategy
Upper airway surgery Oral appliance Weight loss Position therapy
Stimulation devices Pharmacological activation of airway muscles Training
Certain sedatives
Supplemental O_2 CO_2 CA-inhibitors

Fig. 1. Physiologic phenotyping in 69 random patients with OSA and 21 controls. Please note that a single patient may appear in more than one category. CA, carbonic anhydrase. (*Data from* Eckert DJ, White DP, Jordan AS, et al. Defining phenotypic causes of obstructive sleep apnea. Identification of novel therapeutic targets. Am J Respir Crit Care Med 2013;188(8):1002; with permission.)

SPECIFIC PHARMACOLOGIC STRATEGIES EXPLORED IN OSA

A substantial body of literature on drug therapies in OSA is available. As mentioned earlier, most of the trials in OSA are limited in size; however, there are also larger studies that meet more stringent quality criteria. Most studies have addressed the direct interventional effects on sleep-disordered breathing, whereas others focused the effects on OSA following treatment of associated conditions, such as obesity, arterial hypertension, or gastroesophageal reflux disease.

Noradrenaline and Dopamine Mechanisms

The central noradrenergic system is highly state dependent and therefore influenced by sleep as well as arousal mechanisms. The major source of noradrenergic neurons and activity is in the locus coeruleus in the brain stem but there is widespread distribution of adrenergic receptors throughout the brain and spinal cord. Arousals from sleep are associated with periodic activation of autonomic activity, which spills over on cardiovascular and respiratory regulation, importantly in the form of a tonic excitatory influence on hypoglossal motoneurons. This mechanism would provide a rationale for the use of adrenergic agents in OSA. Tricyclic antidepressant drugs increase central adrenergic neuronal activity by inhibition of noradrenaline reuptake. Protriptyline was, in fact, one of the first drugs to be tested in OSA.[38,39] The findings pointed toward improved oxygen saturation in parallel with changes in sleep architecture but this finding was not confirmed in subsequent controlled studies.[40] The studies of protriptyline also suggested that the drug reduces rapid eye movement (REM) sleep.

Recent focus in this field is on the selective norepinephrine reuptake inhibitor atomoxetine. The compound had only moderate effects on the AHI when administered alone[41] but it was speculated that the physiologic limitation of the effect was of muscarinergic nature. In subsequent studies, Taranto-Montemurro and coworkers combined atomoxetine with the antimuscarinergic oxybutynin resulting in a reduction of the AHI by 62% in a pilot trial.[28] Genioglossus muscle responsiveness was reduced along with the reduction of the AHI.[42] A subsequent trial using a combination of the adrenergic drug reboxetine and hyoscine butylbromide recorded an effect of 35%,[29] whereas the combination of reboxetine and oxybutynin lowered the AHI from 49 to 18 in a 7-night placebo controlled trial.[30] A potential limitation of such combinations in OSA patients is the effect on circulatory system (eg, heart rate, blood pressure). A related phase 2, randomized, double-blind, placebo-controlled, parallel-arm dose-finding study was recently completed (clinicaltrials.gov: NCT05071612).

Only a few studies have dealt with dopamine-related mechanisms in OSA. Dopamine is recognized as an inhibitory neurotransmitter in the mammalian carotid body and may, therefore, be involved in respiratory control mechanisms in OSA. Domperidone, a peripherally acting dopamine antagonist, increased the hypercapnic ventilatory response in patients with OSA.[43] An uncontrolled study looking at the combination of domperidone and pseudoephedrine reported beneficial effects on sleepiness and possibly fewer apneas as well as improved oxygenation.[44] However, the observed effects may have been caused by concomitant weight reduction.

Acetylcholine Mechanisms

Drugs that modulate acetylcholinergic activity might theoretically affect OSA by multiple mechanisms. Acetylcholine functions as a neurotransmitter in the peripheral and the central nervous systems. Cholinergic mechanisms regulate autonomic nervous function and constitute the main active neurotransmitter system during REM sleep. Indeed, animal studies have demonstrated a reduction of genioglossal muscle tone after hypoglossal motor nucleus application of compounds that facilitate acetylcholinergic tone.[45] The procholinergic respiratory stimulant nicotine is known to activate upper airway muscle activity in animals but the effects were inconsistent in patients with OSA. Nicotine gum taken at bedtime reduced the AHI in one study[46] but this was not confirmed in 2 subsequent randomized trials exploring the effects of nicotine patches.[47,48] In addition, sleep quality deteriorated after nicotine.[47] Another study on healthy awake participants did not find a consistent increase of genioglossal muscle activity after a transmucosal nicotine patch.[49]

Other studies suggest that increased cholinergic activity may be beneficial and, in fact, reduce OSA. Acetylcholine is known to modulate secretory activity in the upper airway, and this may result in a reduction of airway compliance and reduced collapsibility during sleep. Other indirect evidence demonstrated that a reduced thalamic cholinergic nerve terminal density was associated with OSA severity in patients with multisystem atrophy, potentially as a result of reduced pontine cholinergic mechanisms.[50]

The cholinesterase inhibitory drug physostigmine increases both muscarinic and nicotinic activity by a reduced enzymatic degradation of acetylcholine. A double-blind, placebo-controlled, randomized, crossover trial of infused physostigmine in lean patients with OSA demonstrated a reduction of AHI particularly during REM sleep.[51] Improvement of OSA was also reported in a small randomized controlled study using the orally available cholinesterase inhibitor donepezil administered for 4 weeks.[52] However, a recent study using a single dose of donepezil in OSA patients did not confirm these initial promising findings.[53] There are currently no ongoing studies in this area but future investigations that account for potential intraindividual differences in OSA pathophysiology may result in the identification of a specific therapeutic target for drugs of this class.

Serotonin Modulation

Brainstem raphe nuclei constitute the principal source of central serotonin (5-hydroxytryptamine [5-HT]). Axons from these neurons extend to almost every part of the central nervous system. There are at least 7 different serotonin receptor families that mediate either excitatory or inhibitory neurotransmission. The various receptor subtypes, either G protein-coupled receptors or a ligand-gated ion channel, are located in the central and peripheral nervous systems. Several of these receptors have been intimately associated with different aspects of sleep. There is also a link to other physiologic mechanisms, such as appetite, cognition, respiration, and cardiovascular function. Serotonin modulates activity of several neurotransmitter systems, including glutamate, γ-aminobutyric acid (GABA), dopamine, adrenalin/noradrenalin, and acetylcholine.[54]

Tonic 5-HT input to the hypoglossal motoneurons from the medullary raphe decreases from wakefulness to non-REM sleep to reach a minimum during REM sleep. Monoamino oxidase A-deficient transgenic mice have increased rates of central apnea, which is sharply reduced after the administration of ondansetron or fluoxetine.[55] Hypoglossal nerve firing and genioglossus muscle activity are facilitated by 5-HT, which is reduced during REM sleep.[56] This finding may be physiologically relevant in patients with REM sleep-dependent OSA but would theoretically provide less of a therapeutic window during REM sleep for 5-HT reuptake inhibitors.[57] A recent systemic review on polymorphism of the serotonin transporter gene and the peripheral 5-HT in OSA found that the allele 10 of serotonin transporter gene variable number of tandem repeats and the long/long allele genotype were associated with a higher prevalence of OSA and the L allele with a higher AHI and a longer time with oxygen desaturation during sleep.[58]

The 5-HT2A and 5-HT2C subtypes are the predominant postsynaptic receptors on dilator motor neurons. The 5-HT1A (inhibitory) and 5-HT2 subtypes are found in central respiratory controller areas. Stimulation of these receptors, as well as the 5-HT3 receptor in animal models, induced respiratory inhibition, an effect that may have involved the nodose ganglion.[59] These mechanisms also seem to be determined by species differences and animal preparations. For instance, ondansetron (a 5-HT3 receptor antagonist) reduced sleep-disordered breathing during REM sleep by 54% in an English bulldog model[60] but had no effect in human OSA.[61] Also, serotonin-mediated effects are claimed to be overestimated in vagotomized animal preparation.[62]

Clinical data suggest that selective serotonin reuptake inhibitor drugs might reduce AHI, mainly during non-REM sleep. Fluoxetine reduced AHI by approximately 40% in a small uncontrolled study,[63] and a double-blind controlled study of paroxetine demonstrated a 20% reduction of the AHI during non-REM sleep.[57] Human experimental studies also report an increased genioglossus muscle activity after paroxetine during wake.[64] Indeed, serotonergic medullary raphe activity is particularly low during REM sleep; this could explain a lower effect of this drug class during this sleep phase.[65] A particular focus in this area has been placed on mirtazapine, a drug with 5-HT1 agonistic and 5-HT2/5-HT3 receptor antagonistic properties. Mirtazapine is known to promote slow-wave sleep in men,[66] and animal data suggest that this is accompanied by increased genioglossus activity[67] and, consequently, a reduction of sleep apnea.[68] Early human studies also reported a prominent reduction of OSA[69] but this effect was not confirmed in subsequent randomized controlled trials.[70] Side effects, including sedation and weight gain, limit the usefulness of mirtazapine in OSA.

Hence, although animal data suggest an association between serotonergic mechanisms and control of breathing, there is yet no evidence that these mechanisms have major impact on human sleep apnea.

Carbonic Anhydrase Inhibitors

High loop gain, as previously described, refers to an unstable respiratory control system that responds sharply to only small changes in local P_{CO_2}. Pronounced oscillations may periodically lead to low ventilatory drive and a propensity to airway collapse, particularly in patients with a narrow upper airway. There are data suggesting that carbonic anhydrase (CA) activity, either primarily or secondarily, is increased in patients with OSA in relation to the severity of the condition.[71] In an uncontrolled study, the CA inhibitor acetazolamide was found to cause a marked reduction of loop gain in 12 out of 13 tested subjects. This change was paralleled with a 50% reduction of the AHI.[72] The effect was seen during both REM and non-REM sleep. Other physiologic traits, such as the arousal threshold or upper airway muscle activity, remained unaffected. These data aligned well with previous studies involving CA inhibition. For instance, a placebo-controlled study of acetazolamide in high-altitude induced sleep-disordered breathing demonstrated almost complete restoration of ventilation during sleep, along with an improvement of oxygenation.[73] Another high altitude study addressed subjects with severe sleep apnea off CPAP at 490 m and at altitudes of 1860 m and 2590 m. Exposure to altitude leads to a sharp increase in AHI and periodic hypoxia during sleep, whereas acetazolamide 250 mg twice daily reduced the AHI, improved the oxygen saturation, nocturnal transcutaneous P_{CO_2}, sleep efficiency, and subjective insomnia.[74] In addition, acetazolamide prevented excessive blood pressure elevations at altitude. Other small short-term studies of acetazolamide also demonstrated an almost 50% reduction of central apneas[75] and a 20% reduction of obstructive events.[76]

CA inhibitors improve sleep-disordered breathing via several mechanisms. These include a reduced reabsorption of bicarbonate in the proximal tubule of the kidney, promotion of diuresis, increased cerebral blood flow, and a stimulation of ventilation via metabolic acidosis.[77] Consequently, CA inhibitors induce a left-shift of the hypercapnic/ventilatory response curve, reduce apnea threshold, and stabilize breathing.[78] In addition, emerging data suggest that acetazolamide attenuates the increase in ventilation following arousal from sleep, which further improves ventilatory instability in OSA patients.[79]

CA inhibitors, such as topiramate[27] and zonisamide,[80] have also been shown to reduce OSA, suggesting that the beneficial effect on OSA is drug class-specific (**Fig. 2**). Interestingly, beside effects on the breathing disorder, there are reports on body weight reduction following these drugs, which may add to the overall treatment effect in OSA.[81] According to the newly published European Respiratory Society guideline on non-CPAP therapies for OSA, CA inhibitor use was suggested in randomized controlled trials but not in the clinical practice.[5] Common side effects of CA inhibitors include paresthesia, vertigo, and unpleasant taste.

It is possible that comorbidities linked to OSA may be affected as a result of CA inhibition. Parati and colleagues[82] demonstrated an increased diastolic and mean arterial blood pressure in 21 healthy volunteers receiving placebo exposed to a high altitude. This effect was inhibited in the group of 21 controls receiving acetazolamide 2×250 mg daily. The findings may have implications for blood pressure control in patients with OSA and periodic hypoxemia at sea level. Indeed, a recent trial from our group recruited hypertensive patients with OSA and evaluated the effect on both blood pressure and respiration during sleep in a crossover fashion, comparing CPAP, acetazolamide, and CPAP plus acetazolamide treatment.[83] Following washout of antihypertensive medication, acetazolamide, but not CPAP, significantly

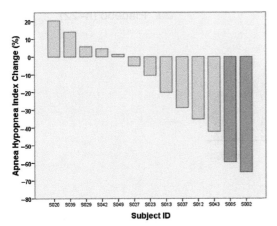

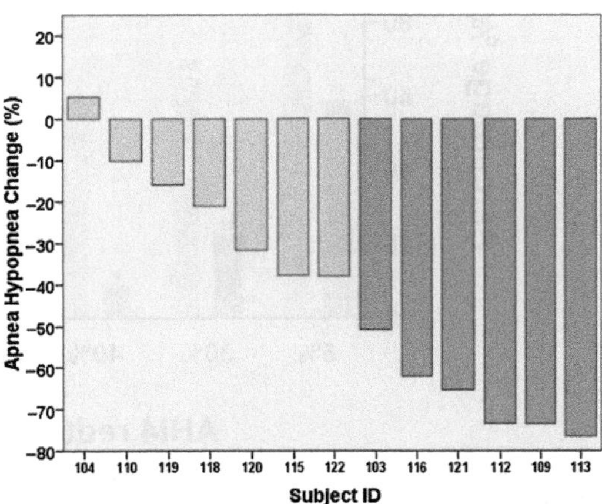

Fig. 2. Reduction of the AHI after 2 different drugs with carbonic anhydrase inhibitory effect, zonisamide (*left*) and acetazolamide (*right*), after a 4-week treatment period. Shown is the relative effect in individual subjects with OSA. Green bars signify subjects reaching an AHI less than 10 or with a 50% AHI reduction. Note the superior effect after acetazolamide because all subjects except one in fact reduced the AHI. The variability in the treatment response may reflect that these subjects have different pathophysiologic traits. ID, identification.

reduced systolic blood pressure and vascular stiffness. Sleep-disordered breathing was reduced with approximately 40%. It is proposed that increased CA activity constitutes a physiologic trait in OSA that contributes to comorbid hypertension.[84]

Finally, sulthiame, a CA inhibitor used for childhood epilepsy, was recently investigated as a treatment of OSA. A recently completed controlled phase II dose-finding trial suggested the drug was tolerated in moderate-to-severe OSA patients with an overall 40% reduction of AHI (3% desaturation/arousal hypopnea criterion) and improved nocturnal oxygenation.[85] Results were comparable when AHI 4% desaturation hypopnea criterion was applied. (**Fig. 3**) A phase IIb/III multicenter randomized, double-blind, placebo-controlled, dose-ranging study is ongoing ClinicalTrials.gov: NCT05236842.

The Γ-aminobutyric Acid-benzodiazepine Receptor Complex

GABA is the main inhibitory neurotransmitter in the central nervous system. This amino acid regulates neuronal excitability by binding to specific transmembrane receptors referred to as the (GABA)-benzodiazepine receptor complex both presynaptically and postsynaptically.[86] This complex has been implicated in the modulation of the arousal threshold in OSA. In addition, episodic hypoxia has been speculated to accelerate the progression of OSA by GABAergic mechanisms via impairment of neural control of upper airway patency and respiratory contractile function.[87] Hence, agonists at this receptor, including various short-acting and long-acting benzodiazepines and benzodiazepine-like drugs, have been regarded as potentially contraindicated in patients with OSA. However, there are data suggesting that a higher arousal threshold in fact may be beneficial in certain patients.[88] Any medication that increases the arousal threshold may have the potential to buy time for the upper airway muscle recruitment and possibly stabilization of airway patency. Eckert and coworkers reported a reduction of the AHI from 31 to 24 in a study administering eszopiclone in patients with moderate-to-severe OSA.[32] The greatest reductions in the AHI occurred in patients with a low arousal threshold. However, several subsequent trials using varies compounds in this class showed only minor effects on sleep apnea severity and inconsistent effects on OSA endotypic traits.[33–35,89–91] These findings suggest that manipulation of the arousal threshold alone may not be sufficient to treat OSA. Nevertheless, hypnotics in combination with other treatment strategies may be found useful in the design of tailored pharmacologic therapies in OSA.[92,93]

Potassium Channel Blockers

Potassium channels are widely distributed ion channels that control a variety of cell functions. Potassium channel blockade has been shown to modulate hypoglossal motoneuron activity and is identified as a potential mechanism for muscle activation in all stages of sleep. Studies in a rat

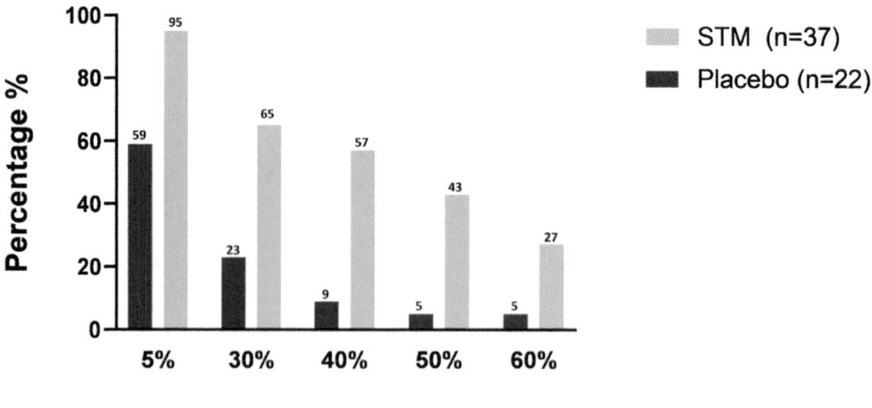

Fig. 3. Proportions of patients with apnea–hypopnea index 4% (≥4% desaturation for hypopnea definition, AHI4) reductions in the sulthiame (200 or 400 mg, STM) and placebo groups. Adapted with permission of the American Thoracic Society. Copyright © 2022 American Thoracic Society. All rights reserved. Figure redrawn from Hedner J, Stenlöf K, Zou D, et al. A randomized controlled clinical trial exploring safety and tolerability of sulthiame in sleep apnea. Am J Respir Crit Care Med 2022;205:1468. The American Journal of Respiratory and Critical Care Medicine is an official journal of the American Thoracic Society. Readers are encouraged to read the entire article for the correct context at DOI: 10.1164/rccm.202109-2043OC. The authors grantee the accuracy of adaptations.

model, using local application, have demonstrated a considerable activation of genioglossal activity.[94] However, administration of a voltage-gated potassium channel blocker 4-aminopyridine caused only a small increase in tonic genioglossus muscle activity during REM sleep in healthy subjects.[95]

In a spontaneously breathing anesthetized pig model, Wirth and coworkers investigated the potassium channel blocker AVE-0118 administered topically in the upper airway.[96] AVE-0118 was found to, with a duration of more than 4 hours, dose-dependently inhibit upper airway collapsibility in a manner that was abolished by upper airway lidocaine anesthesia. Promising data in the study of AVE-0118 (BAY 2253651) led to the first-in-patient randomized, placebo-controlled, parallel group study to investigate the efficacy and safety of BAY 2253651 for the treatment of OSA. However, compared with placebo, a single dose of 100 μg BAY 2253651, applied nasally, did not reduce AHI in patients with moderate-to-severe OSA.[97] A proof of mechanism trial with a chemically related compound (BAY2586116) was recently terminated (EudraCT number: 2020–000520–19). Sensitization of the negative pressure reflex to maintain upper airway patency remains a promising target for pharmacologic treatment of OSA. With proper patient selections and an improved solution for the route of administration, the TASK potassium channel blocker still might provide a desire potential option for OSA patients with upper airway muscle tone deficiency during sleep.

Tetrahydrocannabinols

Animal data suggest that D9-tetrahydrocannabinol might improve spontaneous sleep-disordered breathing presumably by stabilization of autonomic output and reduced serotonin-induced exacerbation of sleep apnea.[98] Dronabinol, an exogenous cannabinoid type 1 and type 2 receptor agonist, at dosages of 2.5 to 10.0 mg daily reduced sleep-disordered breathing in a pilot study of 17 patients with moderate-to-severe OSA.[99] In a subsequent placebo-controlled trial of OSA patients receiving 2.5 or 10.0 mg for up to 6 weeks, the AHI was dose-dependently reduced with approximately 40%, along with a reduced Epworth sleepiness scale score.[100] The maintenance of wakefulness test sleep latency, gross sleep architecture, and overnight oxygenation remained unchanged after therapy.

The potential underlying mechanisms of medical cannabis extracts remain unresolved, and there is no information on possible specific target groups based on physiologic mechanisms considered in OSA. There has been a proof-of-concept study on dronabinol and acetazolamide combination for the treatment of OSA demonstrating favourable results (Australian clinical trials registry: ACTRN12620000916943). Future studies are needed to fully explore the functionality of dronabinol as a treatment of OSA.[101]

Miscellaneous

The respiratory stimulant caffeine is a frequently used xanthine for the treatment of apnea in premature infants. Caffeine reduces, but does not eliminate, apnea. Other xanthines, such as theophylline and aminophylline, are known to influence ventilation by multiple effects, including an antagonistic action on adenosine in the central nervous system. There is also a peripheral effect that involves a stimulation of diaphragm contractility.

OSA was reduced by 20% in an early placebo-controlled trial of theophylline but this was accompanied by a deterioration of sleep quality.[102] Similar, but smaller, reductions of AHI were reported in other trials[103,104] but the residual AHI and CPAP pressure were not significantly affected by sustained-release theophylline in patients with OSA under CPAP treatment.[105] Hence, the effect of xanthines seems to be weak in adult OSA patients.

Several studies have attempted to reduce upper airway compliance by compounds that lower surface tension of liquids in the upper airway lining. These studies are generally small, and the effect size is moderate.[106–108] The effect of fluticasone on nasal airflow resistance-induced reduction of AHI was approximately 25% in patients with mild OSA and coexisting rhinitis.[109] The effect of combination of pseudoephedrine (an α-1 adrenergic agonist) and diphenhydramine (an antihistaminic-antimuscarinic) on OSA severity was recently studied in a placebo-controlled crossover trial. Despite a small improvement in upper airway collapsibility, the drug combination did not improve the AHI.[110]

A different approach is that of various hormone replacement therapies in OSA. For instance, sex-related steroids have been speculated to mediate a protective effect against OSA, which may be related to an oscillation of genioglossus electromyographic activity during the menstrual cycle.[111] Other potential mechanisms include respiratory stimulation, improved chemosensitivity, or a modification of the arousal threshold.[112] However, the clinical utility of hormone replacement has been controversial and studies on OSA patients yield inconsistent results. There is a lack of a cost–benefit assessment that takes potential side effects into account.

The effect of substitution therapy on OSA in hypothyroidism has been previously discussed.[113] Hormone substitution may affect either a ventilator response or structure of the thyroid gland with potential influence in airway patency. Nevertheless, studies in the field are few, restricted in size, and with variable results. Most recommendations favor CPAP in patients with OSA receiving supplementation therapy. Repeat sleep studies may be needed once hypothyroidism has been fully substituted.

TREATMENT ADDRESSING SPECIFIC SYMPTOMS AND COMORBID CONDITIONS IN OSA

Reduction of Daytime Sleepiness in Sleep-Disordered Breathing

Although most daytime somnolence in OSA is eliminated by conventional therapy, there is a subset of patients with residual excessive daytime sleepiness. The exact size of this group remains unknown but at least 12% of CPAP adherent patients are affected.[114] There have been several studies on the efficacy and usefulness of pharmacologic therapy addressing sleepiness in such patients.[115]

The analeptic modafinil, which is widely used on this indication, has multiple pharmacologic effects, including facilitation of monoamine release and promotion of hypothalamic histamine levels, which may be relevant to promotion of wakefulness. Modafinil reduces subjective and objective sleepiness, improves vigilance and quality of life in CPAP-treated OSA patients.[116] The compound has been documented in the context of driving and neurocognitive performance as well as sleepiness in patients with OSA under short-term CPAP withdrawal.[117] Armodafinil, the R-isomer of racemic modafinil, has been documented in a randomized placebo-controlled study of CPAP-adherent patients with OSA.[118] However, an European Medicines Agency pharmacovigilance program has alerted on the link between modafinil and serious skin reactions, especially in children, as well as psychiatric/cardiovascular adverse reactions. This finding has led to a restriction of the recommendation of modafinil outside the use in narcolepsy.

Pitolisant is a novel antagonist/inverse agonist of the histamine H_3-receptor that enhances the activity of histaminergic neurons in the brain. The effect in various conditions, in particular narcolepsy, on excessive diurnal sleepiness has been well documented.[119] Two recent randomized trials have confirmed the effect of pitolisant in OSA patients either refusing CPAP treatment[120] or with residual sleepiness despite good CPAP adherence.[121] The European Medicines Agency recently approved pitolisant for use in OSA patients with residual daytime sleepiness after CPAP or not tolerating CPAP treatment.[122]

Solriamfetol, a selective dopamine and norepinephrine reuptake inhibitor, is another recently approved drug for the treatment of excessive daytime sleepiness in patients with narcolepsy[123] or CPAP-adherent OSA.[124] In a 12-week double-blind randomized placebo-controlled parallel-group trial, solriamfetol 150 mg daily resulted in a

10.7 minutes improvement of wakefulness on the maintenance of wakefulness test and 4.5 units reduction of Epworth sleepiness scale compared with placebo in CPAP-adherent OSA patients with persistent daytime sleepiness.[124] Importantly, CPAP adherence was unaffected by solriamfetol in OSA patients.[125] Side effects were moderately common, most prominently headache in about 10% of studied patients. Solriamfetol was also reported to cause a dose-related increase in blood pressure and heart rate.[124]

Hence, there are pharmacologic strategies that may be considered in the treatment of excessive sleepiness in OSA but drug therapy is still relatively infrequent on this indication. Indirect comparison of these drugs showed variations of improvement after 12 weeks treatment on Epworth sleepiness scale, maintenance of wakefulness test, and clinical global impression of change in OSA patients.[126] Long-term safety and maintenance of efficacy studies are warranted.[127]

Weight Reduction and Sleep-Disordered Breathing

Moderate-to-severe OSA is present in at least 50% of obese patients, and approximately 50% of patients with OSA are obese. A more or less linear relationship between body mass index and OSA severity was described earlier.[128] There is a wealth of weight-reduction study data suggesting that the AHI is reduced by approximately 3% for every 1% of body weight that is lost.[129] In the United States and Europe, at least 6 drugs have been approved for long-term weight management including orlistat, phentermine-topiramate, naltrexone-bupropion, liraglutide, semaglutide, and Tirzepatide.

Protocols that address pharmacologic weight reductions suggest not only that OSA is modifiable by weight loss but also that added metabolic benefits may be achieved in patients with a combination of the 2 conditions. The long-acting glucagon-like peptide-1 receptor agonist liraglutide was investigated in a large-scale sleep apnea study during 32 weeks.[130] During dietary deficit, a dose of 3 mg resulted in a 5.7% weight loss (placebo 1.6%) and 12.2 events per hour reduction of AHI (placebo 6.1 events per hour, baseline 49.2 events per hour) along with an improvement of systolic blood pressure and HbA1c. Another approach includes the combination of phentermine and a CA inhibitor topiramate in obese patients with OSA. In this 28-week placebo-controlled study, body weight dropped by 10.3% (placebo 4.2%), whereas the AHI decreased by 69% (placebo 38%).[27] Again, there were beneficial effects on blood pressure, sleep fragmentation, and sleep quality.

To summarize, there is little doubt that drug-induced weight loss is feasible in obese patients with sleep apnea, and the added beneficial effects on comorbid conditions in these patients may compete with those induced by conventional mechanical therapies such as CPAP.[131,132] A randomized double-blinded placebo controlled trial to evaluate the effect and safety of Tirzepatide in obese sleep apnea patients is ongoing. (ClinicalTrials.gov: NCT05412004).

Antihypertensive Therapy and Obstructive Sleep Apnea

More than 50% of the adult population with sleep apnea, investigated in European sleep laboratories, receive treatment with antihypertensive drugs.[133] In fact, OSA is considered as one of the most prevalent causes of secondary hypertension in middle-aged adults.[134] An experimental study showed that acute changes in systemic blood pressure adversely influenced genioglossus activity.[135] The question has been raised as to whether blood pressure reduction per se, or medications specifically used for the treatment of arterial hypertension, may influence sleep apnea. Few clinical trials have been conducted to address this issue, and the results are inconsistent. Both the angiotensin-converting enzyme inhibitor cilazapril and the β-blocker metoprolol were found to moderately reduce apnea frequency during sleep in an early double-blind trial.[136] However, no effect on AHI was found after the selective β1 blocker celiprolol compared with the placebo in a subsequent study.[137] Another double-blind randomized trial addressing cilazapril reported a marginal reduction of the respiratory disturbance index and the apnea index during non-REM but not during REM sleep.[138] This finding was not confirmed in a controlled trial comparing CPAP and the angiotensin II receptor antagonist valsartan.[139] A randomized study that compared the effect of atenolol, amlodipine, enalapril, hydrochlorothiazide, and losartan in 40 hypertensive patients with OSA found no effect on sleep-disordered breathing by any of the compounds studied, although a better controlled nocturnal blood pressure was achieved after atenolol.[140] Nevertheless, a meta-analysis of 11 studies evaluating the effect of antihypertensive medications on the severity of OSA suggested a small but significant reduction of AHI.[141] The effect is more pronounced with the use of diuretics, suggesting volume control by promoting diuresis[142] or suppressing aldosterone[143] may reduce neck fluid accumulation and thereby lower upper airway collapsibility during sleep in hypertensive patients with OSA.

Gastroesophageal Reflux and Sleep-Disordered Breathing

Gastroesophageal reflux disease is common in patients with OSA.[144] The exact mechanistic relationship between the two conditions is unclear but may, beside common predisposing factors (eg, obesity, alcohol intake) and sleep position,[145] involve the periodic reduction of intrathoracic pressure caused by OSA. Alternatively, acid reflux in gastroesophageal reflux disease may produce arousals and night choking as well as acid-induced long-term pharyngeal tissue swelling, which promotes upper airway obstruction during sleep.

Indeed, AHI decreased from 38 $\pm$ 19 to 29 $\pm$ 12 events/h after 2 to 12 months treatment with the proton pump inhibitor esomeprazole 40 mg daily in patients with gastroesophageal reflux disease and OSA.[146] A small parallel group study using the histamine H2 receptor antagonist nizatidine reported a decrease in the arousal index, but not in the AHI, after 1 month of treatment,[147] whereas omeprazole produced reductions in the apnea index and the AHI by 31% and 25%, respectively, in a preliminary study.[148] These findings were not supported by a more recent study, in which rabeprazole significantly improved objective and subjective measures of sleep quality in patients with OSA and gastroesophageal reflux disease but the AHI remained unchanged.[149]

SUMMARY

There is an unmet need for a drug therapy in OSA. However, previous attempts to identify an omnipotent drug have generally been unsuccessful. There is currently no available pharmacologic alternative to the mechanical therapies generally applied in this condition. Although the general efficacy of a medication may be lower than that seen after CPAP, it should be recognized that a poorer efficacy in comparative terms may be overcome by better compliance or by beneficial effects on comorbidity. In fact, the poor long-term compliance with CPAP actually strengthens the incentive to explore novel drug candidates.

Systematic drug development is a time-consuming process. Many currently available medications have been developed from basic chemistry through early testing and larger-scale clinical trials. This process has not yet been applied in OSA because relevant experimental models of the disorder are lacking. However, we have recently seen an improved understanding of physiologic mechanisms that may accelerate the development of drugs in sleep apnea. These insights have also enabled a more tailored approach to the disorder. Specific phenotypes/endotypes of OSA have been described. Because of better classification of the disease, we may now recognize responders to specific therapies. Pharmacologic treatment in OSA is advancing into a new chapter allowing us to develop adaptive tailored medication strategies for OSA patients in the near future.

CLINICS CARE POINTS

- Phenotyping and physiological endotype characterization enable precision medicine in treatment of sleep disordered breathing.
- Patient-reported outcomes, long term safety and efficacy profiles are important considerations in pharmacotherapy of obstructive sleep apnea.
- Tailored drug therapy may show add-on effects in combination with non-positive airway pressure treatment (eg, oral appliance therapy, upper airway surgery).
- Drug treatment plays a unique role in adaptive, shared-decision making sleep apnea management protocols.

DISCLOSURE

Dr J. Hedner has received funding from Swedish Heart and Lung Foundation, Swedish State Funds for Clinical Research LUA/ALF, ResMed, Philips, Bayer, and Desitin.

REFERENCES

1. Benjafield AV, Ayas NT, Eastwood PR, et al. Estimation of the global prevalence and burden of obstructive sleep apnoea: a literature-based analysis. Lancet Respir Med 2019;7(8):687–98.
2. Dempsey JA, Veasey SC, Morgan BJ, et al. Pathophysiology of sleep apnea. Physiol Rev 2010;90(1):47–112.
3. McNicholas WT, Bonsigore MR, Management Committee of ECAB. Sleep apnoea as an independent risk factor for cardiovascular disease: current evidence, basic mechanisms and research priorities. Eur Respir J 2007;29(1):156–78.
4. Javaheri S, Barbe F, Campos-Rodriguez F, et al. Sleep apnea: Types, mechanisms, and clinical cardiovascular consequences. J Am Coll Cardiol 2017;69(7):841–58.
5. Randerath W, Verbraecken J, de Raaff CAL, et al. European Respiratory Society guideline on non-

CPAP therapies for obstructive sleep apnoea. Eur Respir Rev 2021;30(162). https://doi.org/10.1183/16000617.0200-2021.
6. Hedner J, Zou D. Drug therapy in obstructive sleep apnea. Sleep Med Clin 2018;13(2):203–17.
7. Gaisl T, Haile SR, Thiel S, et al. Efficacy of pharmacotherapy for OSA in adults: a systematic review and network meta-analysis. Sleep Med Rev 2019;46:74–86.
8. Mason M, Welsh EJ, Smith I. Drug therapy for obstructive sleep apnoea in adults. Cochrane Database Syst Rev 2013;(5):CD003002. https://doi.org/10.1002/14651858.CD003002.pub3.
9. Taranto-Montemurro L, Messineo L, Wellman A. Targeting endotypic traits with medications for the pharmacological treatment of obstructive sleep apnea. A review of the current literature. J Clin Med 2019;8(11). https://doi.org/10.3390/jcm8111846.
10. Bosi M, Incerti Parenti S, Sanna A, et al. Non-continuous positive airway pressure treatment options in obstructive sleep apnoea: a pathophysiological perspective. Sleep Med Rev 2021;60:101521. https://doi.org/10.1016/j.smrv.2021.101521.
11. Weaver TE, Grunstein RR. Adherence to continuous positive airway pressure therapy: the challenge to effective treatment. Proc Am Thorac Soc 2008;5(2):173–8.
12. McEvoy RD, Antic NA, Heeley E, et al. CPAP for Prevention of Cardiovascular Events in Obstructive Sleep Apnea. N Engl J Med Sep 8 2016;375(10):919–31. https://doi.org/10.1056/NEJMoa1606599.
13. Grote L, Hedner J, Grunstein R, et al. Therapy with nCPAP: incomplete elimination of sleep related breathing disorder. Eur Respir J 2000;16(5):921–7.
14. Oh A, Grivell N, Chai-Coetzer CL. What is a clinically Meaningful target for positive airway pressure adherence? Sleep Med Clin 2021;16(1):1–10.
15. Kohler M, Bloch KE, Stradling JR. Pharmacological approaches to the treatment of obstructive sleep apnoea. Expert Opin Investig Drugs 2009;18(5):647–56.
16. Radmand R, Chiang H, Di Giosia M. Defining and measuring compliance with oral appliance therapy. J Dent Sleep Med 2021;8(3).
17. McNicholas WT, Bassetti CL, Ferini-Strambi L, et al. Challenges in obstructive sleep apnoea. Lancet Respir Med 2018;6(3):170–2.
18. Pevernagie DA, Gnidovec-Strazisar B, Grote L, et al. On the rise and fall of the apnea-hypopnea index: a historical review and critical appraisal. J Sleep Res 2020;29(4):e13066.
19. Malhotra A, Ayappa I, Ayas N, et al. Metrics of sleep apnea severity: beyond the apnea-hypopnea index. Sleep 2021;44(7). https://doi.org/10.1093/sleep/zsab030.
20. Kulkas A, Tiihonen P, Eskola K, et al. Novel parameters for evaluating severity of sleep disordered breathing and for supporting diagnosis of sleep apnea-hypopnea syndrome. J Med Eng Technol 2013;37(2):135–43.
21. Azarbarzin A, Sands SA, Stone KL, et al. The hypoxic burden of sleep apnoea predicts cardiovascular disease-related mortality: the Osteoporotic Fractures in Men Study and the Sleep Heart Health Study. Eur Heart J 2019;40(14):1149–57.
22. Mazzotti DR, Keenan BT, Lim DC, et al. Symptom subtypes of obstructive sleep apnea Predict Incidence of cardiovascular outcomes. Am J Respir Crit Care Med 2019;200(4):493–506.
23. Suurna MV, Jacobowitz O, Chang J, et al. Improving outcomes of hypoglossal nerve stimulation therapy: current practice, future directions, and research gaps. Proceedings of the 2019 International Sleep Surgery Society Research Forum. J Clin Sleep Med 2021;17(12):2477–87.
24. Randerath W, Bassetti CL, Bonsignore MR, et al. Challenges and perspectives in obstructive sleep apnoea: report by an ad hoc working group of the sleep disordered breathing group of the European respiratory Society and the European sleep research Society. Eur Respir J 2018;52(3). https://doi.org/10.1183/13993003.02616-2017.
25. Eckert DJ, White DP, Jordan AS, et al. Defining phenotypic causes of obstructive sleep apnea. Identification of novel therapeutic targets. Am J Respir Crit Care Med 2013;188(8):996–1004.
26. Eckert DJ. Phenotypic approaches to obstructive sleep apnoea - new pathways for targeted therapy. Sleep Med Rev 2018;37:45–59.
27. Winslow DH, Bowden CH, DiDonato KP, et al. A randomized, double-blind, placebo-controlled study of an oral, extended-release formulation of phentermine/topiramate for the treatment of obstructive sleep apnea in obese adults. Sleep 2012;35(11):1529–39.
28. Taranto-Montemurro L, Messineo L, Sands SA, et al. The combination of atomoxetine and oxybutynin greatly reduces obstructive sleep apnea severity. A randomized, placebo-controlled, double-blind crossover trial. Am J Respir Crit Care Med 2019;199(10):1267–76.
29. Lim R, Messineo L, Grunstein RR, et al. The noradrenergic agent reboxetine plus the antimuscarinic hyoscine butylbromide reduces sleep apnoea severity: a double-blind, placebo-controlled, randomised crossover trial. J Physiol 2021;599(17):4183–95.
30. Perger E, Taranto Montemurro L, Rosa D, et al. Reboxetine Plus Oxybutynin for OSA Treatment: A 1-Week, Randomized, Placebo-Controlled, Double-Blind Crossover Trial. Chest Jan 2022;161(1):237–47. https://doi.org/10.1016/j.chest.2021.08.080.

31. Younes M. Role of arousals in the pathogenesis of obstructive sleep apnea. Am J Respir Crit Care Med 2004;169(5):623–33.
32. Eckert DJ, Owens RL, Kehlmann GB, et al. Eszopiclone increases the respiratory arousal threshold and lowers the apnoea/hypopnoea index in obstructive sleep apnoea patients with a low arousal threshold. Clin Sci (Lond) 2011;120(12): 505–14.
33. Eckert DJ, Malhotra A, Wellman A, et al. Trazodone increases the respiratory arousal threshold in patients with obstructive sleep apnea and a low arousal threshold. Sleep 2014;37(4):811–9.
34. Carter SG, Berger MS, Carberry JC, et al. Zopiclone increases the arousal threshold without impairing genioglossus activity in obstructive sleep apnea. Sleep 2016;39(4):757–66.
35. Carberry JC, Fisher LP, Grunstein RR, et al. Role of common hypnotics on the phenotypic causes of obstructive sleep apnoea: paradoxical effects of zolpidem. Eur Respir J 2017;50(6). https://doi.org/10.1183/13993003.01344-2017.
36. Younes M, Ostrowski M, Thompson W, et al. Chemical control stability in patients with obstructive sleep apnea. Am J Respir Crit Care Med 2001; 163(5):1181–90.
37. Schmickl CN, Landry SA, Orr JE, et al. Acetazolamide for OSA and central sleep apnea: a Comprehensive systematic review and meta-analysis. Chest 2020;158(6):2632–45.
38. Brownell LG, West P, Sweatman P, et al. Protriptyline in obstructive sleep apnea: a double-blind trial. N Engl J Med 1982;307(17):1037–42.
39. Smith PL, Haponik EF, Allen RP, et al. The effects of protriptyline in sleep-disordered breathing. Am Rev Respir Dis 1983;127(1):8–13.
40. Whyte KF, Gould GA, Airlie MA, et al. Role of protriptyline and acetazolamide in the sleep apnea/hypopnea syndrome. Sleep 1988;11(5):463–72.
41. Bart Sangal R, Sangal JM, Thorp K. Atomoxetine improves sleepiness and global severity of illness but not the respiratory disturbance index in mild to moderate obstructive sleep apnea with sleepiness. Sleep Med 2008;9(5):506–10.
42. Taranto-Montemurro L, Messineo L, Azarbarzin A, et al. Effects of the combination of atomoxetine and oxybutynin on OSA endotypic traits. Chest 2020;157(6):1626–36.
43. Osanai S, Akiba Y, Fujiuchi S, et al. Depression of peripheral chemosensitivity by a dopaminergic mechanism in patients with obstructive sleep apnoea syndrome. Eur Respir J 1999;13(2):418–23.
44. Larrain A, Kapur VK, Gooley TA, et al. Pharmacological treatment of obstructive sleep apnea with a combination of pseudoephedrine and domperidone. J Clin Sleep Med 2010;6(2): 117–23.
45. Liu X, Sood S, Liu H, et al. Opposing muscarinic and nicotinic modulation of hypoglossal motor output to genioglossus muscle in rats in vivo. J Physiol 2005;565(Pt 3):965–80.
46. Gothe B, Strohl KP, Levin S, et al. Nicotine: a different approach to treatment of obstructive sleep apnea. Chest 1985;87(1):11–7.
47. Davila DG, Hurt RD, Offord KP, et al. Acute effects of transdermal nicotine on sleep architecture, snoring, and sleep-disordered breathing in nonsmokers. Am J Respir Crit Care Med 1994;150(2):469–74.
48. Zevin S, Swed E, Cahan C. Clinical effects of locally delivered nicotine in obstructive sleep apnea syndrome. Am J Ther 2003;10(3):170–5.
49. Slamowitz DI, Edwards JK, Chajek-Shaul T, et al. The influence of a transmucosal cholinergic agonist on pharyngeal muscle activity. Sleep 2000;23(4):543–50.
50. Gilman S, Chervin RD, Koeppe RA, et al. Obstructive sleep apnea is related to a thalamic cholinergic deficit in MSA. Neurology 2003;61(1):35–9.
51. Hedner J, Kraiczi H, Peker Y, et al. Reduction of sleep-disordered breathing after physostigmine. Am J Respir Crit Care Med 2003;168(10):1246–51.
52. Sukys-Claudino L, Moraes W, Guilleminault C, et al. Beneficial effect of donepezil on obstructive sleep apnea: a double-blind, placebo-controlled clinical trial. Sleep Med 2012;13(3):290–6.
53. Li Y, Owens RL, Sands S, et al. The effect of donepezil on arousal threshold and apnea-hypopnea index. A randomized, double-blind, Cross-over study. Ann Am Thorac Soc 2016;13(11):2012–8.
54. Lipford MC, Ramar K, Liang YJ, et al. Serotnin as a possible biomarker in obstructive sleep apnea. Sleep Med Rev 2016;28:125–32.
55. Real C, Seif I, Adrien J, et al. Ondansetron and fluoxetine reduce sleep apnea in mice lacking monoamine oxidase A. Respir Physiol Neurobiol 2009;168(3):230–8.
56. Neuzeret PC, Sakai K, Gormand F, et al. Application of histamine or serotonin to the hypoglossal nucleus increases genioglossus muscle activity across the wake-sleep cycle. J Sleep Res 2009; 18(1):113–21.
57. Kraiczi H, Hedner J, Dahlof P, et al. Effect of serotonin uptake inhibition on breathing during sleep and daytime symptoms in obstructive sleep apnea. Sleep 1999;22(1):61–7.
58. Maierean AD, Bordea IR, Salagean T, et al. Polymorphism of the serotonin transporter gene and the peripheral 5-hydroxytryptamine in obstructive sleep apnea: what do We Know and what are We looking for? A systematic review of the literature. Nat Sci Sleep 2021;13:125–39.
59. Veasey SC. Serotonin agonists and antagonists in obstructive sleep apnea: therapeutic potential. Am J Respir Med 2003;2(1):21–9.

60. Veasey SC, Chachkes J, Fenik P, et al. The effects of ondansetron on sleep-disordered breathing in the English bulldog. Sleep 2001;24(2):155–60.
61. Stradling J, Smith D, Radulovacki M, et al. Effect of ondansetron on moderate obstructive sleep apnoea, a single night, placebo-controlled trial. J Sleep Res 2003;12(2):169–70.
62. Sood S, Morrison JL, Liu H, et al. Role of endogenous serotonin in modulating genioglossus muscle activity in awake and sleeping rats. Am J Respir Crit Care Med 2005;172(10):1338–47.
63. Hanzel DA, Proia NG, Hudgel DW. Response of obstructive sleep apnea to fluoxetine and protriptyline. Chest 1991;100(2):416–21.
64. Sunderram J, Parisi RA, Strobel RJ. Serotonergic stimulation of the genioglossus and the response to nasal continuous positive airway pressure. Am J Respir Crit Care Med 2000;162(3 Pt 1):925–9.
65. Berry RB, Yamaura EM, Gill K, et al. Acute effects of paroxetine on genioglossus activity in obstructive sleep apnea. Sleep 1999;22(8):1087–92.
66. Aslan S, Isik E, Cosar B. The effects of mirtazapine on sleep: a placebo controlled, double-blind study in young healthy volunteers. Sleep 2002;25(6): 677–9.
67. Berry RB, Koch GL, Hayward LF. Low-dose mirtazapine increases genioglossus activity in the anesthetized rat. Sleep 2005;28(1):78–84.
68. Carley DW, Radulovacki M. Mirtazapine, a mixed-profile serotonin agonist/antagonist, suppresses sleep apnea in the rat. Am J Respir Crit Care Med 1999;160(6):1824–9.
69. Carley DW, Olopade C, Ruigt GS, et al. Efficacy of mirtazapine in obstructive sleep apnea syndrome. *Sleep* Jan 2007;30(1):35–41.
70. Marshall NS, Yee BJ, Desai AV, et al. Two randomized placebo-controlled trials to evaluate the efficacy and tolerability of mirtazapine for the treatment of obstructive sleep apnea. Sleep 2008; 31(6):824–31.
71. Wang T, Eskandari D, Zou D, et al. Increased carbonic anhydrase activity is associated with sleep apnea severity and related hypoxemia. Sleep 2015;38(7):1067–73.
72. Edwards BA, Sands SA, Eckert DJ, et al. Acetazolamide improves loop gain but not the other physiological traits causing obstructive sleep apnoea. J Physiol 2012;590(5):1199–211.
73. Fischer R, Lang SM, Leitl M, et al. Theophylline and acetazolamide reduce sleep-disordered breathing at high altitude. Eur Respir J 2004; 23(1):47–52.
74. Nussbaumer-Ochsner Y, Latshang TD, Ulrich S, et al. Patients with obstructive sleep apnea syndrome benefit from acetazolamide during an altitude sojourn: a randomized, placebo-controlled, double-blind trial. Chest 2012;141(1):131–8.
75. Javaheri S. Acetazolamide improves central sleep apnea in heart failure: a double-blind, prospective study. Am J Respir Crit Care Med 2006;173(2):234–7.
76. Tojima H, Kunitomo F, Kimura H, et al. Effects of acetazolamide in patients with the sleep apnoea syndrome. Thorax 1988;43(2):113–9.
77. Swenson ER, Leatham KL, Roach RC, et al. Renal carbonic anhydrase inhibition reduces high altitude sleep periodic breathing. Respir Physiol 1991;86(3):333–43.
78. Teppema LJ, Boulet LM, Hackett HK, et al. Influence of methazolamide on the human control of breathing: a comparison to acetazolamide. Exp Physiol 2020;105(2):293–301.
79. Edwards BA, Connolly JG, Campana LM, et al. Acetazolamide attenuates the ventilatory response to arousal in patients with obstructive sleep apnea. Sleep 2013;36(2):281–5.
80. Eskandari D, Zou D, Karimi M, et al. Zonisamide reduces obstructive sleep apnoea: a randomised placebo-controlled study. Eur Respir J 2014; 44(1):140–9.
81. Gadde KM, Franciscy DM, Wagner HR 2nd, et al. Zonisamide for weight loss in obese adults: a randomized controlled trial. JAMA 2003;289(14): 1820–5.
82. Parati G, Revera M, Giuliano A, et al. Effects of acetazolamide on central blood pressure, peripheral blood pressure, and arterial distensibility at acute high altitude exposure. Eur Heart J 2013; 34(10):759–66.
83. Eskandari D, Zou D, Grote L, et al. Acetazolamide reduces blood pressure and sleep-disordered breathing in patients with hypertension and obstructive sleep apnea: a randomized controlled trial. J Clin Sleep Med 2018;14(3):309–17.
84. Hoff E, Zou D, Schiza S, et al. Carbonic anhydrase, obstructive sleep apnea and hypertension: effects of intervention. J Sleep Res 2020;29(2):e12956.
85. Hedner J, Stenlof K, Zou D, et al. A Randomized Controlled Clinical Trial Exploring Safety and Tolerability of Sulthiame in Sleep Apnea. Am J Respir Crit Care Med Jun 15 2022;205(12):1461–9. https://doi.org/10.1164/rccm.202109-2043OC.
86. Roy-Byrne PP. The GABA-benzodiazepine receptor complex: structure, function, and role in anxiety. J Clin Psychiatry 2005;66(Suppl 2):14–20.
87. Richter DW, Schmidt-Garcon P, Pierrefiche O, et al. Neurotransmitters and neuromodulators controlling the hypoxic respiratory response in anaesthetized cats. J Physiol 1999;514(Pt 2): 567–78.
88. Eckert DJ, Younes MK. Arousal from sleep: implications for obstructive sleep apnea pathogenesis and treatment. J Appl Phys (1985) 2014;116(3):302–13.
89. Carter SG, Carberry JC, Cho G, et al. Effect of 1 month of zopiclone on obstructive sleep apnoea

severity and symptoms: a randomised controlled trial. Eur Respir J 2018;52(1). https://doi.org/10.1183/13993003.00149-2018.

90. Carter SG, Carberry JC, Grunstein RR, et al. Randomized trial on the effects of high-dose zopiclone on OSA severity, upper airway Physiology, and Alertness. Chest 2020;158(1):374–85.
91. Messineo L, Eckert DJ, Lim R, et al. Zolpidem increases sleep efficiency and the respiratory arousal threshold without changing sleep apnoea severity and pharyngeal muscle activity. J Physiol 2020;598(20):4681–92.
92. Edwards BA, Sands SA, Owens RL, et al. The combination of supplemental oxygen and a hypnotic markedly improves obstructive sleep apnea in patients with a mild to moderate upper airway collapsibility. Sleep 2016;39(11):1973–83.
93. Messineo L, Carter SG, Taranto-Montemurro L, et al. Addition of zolpidem to combination therapy with atomoxetine-oxybutynin increases sleep efficiency and the respiratory arousal threshold in obstructive sleep apnoea: a randomized trial. Respirology 2021;26(9):878–86.
94. Grace KP, Hughes SW, Horner RL. Identification of a pharmacological target for genioglossus reactivation throughout sleep. Sleep 2014;37(1):41–50.
95. Taranto-Montemurro L, Sands SA, Azarbarzin A, et al. Effect of 4-aminopyridine on genioglossus muscle activity during sleep in healthy adults. Ann Am Thorac Soc 2017;14(7):1177–83.
96. Wirth KJ, Steinmeyer K, Ruetten H. Sensitization of upper airway mechanoreceptors as a new pharmacologic principle to treat obstructive sleep apnea: investigations with AVE0118 in anesthetized pigs. Sleep 2013;36(5):699–708.
97. Gaisl T, Turnbull CD, Weimann G, et al. BAY 2253651 for the treatment of obstructive sleep apnoea: a multicentre, double-blind, randomised controlled trial (SANDMAN). Eur Respir J 2021;58(5). https://doi.org/10.1183/13993003.01937-2021.
98. Carley DW, Paviovic S, Janelidze M, et al. Functional role for cannabinoids in respiratory stability during sleep. Sleep 2002;25(4):391–8.
99. Prasad B, Radulovacki MG, Carley DW. Proof of concept trial of dronabinol in obstructive sleep apnea. Front Psychiatry 2013;4:1. https://doi.org/10.3389/fpsyt.2013.00001.
100. Carley DW, Prasad B, Reid KJ, et al. Pharmacotherapy of apnea by Cannabimimetic Enhancement, the PACE clinical trial: effects of dronabinol in obstructive sleep apnea. Sleep 2018;41(1). https://doi.org/10.1093/sleep/zsx184.
101. Ramar K, Rosen IM, Kirsch DB, et al. Medical cannabis and the treatment of obstructive sleep apnea: an American Academy of sleep medicine position Statement. J Clin Sleep Med 2018;14(4):679–81.
102. Mulloy E, McNicholas WT. Theophylline in obstructive sleep apnea. A double-blind evaluation. Chest 1992;101(3):753–7.
103. Saletu B, Oberndorfer S, Anderer P, et al. Efficiency of continuous positive airway pressure versus theophylline therapy in sleep apnea: comparative sleep laboratory studies on objective and subjective sleep and awakening quality. Neuropsychobiology 1999;39(3):151–9.
104. Hein H, Behnke G, Jorres RA, et al. The therapeutic effect of theophylline in mild obstructive sleep Apnea/Hypopnea syndrome: results of repeated measurements with portable recording devices at home. Eur J Med Res 2000;5(9):391–9.
105. Orth MM, Grootoonk S, Duchna HW, et al. Short-term effects of oral theophylline in addition to CPAP in mild to moderate OSAS. Respir Med 2005;99(4):471–6.
106. Jokic R, Klimaszewski A, Mink J, et al. Surface tension forces in sleep apnea: the role of a soft tissue lubricant: a randomized double-blind, placebo-controlled trial. Am J Respir Crit Care Med 1998;157(5 Pt 1):1522–5.
107. Morrell MJ, Arabi Y, Zahn BR, et al. Effect of surfactant on pharyngeal mechanics in sleeping humans: implications for sleep apnoea. Eur Respir J 2002;20(2):451–7.
108. Kirkness JP, Madronio M, Stavrinou R, et al. Relationship between surface tension of upper airway lining liquid and upper airway collapsibility during sleep in obstructive sleep apnea hypopnea syndrome. J Appl Physiol (1985) 2003;95(5):1761–6.
109. Kiely JL, Nolan P, McNicholas WT. Intranasal corticosteroid therapy for obstructive sleep apnoea in patients with co-existing rhinitis. Thorax 2004;59(1):50–5.
110. Taranto-Montemurro L, Sands S, Azarbarzin A, et al. Impact of cold and flu medication on obstructive sleep apnoea and its underlying traits: a pilot randomized controlled trial. Respirology 2021;26(5):485–92.
111. Popovic RM, White DP. Upper airway muscle activity in normal women: influence of hormonal status. J Appl Physiol (1985) 1998;84(3):1055–62.
112. Martins FO, Conde SV. Gender differences in the context of obstructive sleep apnea and metabolic diseases. Front Physiol 2021;12:792633.
113. Hedner J, Grote L, Zou D. Pharmacological treatment of sleep apnea: current situation and future strategies. Sleep Med Rev 2008;12(1):33–47.
114. Gasa M, Tamisier R, Launois SH, et al. Residual sleepiness in sleep apnea patients treated by continuous positive airway pressure. J Sleep Res 2013;22(4):389–97.

115. Javaheri S, Javaheri S. Update on persistent excessive daytime sleepiness in OSA. Chest 2020;158(2):776–86.
116. Chapman JL, Vakulin A, Hedner J, et al. Modafinil/armodafinil in obstructive sleep apnoea: a systematic review and meta-analysis. Eur Respir J 2016;47(5):1420–8.
117. Williams SC, Marshall NS, Kennerson M, et al. Modafinil effects during acute continuous positive airway pressure withdrawal: a randomized crossover double-blind placebo-controlled trial. Am J Respir Crit Care Med 2010;181(8):825–31.
118. Roth T, White D, Schmidt-Nowara W, et al. Effects of armodafinil in the treatment of residual excessive sleepiness associated with obstructive sleep apnea/hypopnea syndrome: a 12-week, multicenter, double-blind, randomized, placebo-controlled study in nCPAP-adherent adults. Clin Ther 2006;28(5):689–706.
119. Dauvilliers Y, Bassetti C, Lammers GJ, et al. Pitolisant versus placebo or modafinil in patients with narcolepsy: a double-blind, randomised trial. Lancet Neurol 2013;12(11):1068–75.
120. Dauvilliers Y, Verbraecken J, Partinen M, et al. Pitolisant for daytime sleepiness in patients with obstructive sleep apnea who Refuse continuous positive airway pressure treatment. A randomized trial. Am J Respir Crit Care Med 2020;201(9):1135–45.
121. Pepin JL, Georgiev O, Tiholov R, et al. Pitolisant for residual excessive daytime sleepiness in OSA patients adhering to CPAP: a randomized trial. Chest 2021;159(4):1598–609.
122. Available at: https://www.ema.europa.eu/en/medicines/human/EPAR/ozawade. Accessed January 06 2022.
123. Thorpy MJ, Shapiro C, Mayer G, et al. A randomized study of solriamfetol for excessive sleepiness in narcolepsy. Ann Neurol 2019;85(3):359–70.
124. Schweitzer PK, Rosenberg R, Zammit GK, et al. Solriamfetol for excessive sleepiness in obstructive sleep apnea (TONES 3). A randomized controlled trial. Am J Respir Crit Care Med 2019;199(11):1421–31.
125. Schweitzer PK, Mayer G, Rosenberg R, et al. Randomized controlled trial of solriamfetol for excessive daytime sleepiness in OSA: an analysis of subgroups adherent or Nonadherent to OSA treatment. Chest 2021;160(1):307–18.
126. Ronnebaum S, Bron M, Patel D, et al. Indirect treatment comparison of solriamfetol, modafinil, and armodafinil for excessive daytime sleepiness in obstructive sleep apnea. J Clin Sleep Med 2021;17(12):2543–55.
127. Malhotra A, Shapiro C, Pepin JL, et al. Long-term study of the safety and maintenance of efficacy of solriamfetol (JZP-110) in the treatment of excessive sleepiness in participants with narcolepsy or obstructive sleep apnea. Sleep 2020;43(2). https://doi.org/10.1093/sleep/zsz220.
128. Young T, Palta M, Dempsey J, et al. The occurrence of sleep-disordered breathing among middle-aged adults. N Engl J Med 1993;328(17):1230–5.
129. Young T, Peppard PE, Gottlieb DJ. Epidemiology of obstructive sleep apnea: a population health perspective. Am J Respir Crit Care Med 2002;165(9):1217–39.
130. Blackman A, Foster GD, Zammit G, et al. Effect of liraglutide 3.0 mg in individuals with obesity and moderate or severe obstructive sleep apnea: the SCALE Sleep Apnea randomized clinical trial. Int J Obes (Lond) 2016;40(8):1310–9.
131. Drager LF, Brunoni AR, Jenner R, et al. Effects of CPAP on body weight in patients with obstructive sleep apnoea: a meta-analysis of randomised trials. Thorax 2015;70(3):258–64.
132. Herculano S, Grad GF, Drager LF, et al. Weight gain induced by continuous positive airway pressure in patients with obstructive sleep apnea is mediated by fluid accumulation: a randomized crossover controlled trial. Am J Respir Crit Care Med 2021;203(1):134–6.
133. Hedner J, Grote L, Bonsignore M, et al. The European Sleep Apnoea Database (ESADA): report from 22 European sleep laboratories. Eur Respir J 2011;38(3):635–42.
134. Williams B, Mancia G, Spiering W, et al. ESC/ESH Guidelines for the management of arterial hypertension. Eur Heart J 2018;39(33):3021–104.
135. Garpestad E, Basner RC, Ringler J, et al. Phenylephrine-induced hypertension acutely decreases genioglossus EMG activity in awake humans. J Appl Physiol (1985) 1992;72(1):110–5.
136. Mayer J, Weichler U, Herres-Mayer B, et al. Influence of metoprolol and cilazapril on blood pressure and on sleep apnea activity. J Cardiovasc Pharmacol 1990;16(6):952–61.
137. Planes C, Foucher A, Leroy M, et al. Effect of celiprolol treatment in hypertensive patients with sleep apnea. Sleep 1999;22(4):507–13.
138. Grote L, Wutkewicz K, Knaack L, et al. Association between blood pressure reduction with antihypertensive treatment and sleep apnea activity. Am J Hypertens 2000;13(12):1280–7.
139. Pepin JL, Tamisier R, Barone-Rochette G, et al. Comparison of continuous positive airway pressure and valsartan in hypertensive patients with sleep apnea. Am J Respir Crit Care Med 2010;182(7):954–60.
140. Kraiczi H, Hedner J, Peker Y, et al. Comparison of atenolol, amlodipine, enalapril, hydrochlorothiazide, and losartan for antihypertensive treatment

in patients with obstructive sleep apnea. Am J Respir Crit Care Med 2000;161(5):1423–8.
141. Khurshid K, Yabes J, Weiss PM, et al. Effect of antihypertensive medications on the severity of obstructive sleep apnea: a systematic review and meta-analysis. J Clin Sleep Med 2016;12(8):1143–51.
142. Kasai T, Bradley TD, Friedman O, et al. Effect of intensified diuretic therapy on overnight rostral fluid shift and obstructive sleep apnoea in patients with uncontrolled hypertension. J Hypertens 2014;32(3):673–80.
143. Gaddam K, Pimenta E, Thomas SJ, et al. Spironolactone reduces severity of obstructive sleep apnoea in patients with resistant hypertension: a preliminary report. J Hum Hypertens 2010;24(8):532–7.
144. Wu ZH, Yang XP, Niu X, et al. The relationship between obstructive sleep apnea hypopnea syndrome and gastroesophageal reflux disease: a meta-analysis. Sleep Breath 2019;23(2):389–97.
145. Schuitenmaker JM, van Dijk M, Oude Nijhuis RAB, et al. Associations between sleep position and nocturnal gastroesophageal reflux: a study using Concurrent monitoring of sleep position and Esophageal pH and Impedance. Am J Gastroenterol 2022;117(2):346–51.
146. Friedman M, Gurpinar B, Lin HC, et al. Impact of treatment of gastroesophageal reflux on obstructive sleep apnea-hypopnea syndrome. Ann Otol Rhinol Laryngol 2007;116(11):805–11.
147. Ing AJ, Ngu MC, Breslin AB. Obstructive sleep apnea and gastroesophageal reflux. Am J Med 2000;108(Suppl 4a):120S–5S.
148. Senior BA, Khan M, Schwimmer C, et al. Gastroesophageal reflux and obstructive sleep apnea. Laryngoscope 2001;111(12):2144–6.
149. Orr WC, Robert JJ, Houck JR, et al. The effect of acid suppression on upper airway anatomy and obstruction in patients with sleep apnea and gastroesophageal reflux disease. J Clin Sleep Med 2009;5(4):330–4.

Drug-Induced Insomnia and Excessive Sleepiness

Ann Van Gastel, MD[a,b,*]

KEYWORDS

• Drugs • Medication • Psychotropic • Nonpsychotropic • Sleep • Insomnia • Sedation • Sleepiness

KEY POINTS

- Undesirable side effects of insomnia and/or sleepiness may occur with many prescribed drugs, psychotropics as well as nonpsychotropics.
- These central nervous system effects can be explained by the interactions of a drug with any of the numerous neurotransmitters and receptors that are involved in sleep and wakefulness.
- A close—sometimes bidirectional—relationship between disease and (disturbed) sleep/wakefulness is often present. Drug effects may increase the complexity of this interaction.
- Effects of disease and/or drugs on sleep and wakefulness may create a vicious circle, influencing health and quality of life.
- Direct and indirect effects of drugs on the disease as well as on sleep and wakefulness need to be weighed.

INTRODUCTION

Sleep and waking function are closely connected in a 24-hour rhythm. The central nervous system (CNS) structures involved in the promotion of the waking state include neurons containing serotonin (5-HT), norepinephrine (NE), dopamine (DA), acetylcholine (ACh), histamine (HA), orexin (OX), and glutamate (GLU). Selective activation of either DA receptor D_1 or D_2; 5-HT receptors 5-HT_1,5-HT_{2A}, 5-HT_{2C}, 5-HT_6, and 5-HT_7 ; NE α_1 receptor; HA H_1 receptor; ACh m_1 receptor; OX OX_1 and OX_2 receptors; or GLU AMPA, kainate and NMDA receptors increases wake and reduces non-rapid eye movement (REM) and REM sleep.[1] Neurons that constitute the non-REM sleep-inducing system contain γ-aminobutyric acid (GABA) and galanin and inhibit cells involved in the promotion of wake. Somnogens, including adenosine, prostaglandin D_2, nitric oxide, and cytokines, also promote sleep, mainly non-REM sleep, in humans.[2] The REM sleep induction regions include predominantly glutamatergic neurons.[3]

Many drugs have the potential to disrupt sleep and waking function due to their pharmacologic effects at any of the numerous receptors and neurotransmitters involved in sleep–wake regulation. As such, insomnia and/or daytime sleepiness are common side effects of psychotropic as well as nonpsychotropic medication. The lipophilicity, which determines the easiness with which a drug crosses the blood–brain barrier (BBB), and the receptor binding profile determine its possible CNS effects.

There are some general considerations to take into account. First, there can be beneficial as well as adverse effects of drugs on sleep and

There are no conflicts of interest. There are no funding sources.
Sleep Med Clin 13 (2018) 147-159 https://doi.org/10.1016/j.jsmc.2018.02.001 1556-407X/18/

[a] Multidisciplinary Sleep Disorders Centre and University Department of Psychiatry, Antwerp University Hospital, Drie Eikenstraat 655, 2650 Edegem, Antwerp, Belgium; [b] Faculty of Medicine and Health Sciences, Collaborative Antwerp Psychiatric Research Institute (CAPRI), University of Antwerp (UA), Campus Drie Eiken, Universiteitsplein 1, 2610 Wilrijk, Antwerp, Belgium
* Drie Eikenstraat 655, 2650 Edegem, Antwerp, Belgium.
E-mail address: Ann.Van.Gastel@uza.be

Sleep Med Clin 17 (2022) 471–484
https://doi.org/10.1016/j.jsmc.2022.06.011
1556-407X/22/

wakefulness (**Table 1**). The effects may be desired when a drug is prescribed with the goal of creating sleep (eg, hypnotics) or alertness (eg, stimulants). When the desired effects go on too long, however, they become undesired; for example, hangover effects of hypnotics or insomnia complaints provoked by a stimulant. Second, knowing how a good sleep is necessary for optimal functioning and well-being, drug effects may have far-reaching consequences. Effects on sleep quality or on sleep duration also affect daytime functioning. When a patient presents with daytime sleepiness, it may be either a direct effect of a drug or an indirect effect as the consequence of a disturbed sleep. Third, the mechanisms by which (un)wanted effects occur vary. They may directly affect the CNS (e.g. drugs that stimulate the serotonergic system may disrupt sleep) or indirectly (e.g. causing or aggravating conditions that disturb sleep such as restless legs syndrome [RLS] or periodic limb movement disorder [PLMD]). The effects may be more or less obvious when sleep is interrupted by periods of wakefulness than when sleep architecture as registered by polysomnography is disturbed. Finally, the effects can be present in cases of administration of a drug (e.g. sedative effect) or withdrawal of a drug (e.g. rebound insomnia).

In this article, several classes of pharmacologic agents and individual drugs are discussed, mainly regarding their effects of inducing or aggravating insomnia and/or daytime somnolence. Due to the overlap of terms used in studies and in clinical practice, the terms, *sedation*, *(daytime) sleepiness*, and *(hyper-)somnolence*, are used interchangeably.

ANTIDEPRESSANTS

Antidepressants (ADs) are mainly used for the treatment of depression. Some ADs are also used in other conditions such as anxiety disorders, obsessive-compulsive disorder, eating disorders, and primary headache disorder, or in the treatment of chronic pain. Sedating ADs are used off-label for the treatment of chronic insomnia. ADs may alter sleep patterns both indirectly (i.e. by their effect on an underlying depression and the associated sleep abnormalities) and through direct effects on sleep. A close, bidirectional relationship between insomnia and depression is clearly demonstrated.[4]

ADs can be divided into 3 main classes, according to their major action mechanism.[5] The largest group of ADs consists of monoamine reuptake inhibitors. These agents increase the amount of monoamines in the synapse by inhibiting mainly the reuptake of serotonin and/or NE. Monoamine oxidase inhibitors (MAOIs) also increase the level of serotonin and/or NE (and to a lesser extent DA) by preventing breakdown by the monoamine oxidase (MAO) enzyme. A third diverse group of compounds has complex effects on monoamine mechanisms but shares the ability to block 5-HT_2 receptors.

Depending on their acute pharmacologic properties, effects of ADs on sleep and daytime alertness are variable. Acute effects of ADs on sleep not only are reflected in patients' subjective complaints but also can be demonstrated in studies with PSG.[6]

Monoamine Reuptake Inhibitors

The monoamine reuptake inhibitors class of ADs includes tricyclic ADs (TCAs) and the newer, more selective reuptake inhibitors, which also potently inhibit the presynaptic uptake of serotonin and/or NE and/or DA but exert relatively weak effects on other neurotransmitter/receptor systems.

Tricyclic Antidepressants

TCAs inhibit the reuptake of both serotonin and NE but TCAs are nonspecific monoamine reuptake inhibitors. They also have antagonist activities at a variety of neurotransmitter receptors, such as NE α_1, HA $H_1$and ACh receptors, which are associated with many side effects, including sedative effects. TCAs demonstrate wide intraclass variability with respect to effects on nocturnal sleep and daytime sleepiness. Tertiary amine TCAs (e.g. amitriptyline and trimipramine) tend to be more sedating, whereas secondary amine TCAs (desipramine and nortriptyline) tend to be more activating.[7] The TCA doxepin is Food and Drug Administration approved for the treatment of maintenance insomnia in very low doses of 3 mg and 6 mg. These low doses are presumed to promote sleep by antagonizing only the HA-based arousal pathways without any other receptor effects.[8]

Selective Serotonin Reuptake Inhibitors

Selective serotonin reuptake inhibitors (SSRIs), such as (es)citalopram, fluoxetine, fluvoxamine, paroxetine, and sertraline, potently inhibit the presynaptic uptake of serotonin while exerting relatively weak effects on other neurotransmitter/receptor systems. Based on data from a Food and Drug Administration study register,[6,7] the highest rates of treatment-emergent insomnia and somnolence with SSRIs were found in patients suffering from obsessive-compulsive disorder treated with high-dose fluvoxamine, 31% and 27%, respectively. The lowest rate of treatment-

Table 1
Drug-induced adverse effects of insomnia or sleepiness with possible mechanism of action

Drug Class or Individual Drug	Induced Sleep–Wake Disturbance	Possible Mechanism of Action
ANTIDEPRESSANTS		
Sedating TCA (e.g. amitriptyline,doxepin)	Sleepiness	Antagonism at NE α_1, HA H_1, and ACh receptors
Activating TCA	Insomnia	Inhibition of serotonin and NE reuptake
SSRI	Insomnia	Inhibition of serotonin and NE reuptake
SNRI	Insomnia	Inhibition of serotonin and NE reuptake
Bupropion	Insomnia	Inhibition of NE and DA reuptake
MAOI	Insomnia	Inhibition of MAO enzyme
Atypical sedating AD (e.g. trazodone, mirtazapine)	Sleepiness	Antihistaminergic effect, 5-HT_2- receptor antagonism
ANTIPSYCHOTICS		
First generation	Mostly sleepiness, insomnia also reported	Antagonism at NE α_1, HA H_1, ACh, and DA receptors
Second generation, e.g. clozapine, olanzapine, quetiapine	Variable effects Sleepiness	DA-receptor and 5-HT-receptor antagonism; effects at other receptors vary for each agent
ANTIEPILEPTICS	Mostly sleepiness	Decreased neuronal excitation by variable mechanisms
ANTIPARKINSONIAN AGENTS		
DA replacement drugs	Low-dose sleepiness, high-dose insomnia	DA-receptor agonism
ANALGETICS		
NSAIDs		Prostaglandin synthesis inhibition
Opioids	Sleepiness	μ-opioid and κ-opioid receptor agonism
Triptans	Sleepiness?	5-HT_1-receptor antagonism
ANTIHISTAMINES		
First generation	Sleepiness	Antagonism at HA H_1 receptor
Second generation	None to mild sleepiness	None to little BBB transport
CARDIOVASCULAR DRUGS		
β-Blocking agents	Insomnia	β receptor and 5-HT-receptor antagonism; melatonin suppression
β-blocking and α_1-blocking agents	Insomnia, also sleepiness reported	β and 5-HT receptor antagonism; melatonin suppression; α_1-receptor antagonism
α_1 Antagonists		α_1-receptor antagonism
α_2 Agonist		α_2-receptor stimulation
Angiotensin Converting Enzyme Inhibitors		Interfering dry cough

(*continued on next page*)

Table 1
(*continued*)

Drug Class or Individual Drug	Induced Sleep–Wake Disturbance	Possible Mechanism of Action
Angiotensin receptor blockers		?
Loop diuretics	Insomnia	Nocturia
CORTICOSTEROIDS	Insomnia, sleepiness also reported	Multiple effects on HPA-axis; effects on cytokines
THEOPHYLLINE	Insomnia?	Adenosine antagonist

emergent insomnia complaints (less than 2%) was reported with citalopram. The average prevalence of treatment-emergent insomnia in clinical trials with SSRI was 17% compared with 9% of patients randomized to the placebo arm. The average rate of treatment-emergent somnolence in patients treated with SSRI amounted to 16% compared with 8% of patients receiving placebo.[6,7]

Serotonin-Norepinephrine Reuptake Inhibitors

Venlafaxine and duloxetine are serotonin-NE reuptake inhibitors (SNRIs). They are associated with frequent subjective complaints of insomnia and daytime somnolence as well as vivid dreams.[7] In clinical trials with SNRIs, both treatment-emergent insomnia and somnolence were the most frequent (both equal to 24%) in patients with generalized anxiety disorders treated with venlafaxine. Treatment-emergent insomnia was reported on average in 13% of SNRI-treated patients compared with 7% of the placebo arm. Treatment-emergent somnolence was reported on average in 10% of SNRI-treated patients in comparison to 5% of patients receiving placebo.[7]

Norepinephrine Reuptake Inhibitor

Reboxetine is the only available NE reuptake inhibitor (NRI). There is a dearth of studies reporting the incidence of side effects of insomnia/hypersomnolence with reboxetine.[9]

Norepinephrine-Dopamine Reuptake Inhibitor

Bupropion is the only representative exerting NE and DA reuptake inhibitor (NDRI). Besides its approval as an AD, it is also registered in the United States as an aid for smoking cessation and seasonal affective disorder.

Bupropion is associated with reports of insomnia in patients treated for depression and seasonal affective disorder, with rates ranging from 11% to 20% depending on the dose, formulation, and condition treated.[7] Bupropion is one of the few ADs that shortens REM latency and increases total REM sleep time.[10] This finding is in contrast to most other ADs, which are prominent suppressants of REM sleep.[11]

Monoamine Oxidase Inhibitors

Drugs belonging to this class of ADs act as MAOIs. They deactivate MAO irreversibly (eg, phenelzine and tranylcypromine) or reversibly (moclobemide). Treatment with MAOIs is associated with frequent complaints of insomnia.[7]

5-HT$_2$ Antagonists

This class of ADs constitutes a diverse group of drugs (mirtazapine, mianserine, trazodone, and agomelatine), which share the ability to block 5-HT$_2$ receptors.

In clinical studies with mirtazapine, 54% of patients reported hypersomnolence compared with 18% of patients in the placebo arm. Mirtazapine produces predominantly antihistaminergic effects at lower doses (<30 mg/d) compared with increasingly predominant noradrenergic effects at higher doses.[6]

In clinical studies with trazodone, the reported prevalence of treatment-emergent insomnia complaints in patients with major depressive disorder was very low (less than 2%) but the rate of treatment-emergent somnolence was very high: 46% in patients treated with trazodone compared with 19% of patients receiving placebo. It is common knowledge in clinical practice that the use of trazodone as an AD is often limited by its tendency to produce daytime somnolence. In that respect, it is often used, at low doses, as a sleep aid although this effect has not been well studied.[7]

Agomelatine is a nonsedative AD drug exerting agonistic action at melatonergic M_1 and M_2

receptors and antagonistic action at serotonergic 5-HT2c receptors.

In summary, ADs are associated with different insomnia and somnolence rates, with class-specific or drug-specific effects depending on their mechanisms of action. Some ADs may deteriorate sleep quality mainly due to activation of serotonergic 5-HT_2 receptors and increased noradrenergic and dopaminergic neurotransmission. Among them, most prominent are SNRIs, NRIs, NDRIs, MAOIs, SSRIs, and activating TCAs. However, ADs with antihistaminergic action, such as sedating TCAs, mirtazapine, and mianserine, or strong antagonistic action at serotonergic 5-HT2 receptors, such as trazodone, quickly improve sleep.[6]

In a meta-analysis of occurring insomnia and somnolence with 14 newer, more selective acting ADs during the treatment of major depression, the highest incidence of insomnia was found for bupropion and desvenlafaxine. Agomelatin was the only AD with a lower likelihood of inducing insomnia than placebo. Fluvoxamine and mirtazapine showed the highest frequency of somnolence. Bupropion induced somnolence to a lower extent than placebo.[9]

Most ADs with strong serotonergic action can cause or exacerbate restless legs or periodic limb movements and may cause insomnia and/or hypersomnolence indirectly through these effects.

Withdrawal effects that occur after long-term treatment with most ADs include insomnia, nightmares, and excessive dreaming related to REM rebound.[12]

ANTIPSYCHOTICS

Antipsychotics (APs) are mainly used for the treatment of psychotic disorders and schizophrenia.

APs are divided into typical, or first-generation, APs (FGAs) and the newer atypical, or second-generation, APs (SGAs).[13] Some of the newer atypical APs are also approved for the treatment of bipolar disorder or as an adjunctive treatment of major depression. APs have direct effects on sleep as well as the ability to promote sleep by attenuating symptoms that interfere with sleep, such as psychosis and agitation.

AP effects are mainly exerted by DA receptor antagonism. Many FGAs also exert effects on various monoamines as well as on HA, ACh, and/or NE α_1 receptors. These effects may increase the likelihood of somnolence.[7] FGAs are associated with side effects of extrapyramidal symptoms (EPs) at clinically AP effective dosages. The SGAs—also described as serotonin-DA antagonists—differ from FGAs by their higher ratio interactions with serotonin receptor subtypes, notably the 5-HT_{2A} subtype, as well as with other neurotransmitter systems. All SGAs have different chemical structures, receptor affinities, and side-effect profiles, which are hypothesized to account for the distinct tolerability profiles associated with each of them. SGAs cause fewer EPs but have the propensity to cause weight gain, lipid elevations, and diabetes.[13]

First-Generation Antipsychotics

Among the FGAs, very high rates of somnolence are reported for chlorpromazine (33%) and thioridazine (35%–57%), as well as for haloperidol (23%). Insomnia/disturbed sleep is also reported with haloperidol and thioridazine by approximately one-quarter of patients.[14]

Second-Generation Antipsychotics

The highest rate of somnolence, in 52% of patients, is reported for clozapine. Insomnia/disturbed sleep was reported in only 4% of patients.[14] Somnolence was also frequently reported with risperidone (30%) and olanzapine (29%) and moderately frequent with quetiapine and ziprasidone (16%). Although ziprasidone and quetiapine are expected to be sedating given their pharmacologic profiles, they seem less sedating than other drugs, possibly because of their short half-lives. Aripiprazole is least sedating (12%).[14]

In a study comparing somnolence associated with asenapine, olanzapine, risperidone, and haloperidol relative to placebo, only asenapine and olanzapine had significantly higher rates of somnolence relative to placebo.[15]

Objective measures of daytime sleepiness are rare. Both clozapine and olanzapine, however, reduce multiple sleep latency test (MSLT) results in schizophrenic patients.[16] A placebo-controlled study showed increased Epworth sleepiness scale scores with quetiapine but not with lurasidone in patients with acute schizophrenia.[17]

Among the SGAs, insomnia is highest, with aripiprazole reported in approximately one-quarter of patients. Insomnia is also reported with risperidone (17%) and olanzapine (18%) and in 9% of patients with quetiapine and ziprasidone. Suggested possible mechanisms for this reported insomnia include 5-HT_{1A}-receptor agonism and RLS symptoms secondary to dopaminergic antagonism. Moreover, the 5 agents with the highest incidence of EPs—haloperidol, thioridazine, aripiprazole, risperidone, and olanzapine—have the 5 highest rates of sleep disturbance.[14]

In a 14-day randomized controlled trial PSG study evaluating the effects of paliperidone extended release in patients with schizophrenia-related insomnia, an improved sleep architecture and sleep continuity was found.[18] In another trial, single arm, with longer duration, insomnia was the most common adverse event, occurring in 17.9% of patients treated with paliperidone.[19]

A low-dose quetiapine is increasingly used off-label for the treatment of chronic insomnia. Quetiapine exhibits strong H_1-receptor antagonism and moderate affinity for $5\text{-}HT_{2A}$ receptors. Antagonism at these sites is thought to be responsible for sedative effects of quetiapine.[7] In an open-label pilot study,[20] 18 adults with insomnia were treated with quetiapine, 25 mg at bedtime, with dosages increased to 50 mg in 7 patients and 75 mg in 1 patient. There were improvements in subjective and objective sleep parameters after 2 weeks that continued at 6 weeks. Transient morning hangover was a frequently reported adverse effect.

ANTIEPILEPTICS

The mechanism of action of antiepileptic drugs (AEDs) is via facilitation of GABA, sodium and calcium channel inhibition, inhibition of glutaminergic transmission, or other unknown mechanisms.[21] In addition to the treatment of epilepsy, several AEDs are used in other diseases, for example, in bipolar disorders or chronic pain conditions. Topiramate is used for the treatment of sleep-related eating disorder.

Antiepileptic Drugs in the Treatment of Epilepsy

Sleep and epilepsy have reciprocal effects because sleep is a strong modulator of epileptic activity. Most seizures occur during non-REM sleep; seizures are rare in REM sleep.

Poor sleep quality or quantity induces worsened seizure control, which in turn deteriorates sleep. Hence, a vicious circle is established.[22] Sleep disruption may be caused by seizures, anticonvulsants, or a coexisting sleep disorder. Patients with epilepsy are particularly sensitive to the adverse effects of sleep disruption.[23] In addition, most AEDs affect sleep architecture. These effects may be mediated by mechanism of action or may be indirectly due to treatment effects on epileptic phenomena.[24] Moreover, sleep disorders are common in epilepsy, and many of them have a higher prevalence in patients with epilepsy than in the general population. Treatment of them may improve seizure control. In adults with epilepsy, 40% to 55% of patients had insomnia, whereas 28% to 48% of patients with epilepsy reports daytime sleepiness.[22]

Sleepiness is one of the most commonly reported adverse effects of AEDs. In general, drugs acting on GABAergic neurotransmission (benzodiazepines, barbiturates, tiagabine, and vigabatrin) have the highest reported incidence of sleepiness or fatigue, amounting to 15% to 30% or more.[25] Placebo-controlled trials showed no difference between tiagabine and placebo in the incidence of sedation but open-label long-term studies showed a 25% incidence of sedation with tiagabine.[26] Drugs acting primarily through sodium channel blockade (carbamazepine and phenytoin) show an incidence of sedation of 5% to 10%.[25] Drugs acting via calcium blockade or with multiple mechanisms of action show varying incidence of sedation: rates of 5% to 15% were reported for gabapentin (GBP), lamotrigine, pregabalin (PGB), and zonisamide. For levetiracetam and topiramate, sedation incidence of 15% to 27% was reported.[25]

Insomnia has been reported with lamotrigine.[27]

Compared with healthy controls or untreated patients with epilepsy, patients on phenobarbital, carbamazepine, phenytoin, or valproate have shown increased sleepiness on MSLT or decreased alertness on a maintenance of wakefulness test.[28]

In a review of objective sleep metrics,[24] daytime sleepiness was found not changed by topiramate, lamotrigine, zonisamide, and vigabatrin in patients with epilepsy but was increased by phenobarbital. Daytime sleepiness was unchanged at 1000 mg daily dose for levetiracetam but increased at 2000 mg daily dose. Other studies showed subjective sleepiness with zonisamide[29] and topiramate.[30] The not straightforward results from different studies may be related to several factors. Patients with epilepsy report increased sleepiness, so it is possible that this was attributed to treatment. Moreover, patients who reported sleepiness subjectively may not have objective sleepiness.[24]

In reports of impaired driving, the use of anticonvulsants has been associated with an almost doubled risk of collision rate. Some studies in epileptic patients, however, have commented on the benefit of therapy. Because preventing seizures on the road reduce the incidence of collision, optimal therapy is the key. A large multicenter study discovered higher crash rates in patients not taking their AEDs appropriately compared with medication-adherent patients. This highlights the complex relationships between disease and risks as well as pharmacotherapy and risks. So considering driving ability in epileptic patients, outweighing the decreased risk of collusion against possible sedative effects of AEDs is essential.[31]

Antiepileptic Drugs in the Treatment of Other Disorders

GBP and PGB are newer antiepileptic agents that share some aspects of their mechanism of action. They are presumed to work via the $\alpha_2\delta$ S unit of voltage-gated calcium channels, binding to which reduces calcium influx that decreases the release of several excitatory neurotransmitters.[21] GBP and PGB are approved for the treatment of neuropathic pain. Sedation is reported to occur in 15% to 25% of patients using these drugs to treat neuropathic pain.[28] GBP and PGB also are a recognized treatment of RLS/PLMD.[32] PGB is also indicated for the treatment of generalized anxiety disorder.

ANTIPARKINSON DRUGS

The primary treatment of Parkinson disease (PD) is DA replacement. Levodopa and DA agonists (e.g. pramipexole, ropinirole, and rotigotine) are the principal drugs used. Adjunctive treatments include, among others, dopamine decarboxylase inhibitors (carbidopa and benserazide), which prevent peripheral conversion of levodopa to DA; catechol-O-methyltransferase inhibitors (entacapone and tolcapone), which prolong the duration of the effect of levodopa; and MAO-B inhibitors (selegiline and rasagiline), which block the breakdown of DA.[33]

Sleep disorders are among the most common nonmotor manifestations in PD. Most frequently reported are insomnia, REM sleep behavior disorder, RLS, sleep-disordered breathing, and excessive daytime sleepiness (EDS).[34] Multiple causes for these sleep-related complaints are possible: abnormalities in sleep–wake regulation caused by the disease; motor symptoms, such as rigidity, tremor, dystonia, and poor bed mobility; other sleep disorders; concurrent medical or psychiatric illness; or the medications used for the treatment. As such, it is difficult to determine whether changes in sleep and waking behavior after drug administration are due to the direct effects of a drug or the indirect effects of a drug on the disease.[25]

It is suggested that low doses of dopaminergic medications tend to improve sleep whereas higher doses are likely to disrupt sleep.[34] An increased risk of insomnia compared with placebo was reported in randomized controlled trials for DA agonists, for DA agonist withdrawal, for selegiline and rasagiline (although some data suggest otherwise for rasagiline), and for entacapone. Higher total levodopa equivalent dose and levodopa equivalent dose contributed by DA agonists have been associated with worse measures of subjective and objective sleep in PD. Benefits on motor symptoms have to be weighed against risks of worsening insomnia due to dopaminergic stimulation. Drug-related improvement in PD symptoms may outweigh the sleep-disrupting effects of the drug, resulting in an improvement in sleep overall. Additionally, sleep dysfunction can be associated with and influence motor and nonmotor symptoms in this patient population.[35]

EDS is also common among patients with PD. EDS is more likely to affect patients with advanced PD.[35] Several studies also support a relationship between dopaminergic therapy and EDS. Levodopa equivalent dose independently predicts subjective sleepiness and subjective sleepiness correlated with the use of DA agonists. Sudden-onset sleep episodes are more likely among patients on DA agonists. However, some studies do not support a relationship between dopaminergic therapy and EDS.[35] No increased EDS compared with placebo was shown for rasagiline. In an open-label study, selegiline in combination with reduction or discontinuation of DA agonists led to the reduction or resolution of somnolence in 94% subjects with EDS.

ANALGESICS

In patients with chronic pain, a vicious circle often develops, with pain disrupting sleep and poor sleep further exacerbating pain.[4] Improving sleep quantity and quality in patients with pain may break this vicious circle and as a consequence enhance a patient's overall health and quality of life. Therefore, when using an analgetic, it seems important to know the effects on sleep.[21]

Nonsteroidal Anti-inflammatory Drugs

Nonsteroidal anti-inflammatory drugs (NSAIDs) are among the most commonly used analgesics.

Their therapeutic action is largely due to the inhibition of the 2 isoenzymes of cyclo-oxygenase (COX), COX-1 and COX-2, which are important for the production of prostaglandins. Prostaglandins play a role in regulation of sleep and wakefulness.[36] Prostaglandin D_2 increases proportionately with increased duration of wake and may be involved in sleep initiation.[37] Proposed possible underlying mechanisms of sleep disruption after NSAID intake may relate to the direct and indirect consequences of inhibiting prostaglandin synthesis, including decrease of prostaglandin D_2, reduced melatonin secretion, and modification of body temperature.[38,39]

PSG studies about the influence of NSAIDs on sleep are limited and results are mixed. In healthy patients, acetaminophen does not seem to change sleep structure. For ibuprofen and aspirin, no effects[40] to delayed sleep onset, increased wake after sleep onset, increased stage 2 sleep, decreased slow-wave sleep, and reduced sleep efficiency[39,41] were reported. A study on the effect of tenoxicam on patients with rheumatoid arthritis reported improvement in pain but no changes in PSG parameters during 90 days of treatment.[42] A trial on women with dysmenorrhea treated with therapeutic doses of diclofenac reported subjective and objective improvement in sleep, including sleep quality, sleep efficiency, REM sleep, and a reduction of stage 1 sleep.[43]

Opioids

Opioids are used as major analgetics. Their effects are mediated by specific opioid receptors of which major types are described: mu (μ), kappa (κ), and delta (Δ).[36] Centrally occurring opioids bind to these receptors to exert control over various biological systems, including pain regulation and the sleep–wake cycle. The effect of opioids on the sleep–wake cycle is believed controlled by opioid receptors, their indirect actions on GABAergic transmission, and other neurotransmitter systems and neuromodulators, such as adenosine. One of the mechanisms by which opioids are said to disrupt sleep is through their effects on the availability of adenosine in sites that are important in REM and non-REM sleep.[44]

Somnolence is a common side effect of opioid medication.[28] It varies with used dose, duration of use, age, and underlying disease.[28] The sedative effects may lead to the impression that they promote sleep. On the contrary, opioids have been shown to decrease both REM sleep and SWS in the postoperative period as well as in chronic opiate use and abuse.[45,46] Increased nocturnal awakenings have also been shown.

Nevertheless, the strong analgesic properties of these drugs permit sleep in people who are otherwise unable to sleep, such as those with chronic pain syndromes or severe RLS.

Triptans

Triptans are used for the treatment of migraine and cluster headache. They exert their therapeutic action via agonist effects at the 5-HT_1 receptor.[47]

Reported somnolence is highest with the more lipophilic triptans with active metabolites, such as eletriptan, zolmitriptan, and rizatriptan. Reported somnolence is lowest with less lipophilic triptans without active metabolites, such as sumatriptan, almotriptan, and naratriptan.[48]

Different opinions exist over whether the reported somnolence is the result of the effects of a drug on the serotonergic system (less likely because serotonin is mostly a wake-promoting neurotransmitter) or reflects a symptom of the wider migraine attack.[47] This was illustrated by pooled data from 7 placebo-controlled trials of triptan use in acute migraine. Higher rates of somnolence were shown in responders than nonresponders, whereas similar rates of somnolence were shown in patients who responded to either active treatment or placebo. It is suggested that this must be due, at least to a significant part, to headache relief and unmasking of somnolence as a symptom of the syndrome of a migraine attack, rather than just a side effect of treatment.[49]

H1 antihistamines

HA is widely present throughout the body and the CNS. In most tissues, HA is stored in mast cells, which mediate allergic responses. In the CNS, HA serves as a neurotransmitter promoting wakefulness. Different types of HA receptors have been described. H_1 antihistamines are the mainstay in the treatment of allergic disorders.[50]

The first-generation H_1 antihistamines have much stronger sedative effects than the second-generation H1 antihistamines. The first-generation H_1 antagonists (e.g. chlorpheniramine, diphenhydramine, and hydroxyzine) are lipophilic molecules that can easily permeate the BBB. The second-generation H_1 antihistamines (e.g. bilastine, ebastine, and fexofenadine) are more hydrophilic molecules that do not easily enter the CNS and have as such no (or less) effect on wakefulness. Among second-generation H_1 antihistamines, cetirizine shows a more noticeable sedative effect than others. Central H_1-receptor occupancy varies from almost negligible (e.g. fexofenadine) to 30% for cetirizine.[51] According to brain H_1-receptor occupancy, antihistamines might objectively be classified into 3 categories of sedating, less sedating, and nonsedating antihistamines.[52] Nonsedating antihistamines should be preferentially used whenever possible because most are equally efficacious, whereas adverse effects of sedating antihistamines can be serious.[52]

Because of the sedative side effects, H_1 antagonists are used off-label for the treatment of insomnia. These agents are varyingly effective and may result in daytime sleepiness.

CARDIOVASCULAR DRUGS

β-Adrenergic Blocking Agents

β-Adrenergic blocking drugs are widespread used for a variety of diseases, cardiovascular as well as noncardiovascular, such as migraine, posttraumatic stress disorder, and anxiety disorders. Reported side effects include tiredness, insomnia, and vivid dreams, which may manifest as frank nightmares in some.[53] Several features of β-blocking agents seem to play a role in these CNS side effects. A higher lipophilicity carries a higher risk of entrance in the CNS but other characteristics such as high β_2 and/or 5-HT-receptor occupancy also seem important in potentially causing sleep disruption. Considering all these pharmacologic features, it is suggested that bisoprolol, atenolol, betaxolol, acebutolol, nebivolol, and nadolol involve the lowest risk for insomnia, and sotalol, timolol, pindolol, and carvedilol carry a moderate risk for insomnia, whereas the highest risk for insomnia is borne by labetalol, metoprolol, and propranolol.[25]

β-Blocking agents also inhibit melatonin production by blocking sympathetic signaling to the pineal gland.[54–56] Because the pineal gland is located outside the BBB, both lipophilic (such as propranolol) and hydrophilic (such as atenolol) β-blocking agents suppress melatonin, leading to a reduced circadian signal to initiate sleep, which may help explain the insomnia associated with β-blocker use.[47] An acute study in healthy subjects showed that melatonin supplementation to the β-blocker restores sleep. A 3-week study reported that melatonin supplementation in hypertensive patients chronically treated with β-blockers improved sleep quality.[57]

β-Blockers that have vasodilatating properties through α_1 blockade, for example, carvedilol and labetalol, also are associated with fatigue and somnolence.[25]

α_1 Antagonists

Prazosin is increasingly used off-label to treat nightmares in patients with posttraumatic stress disorder. Insomnia and hallucinations are listed as some of the rare side effects of prazosin by the manufacturer. Low-dose prazosin was associated with nightmares and sleep disturbances in a case report of an elderly patient without previously diagnosed mental illness or coexisting environmental risk factors for nightmares.[58]

α_2-Adrenergic Agonists

For the central-acting antihypertensives, clonidine and methyldopa, sedation is a common side effect, occurring in 30% to 75% of patients. The severity seems to diminish with time. There are also reports of insomnia and nightmares with these drugs.[25]

Angiotensin-Converting Enzyme Inhibitors

A low incidence of central side effects (eg, captopril and cilazapril) is reported.[25] Indirectly, sleep disturbance can be initiated or aggravated because angiotensin-converting enzyme inhibitors can precipitate a dry, irritating cough, which may interfere with sleep.[25] Spirapril was associated with insomnia at high doses of 6 mg.[59] Ramipril improved subjective sleep reports in heart failure patients.[60]

Angiotensin Receptor Blockers

In patients receiving losartan, more adverse effects, including insomnia, were reported, compared with controls who were taking angiotensin-converting enzyme inhibitors or calcium channel blockers.[61]

Loop Diuretics

Research of the effects of loop diuretics on sleep is scarce. Diuretic intake, however, is often associated with nocturia, which may result in sleep fragmentation.[62] However, it was indicated by preliminary work that administration of loop diuretics may improve OSA by reducing peripharyngeal edema.[63]

Statins

Placebo-controlled studies of lovastatin, pravastatin,[64] and simvastatine[65] showed no increased sleep disturbance.

CORTICOSTEROIDS

Corticosteroids, effectors of the hypothalamic pituitary-adrenal axis (HPA) system, elicit their actions through binding to 2 types of intracellular receptors located in the CNS, the mineralocorticoid receptors and the glucocorticoid receptors. Glucocorticoid receptors are widely distributed in the CNS,[66] including anatomic regions implicated in the control of sleep and waking. Corticosteroids are used in a wide medical array. Adverse drug reactions to corticosteroids are known to be associated with the way of administration, the size of the dose, chemical properties, and the length of time for which a drug is prescribed.[67] Behavioral alterations are commonly associated with elevated levels of cortical steroids. Sleep disturbances are recognized as a prominent symptom among these behavioral alterations.[66]

Knowing the link between chronic insomnia and cortisol,[68,69] an association between corticoid administration and insomnia could be expected. The results of objective studies, however, seem inconsistent. In a large study with the use of high-dose prednisolone versus placebo for optic neuritis, 53% of patients treated with prednisolone for optic neuritis reported sleep disturbance compared with 20% on placebo.[70] Otherwise, clinical trials on intranasal corticosteroids report that the improved nasal congestion is associated with improved quality of life, with better sleep and reduced fatigue.[71] Dexamethasone has been shown to increase alertness[66] as well as increase slow-wave sleep.[67] In clinical studies of children with acute lymphoblastic leukemia treated with corticosteroids, both insomnia and hypersomnia are reported as adverse side effects attributed to dexamethasone.[72] Several mediating mechanisms may explain these apparently contradictory research and clinical findings noted in different studies of the effects of corticosteroids and sleep.

Corticosteroids affect sleep at multiple levels of the nervous system.[66,67,73] On the one hand corticosteroids can cause a direct increase in alertness. On the other hand corticosteroids inhibit the release of corticotropin-releasing hormone (CRH) by the HPA axis feedback loop. CRH activates the locus coeruleus-NE system, thereby increasing wakefulness. This indirect CRH inhibition decreases wakefulness and increases slow-wave sleep.[72]

Another potential mechanism for the effects of dexamethasone on sleep involves inflammatory cytokines. Tumor necrosis factor (TNF)-α, interleukin (IL)-1, and IL-6 are important in sleep regulation,[74] and they are associated with daytime sleepiness. TNF-α, IL-1, and IL-6 have been identified as mediators of sickness syndrome in human and animal studies, and they are believed important factors mediating fatigue.[75]

THEOPHYLLINE

Theophylline, related in chemical structure and pharmacologic action to caffeine, is mainly used in the treatment of asthma and chronic obstructive pulmonary disease. Several mechanisms of action have been suggested to explain the effectiveness of theophylline. Adenosine receptor antagonism is believed responsible for some of the CNS side effects, including insomnia and restlessness.[76]

The effect of theophylline on sleep quality and cognitive performance in patients has been the subject of controversy. Two almost identical studies were undertaken to examine the direct effects of theophylline on sleep quality and cognitive performance, without confounding effects from bronchodilatation, in healthy subjects.[77] In 1 study, it was shown that theophylline does not affect sleep quality or cognitive performance in normal adults,[78] whereas, on the contrary, an increased number of arousals and reduced total sleep time were shown in the other study.[79] Dose-dependent increase in MSLT latency and performance was noted with a short-term administration of theophylline in healthy persons.[80] Theophylline-associated sleep disturbances were shown in children with cystic fibrosis.[81] A meta-analysis of 12 studies of theophylline, however, did not indicate impairment in cognition or behavior.[82]

Impaired quality of sleep is common among patients with bronchial asthma[83] and chronic obstructive pulmonary disease.[84] Overall, notwithstanding the—in some studies—reported negative effects of theophylline on sleep architecture, the positive effects on sleep of ameliorated respiration at night presumably outweigh the minimal negative effects on sleep architecture.

DISCUSSION

When choosing a pharmacologic agent for a patient, the adverse-effect profile is the most important consideration after the main therapeutic effect.[85] Awareness of possible side effects such as disturbed sleep and/or daytime sleepiness is important to adapt treatment and reach optimal results for every patient. Besides the importance for health and quality of life, effects on sleep or waking function can be a potential source of noncompliance. Nevertheless, although direct negative effects on sleep or waking function may show themselves in healthy persons, the resulting effects of drugs in patients may not be straightforward. As described previously, the positive effects of theophylline on nighttime respiration in patients presumably outweigh the negative effects on sleep architecture described in healthy persons. As in many conditions, a close bidirectional relationship between disease and sleep exists; drug effects may lead this vicious circle in both ways. In the bidirectional connection between, for example, sleep and pain, direct negative effects of opioids on sleep may be present but indirect effects (ameliorating sleep by reducing pain during the night) may be clinically more important and set an important upward trend for the patient. Vice versa, as, for example, in the bidirectional relationship between insomnia and depression, unwanted drug effects may be further complicating this interaction, for example, aggravating insomnia in an otherwise positive AD response. Disease, sleep disturbances, and medication may also interact for example, in epilepsy, where sleep disruption may be caused by seizures, by anticonvulsants, or by coexisting sleep disorders, any of which may have an adverse impact on daily functioning. Moreover, benefits gained in reducing one sleep problem may be offset by causing or exacerbating another sleep problem.[86] For example, loop diuretics have been associated with decreases in OSA severity. A side effect of diuretic administration, however, is nocturia. Given the entanglement between sleep, health, and quality of life, awareness of effects of drugs on sleep is essential. A vigilant clinician is needed to optimize treatment to the need of the patient.

CLINICS CARE POINTS

- When choosing a pharmacological agent for a patient, the adverse-effect profile is the most important consideration after the main therapeutic effect.
- Given the entanglement between sleep, health and quality of life, awareness of effects of drugs on sleep/wakefulness is essential.
- By the numerous neurotransmitters and receptors that are involved in sleep and wakefulness, almost any drug that crosses the blood-brain barrier may influence sleep and waking behaviour.
- A close - sometimes bidirectional - relationship between disease and (disturbed) sleep/wakefulness is often present e.g. chronic pain, depression, ... Drug effects may increase the complexity of this interaction and may lead this vicious circle in both ways.
- Direct and indirect effects of drugs on the disease as well as on sleep and wakefulness need to be outweighed.
- Besides the importance for health and quality of life, effects on sleep or waking function can be a potential source of non-compliance.

REFERENCES

1. Monti JM. The effect of second-generation antipsychotic drugs on sleep parameters in patients with unipolar or bipolar disorder. Sleep Med 2016;23:89–96.
2. Monti JM. The neurotransmitters of sleep and wake, a physiological reviews series. Sleep Med Rev 2013;17:313–5.
3. Luppi PH, Clement O, Fort P. Paradoxical (REM) sleep genesis by the brainstem is under hypothalamic control. Curr Opin Neurobiol 2013;23:1–7.
4. Sateia MC, Buysse DJ. Insomnia diagnosis and treatment. 1st edition. London: Informa healthcare; 2010.
5. Wilson S, Argyropoulos S. Antidepressants and sleep: a qualitative review of the literature. Drugs 2005;65(7):927–47.
6. Wichniak A, Wierzbicka A, Walecka M, et al. Effects of antidepressants on sleep. Curr Psychiatry Rep 2017;19(9):63.
7. Doghramji K, Jangro WC. Adverse effects of psychotropic medications on sleep. Psychiatr Clin North Am 2016;39(3):487–502.
8. Roth T, Rogowski R, Hull S, et al. Efficacy and safety of doxepin 1 mg, 3 mg, and 6 mg in adults with primary insomnia. Sleep 2007;30(11):1555–61.
9. Alberti S, Chiesa A, Andrisano C, et al. Insomnia and somnolence associated with second-generation antidepressants during the treatment of major depres sion: a meta-analysis. J Clin Psychopharmacol 2015;35(3):296–303.
10. Nofzinger EA, Reynolds CF 3rd, Thase ME, et al. REM sleep enhancement by bupropion in depressed men. Am J Psychiatry 1995;152(2):274–6.
11. Holshoe JM. Antidepressants and sleep: a review. Perspect Psychiatr Care 2009;45(3):191–7.
12. Haddad PM. Antidepressant discontinuation syndromes. Drug Saf 2001;24(3):183–97.
13. Sadock BJ, Sadock VA, Ruiz P. Kaplan and Sadock's synopsis of psychiatry. Behavioral sciences/clinical psychiatry. 11th edition. Philadelphia: Wolters Kluwer; 2015.
14. Krystal AD, Goforth HW, Roth T. Effects of antipsychotic medications on sleep in schizophrenia. Int Clin Psychopharmacol 2008;23(3):150–60.
15. Gao K, Mackle M, Cazorla P, et al. Comparison of somnolence associated with asenapine, olanzapine, risperidone, and haloperidol relative to placebo in patients with schizophrenia or bipolar disorder. Neu-ropsychiatr Dis Treat 2013;9:1145–57.
16. Kluge M, Himmerich H, Wehmeier PM, et al. Sleep propensity at daytime as assessed by Multiple Sleep Latency Tests (MSLT) in patients with schizophrenia increases with clozapine and olanzapine. Schizophr Res 2012;135(1–3):123–7.
17. Loebel AD, Siu CO, Cucchiaro JB, et al. Daytime sleepiness associated with lurasidone and quetiapine XR: results from a randomized double-blind, placebo-controlled trial in patients with schizophrenia. CNS Spectr 2014;19(2):197–205.
18. Luthringer R, Staner L, Noel N, et al. A double-blind, placebo-controlled, randomized study evaluating the effect of paliperidone extended-release tablets on sleep architecture in patients with schizophrenia. Int Clin Psychopharmacol 2007;22(5):299–308.
19. Ücok A, Saka MC, Bilici M. Effects of paliperidone extended release on functioning level and symptoms of patients with recent onset schizophrenia: an open-label, single-arm, flexible-dose, 12-months follow-up study. Nord J Psychiatry 2015;69(6):426–32.

20. Wiegand MH, Landry F, Bruckner T, et al. Quetiapine in primary insomnia: a pilot study. Psychopharmacology (Berl) 2008;196(2):337–8.
21. Bohra MH, Kaushik C, Temple D, et al. Weighing the balance: how analgesics used in chronic pain influence sleep? Br J Pain 2014;8(3):107–18.
22. Jain SV, Kothare SV. Sleep and epilepsy. Semin Pediatr Neurol 2015;22(2):86–92.
23. Bazil CW. Nocturnal seizures and the effects of anticonvulsants on sleep. Curr Neurol Neurosci Rep 2008;8(2):149–54.
24. Jain SV, Glauser TA. Effects of epilepsy treatments on sleep architecture and daytime sleepiness: an evidence-based review of objective sleep metrics. Epilepsia 2014;55(1):26–37.
25. Schweitzer PK, Randazzo AC. Drugs that disturb sleep and wakefulness. In: Kryger MH, Roth T, Dement WC, editors. Principles and practice of sleep medicine. 6th edition. Philadelphia: Elsevier; 2017. p. 480–98.
26. Vossler DG, Morris GL 3rd, Harden CL, et al. Post marketing Antiepileptic Drug Survey (PADS) Group Study Investigators. Tiagabine in clinical practice: effects on seizure control and behavior. Epilepsy Behav 2013;28(2):211–6.
27. Sadler M. Lamotrigine associated with insomnia. Epilepsia 1999;40(3):322–5.
28. Schweitzer PK. Excessive sleepiness due to medications and drugs. In: Thorpy MJ, Billiard M, editors. Sleepiness: causes, consequences and treatment. United Kingdom: Cambridge University Press; 2011. p. 386–98.
29. Leppik IE. Zonisamide. Epilepsia 1999;40(Suppl. 5): S23–9.
30. Glauser TA. Topiramate. Epilepsia 1999;40(Suppl. 5):S71–80.
31. Hetland A, Carr DB. Medications and impaired driving. Ann Pharmacother 2014;48(4):494–506.
32. Garcia-Borreguero D, Kohnen R, Silber MH, et al. The long-term treatment of restless legs syndrome/Willis-Ekbom disease: evidence-based guidelines and clinical consensus best practice guidance: a report from the International Restless Legs Syndrome Study Group. Sleep Med 2013;14(7):675–84.
33. Connolly BS, Lang AE. Pharmacological treatment of Parkinson disease: a review. JAMA 2014;311(16): 1670–83.
34. Videnovic A, Golombek D. Circadian and sleep disorders in Parkinson's disease. Exp Neurol 2013;243: 45–56.
35. Chahine LM, Amara AW, Videnovic A. A systematic review of the literature on disorders of sleep and wakefulness in Parkinson's disease from 2005 to 2015. Sleep Med Rev 2017;35:33–50.
36. Schug SA, Garrett WR, Gillespie G. Opioid and non-opioid analgesics. Best Pract Res Clin Anaesthesiol 2003;17(1):91–110.
37. Datta S, Maclean RR. Neurobiological mechanisms for the regulation of mammalian sleep-wake behavior: reinterpretation of historical evidence and inclusion of contemporary cellular and molecular evidence. Neurosci Biobehav Rev 2007;31(5):775–824.
38. Horne JA. Aspirin and nonfebrile waking oral temperature in healthy men and women: links with SWS changes. Sleep 1989;12:516–21.
39. Murphy PJ, Badia P, Myers BL, et al. Nonsteroidal anti-inflammatory drugs affect normal sleep patterns in humans. Physiol Behav 1994;55(6):1063–6.
40. Gengo F. Effects of ibuprofen on sleep quality as measured using polysomnography and subjective measures in healthy adults. Clin Ther 2006;28(11): 1820–6.
41.. Horne JA, Percival JE, Traynor JR. Aspirin and human sleep. Electroencephalogr Clin Neurophysiol 1980;49(3–4):409–13.
42. Lavie P, Nahir M, Lorber M, et al. Nonsteroidal anti inflammatory drug therapy in rheumatoid arthritis patients. Lack of association between clinical improvement and effects on sleep. Arthritis Rheum 1991;34:655–9.
43. Lacovides S, Avidon I, Bentley A, et al. Diclofenac potassium restores objective and subjective measures of sleep quality in women with primary dysmenorrhea. Sleep 2009;32(8):1019–26.
44. Moore JT, Kelz MB. Opiates, sleep, and pain: the adenosinergic link. Anesthesiology 2009;111(6): 1175–6.
45. Cronin AJ, Keifer JC, Davies MF, et al. Postoperative sleep disturbance: influences of opioids and pain in humans. Sleep 2001;24:39–44.
46. Onen SH, Onen F, Courpron P, et al. How pain and analgesics disturb sleep. Clin J Pain 2005;21(5): 422–31.
47. Nesbitt AD. Headache, drugs and sleep. Cephalalgia 2014;34(10):756–66.
48. Dodick DW, Martin V. Triptans and CNS side-effects: pharmacokinetic and metabolic mechanisms. Cephalalgia 2004;24(6):417–24.
49. Goadsby PJ, Dodick DW, Almas M, et al. Treatment-emergent CNS symptoms following triptan therapy are part of the attack. Cephalalgia 2007;27(3): 254–62.
50. Hu Y, Sieck DE, Hsu WH. Why are second- generation H1-antihistamines minimally sedating? Eur J Pharmacol 2015;765:100–6.
51. Tashiro M, Sakurada Y, Iwabuchi K, et al. Central effects of fexofenadine and cetirizine: measurement of psychomotor performance, subjective sleepiness, and brain histamine H1-receptor occupancy using 11C-doxepin positron emission tomography. J Clin Pharmacol 2004;44(8):890–900.
52. Yanai K, Yoshikawa T, Yanai A, et al. The clinical pharmacology of non-sedating antihistamines. Phar Macol Ther 2017;178:148–56.

53. Pagel JF, Helfter P. Drug induced nightmares - an etiology based review. Hum Psychopharmacol 2003;18(1):59–67.
54. Arendt J, Bojkowski C, Franey C, et al. Immunoassay of 6-hydroxymelatonin sulfate in human plasma and urine: abolition of the urinary 24-hour rhythm with atenolol. J Clin Endocrinol Metab 1985;60:1166–73.
55. Nathan PJ, Maguire KP, Burrows GD, et al. The effect of atenolol, a beta1-adrenergic antagonist, on nocturnal plasma melatonin secretion: evidence for a dose-response relationship in humans. J Pineal Res 1997;23:131–5.
56. Stoschitzky K, Sakotnik A, Lercher P, et al. Influence of beta-blockers on melatonin release. Eur J Clin Pharmacol 1999;55(2):111–5.
57. Scheer FA, Morris CJ, Garcia JI, et al. Repeated melatonin supplementation improves sleep in hypertensive patients treated with beta-blockers: a randomized controlled trial. Sleep 2012;35(10): 1395–402.
58. Kosari S, Naunton M. Sleep disturbances and nightmares in a patient treated with prazosin. J Clin Sleep Med 2016;12(4):631–2.
59. Kantola I, Terént A, Honkanen T, et al. Efficacy and safety of spirapril, a new ace-inhibitor, in elderly hy pertensive patients. Eur J Clin Pharmacol 1996; 50(3):155–9.
60. Gundersen T, Wiklund I, Swedberg K, et al. Effects of 12 weeks of ramipril treatment on the quality of life in patients with moderate congestive heart failure: results of a placebo-controlled trial. Ramipril Study Group. Cardiovasc Drugs Ther 1995;9(4):589–94.
61. Samizo K, Kawabe E, Hinotsu S, et al. Comparison of losartan with ACE inhibitors and dihydropyridine calcium channel antagonists: a pilot study of prescription-event monitoring in Japan. Drug Saf 2002;25(11):811–21.
62. Riegel B, Moser DK, Anker SD, et al. State of the science: promoting self-care in persons with heart fail ure: a scientific statement from the American Heart Association. Circulation 2009;120(12):1141–63.
63. Bucca CB, Brussino L, Battisti A, et al. Diuretics in obstructive sleep apnea with diastolic heart failure. Chest 2007;132(2):440–6.
64. Ehrenberg BL, Lamon-Fava S, Corbett KE, et al. Comparison of the effects of pravastatin and lovastatin on sleep disturbance in hypercholesterolemic subjects. Sleep 1999;22(1):117–21.
65. Keech AC, Armitage JM, Wallendszus KR, et al. Absence of effects of prolonged simvastatin therapy on nocturnal sleep in a large randomized placebo-controlled study. Oxford Cholesterol Study Group. Br J Clin Pharmacol 1996;42(4):483–90.
66. Meixner R, Gerhardstein R, Day R, et al. The alerting effects of dexamethasone. Psychophysiology 2003; 40(2):254–9.
67. Friess E, Tagaya H, Grethe C, et al. Acute cortisol administration promotes sleep intensity in man. Neuropsychopharmacology 2004;29(3):598–604.
68. Vgontzas AN, Bixler EO, Lin HM, et al. Chronic insomnia is associated with nyctohermeral activation of the hypothalamic-pituitary-adrenal axis: clinical implications. J Clin Endocrinol Metab 2001;86(8): 3787–94.
69. Rodenbeck A, Huether G, Ruther E, et al. Interactions between evening and nocturnal cortisol secretion and sleep parameters in patients with severe chronic primary insomnia. Neurosci Lett 2002; 324(2):159–63.
70. Chrousos GA, Kattah JC, Beck RW, et al. Side effects of glucocorticoid treatment. Experience of the optic neuritis treatment trial. JAMA 1993;269(16): 2110–2.
71. Lunn M, Craig T. Rhinitis and sleep. Sleep Med Rev 2011;15(5):293–9.
72. Rosen G, Harris AK, Liu M, et al. The effects of Dexamethasone on sleep in young children with Acute Lymphoblastic Leukemia. Sleep Med 2015; 16(4):503–9.
73. Steiger A. Sleep and the hypothalamo-pituitary-adrenocortical system. Sleep Med Rev 2002;6: 125–38.
74. Krueger K, Rector D, Churchill L. Sleep and cytokines. Sleep Med Clin 2007;2(2):161–9.
75. Bryant P, Trinder J, Curtis N. Sick and tired: does sleep have a vital role in the immune system? Nat Rev Immunol 2004;4:457–67.
76. Vassallo R, Lipsky JJ. Theophylline: recent advances in the understanding of its mode of action and uses in clinical practice. Mayo Clin Proc 1998; 73(4):346–54.
77. Smith PL, Schwartz AR. The effect of theophylline on sleep in normal subjects. Chest 1993;103(1): 5–6.
78. Fitzpatrick MF, Engleman HM, Boellert F, et al. Effect of therapeutic theophylline levels on the sleep quality and daytime cognitive performance of normal subjects. Am Rev Respir Dis 1992;145(6): 1355–8.
79. Kaplan J, Fredrickson PA, Renaux SA, et al. Theophylline effect on sleep in normal subjects. Chest 1993; 103(1):193–5.
80. Roehrs T, Merlotti L, Halpin D, et al. Effects of theophylline on nocturnal sleep and daytime sleepiness/alertness. Chest 1995;108(2):382–7.
81. Avital A, Sanchez I, Holbrow J, et al. Effect of theophylline on lung function tests, sleep quality, and nighttime SaO2 in children with cystic fibrosis. Am Rev Respir Dis 1991;144(6):1245–9.
82. Stein MA, Krasowski M, Leventhal BL, et al. Behavioral and cognitive effects of methylxanthines. A meta-analysis of theophylline and caffeine. Arch Pediatr Adolesc Med 1996;150(3):284–8.

83. Janson C, Gislason T, Boman G, et al. Sleep disturbances in patients with asthma. Respir Med 1990; 84(1):37–42.
84. Mulloy E, McNicholas WT. Theophylline improves gas exchange during rest, exercise, and sleep in severe chronic obstructive pulmonary disease. Am Rev Respir Dis 1993;148(4 Pt 1):1030–6.
85. Novak M, Shapiro CM. Drug-induced sleep disturbances. Focus on nonpsychotropic medications. Drug Saf 1997;16(2):133–49.
86. Jiménez JA, Greenberg BH, Mills PJ. Effects of heart failure and its pharmacological management on sleep. Drug Discov Today Dis Models 2011;8(4): 161–6.

Pharmacologic Management of Excessive Daytime Sleepiness

Taisuke Ono, MD, PhD[a,b,*], Shinichi Takenoshita, MD, MPH[a], Seiji Nishino, MD, PhD[a]

KEYWORDS

- Stimulants • Excessive daytime sleepiness (EDS) • Narcolepsy • Idiopathic hypersomnia
- Modafinil • Sodium oxybate • Pitolisant • Solriamfetol

KEY POINTS

- Excessive daytime sleepiness (EDS) is related to medical and social problems, including mental disorders, physical diseases, poor quality of life, and so forth.
- Several different types of stimulants (or wake-promoting compounds) are available to treat EDS, and a variety of new drugs are under development.
- The side effects of some of the stimulants are potent, and careful selection and management are required.

Abbreviations	
EDS	Excessive daytime sleepiness
ICSD-3	International Classification of Sleep Disorders, Third Edition
CSF	Cerebrospinal fluid
MSL	Mean sleep latency
MSLT	multiple sleep latency test
nPS	Gnocturnal polysomnogram
SOREMP	Sleep onset REM period
MWT	Maintenance of wakefulness test
CNS	Central nervous system
AASM	American Academy of Sleep Medicine
FDA	Food and Drug Administration
DAT	Dopamine transporter
DA	Dopamine
NE	Norepinephrine
GHBG-	hydroxybutyrate
GABAG-	aminobutyric acid
LC	Locus Coeruleus

Sleep Med Clin 12 (2017) 461-478 https://doi.org/10.1016/j.jsmc.2017.03.019. 1556-407X/17/© 2017 Elsevier Inc.

[a] Sleep and Circadian Neurobiology Laboratory, Department of Psychiatry and Behavioral Sciences, Stanford University School of Medicine, Palo Alto, CA, USA; [b] Department of Geriatric Medicine, Kanazawa Medical University School of Medicine, Ishikawa, Japan

* Corresponding author. 3155 Porter Drive, Room 2141, Palo Alto, CA 94304.
E-mail address: taisukeo@kanazawa-med.ac.jp

Sleep Med Clin 17 (2022) 485–503
https://doi.org/10.1016/j.jsmc.2022.06.012
1556-407X/22/

RCT	Randomized Control Trial
BBB	Blood–brain barrier
PG	Protaglandin
DP1	PGD2 receptor
TRH	Thyrotropin-releasing hormone

INTRODUCTION

Excessive daytime sleepiness (EDS) is defined as "irresistible sleepiness in a situation when an individual would be expected to be awake, and alert."[1] EDS has been a big concern not only from a medical but also from a public health point of view. According to recently published articles, the prevalence of patients who suffer from EDS is approximately 20% in the world.[2–4] Patients with EDS have the possibility of falling asleep even when they should wake up and concentrate, for example, when they drive, play sports, or walk outside. Subjects who have EDS encounter a lower quality of life and have a higher odds ratio of developing a mental disorder, cognitive impairment, and motor vehicle accidents.[5–8]

Although nonpharmacologic treatments (ie, napping and work accommodations) are often helpful, a large majority of the diagnosed patients reported using pharmacologic therapies, mostly stimulant medications.[9]

Historically, EDS was also a large concern in the military. Many countries let soldiers take stimulants when they were engaged in military service in World War II. Currently, preventing sleepiness caused by sleep deprivation is still a major research project by the Defense Advanced Research Projects Agency in the United States.

In 1931, the first stimulant (ie, amphetamine) was applied to treat EDS associated with narcolepsy.[10] Since then, many new stimulants have been developed to treat EDS, and many patients received benefits. Stimulants, however, are drugs with strong side effects (ie, sympathomimetic) and addiction potential and these treatments are mostly symptomatic; they improve the level of alertness by simply suppressing sleepiness.

Abuse potential of stimulants is a problem, especially when diagnoses of hypersomnia are loosely made, and this is particularly true for narcolepsy, where stimulant abuse is rare among patients with well-defined narcolepsy.[11–14] In this article, clinical characteristics of common hypersomnias and pharmacologic treatments of each hypersomnia are described. New treatment options under development for treating EDS associated with these hypersomnia are also discussed. The hypersomnias focused on in this article are narcolepsy type 1, narcolepsy type 2, idiopathic hypersomnia, and hypersomnia due to a medical disorder, defined in the *International Classification of Sleep Disorders, Third Edition (ICSD-3).*

TYPES OF HYPERSOMNIAS

According to the *ICDS-3,* published in 2014, diseases that result from EDS are listed as narcolepsy type 1, narcolepsy type 2, idiopathic hypersomnia, Kleine–Levin syndrome, hypersomnia due to a medical disorder, hypersomnia due to a medication or substance, hypersomnia associated with a psychiatric disorder, and insufficient sleep syndrome.[15]

This review covers the pharmacologic treatments of EDS associated with narcolepsy type 1, narcolepsy type 2, idiopathic hypersomnia, and hypersomnia due to a medical disorder, because relatively consistent guidelines for the pharmacotherapy of these diseases are available. The diagnostic criteria of these hypersomnias are summarized in **Fig. 1**. For the treatment of Kleine–Levin syndrome and other hypersomnias, see the article by Arnulf.[16]

NARCOLEPSY

Symptoms of Narcolepsy

Narcolepsy is a syndrome characterized by "EDS that is typically associated with cataplexy and other [rapid eye movement] REM sleep phenomena such as sleep paralysis and hypnagogic hallucinations."[17] The prevalence of narcolepsy with cataplexy has been examined in many studies and falls between 25 and 50 per 100,000 people (0.025%-0.05%).[18,19] The onset of the disease is most often seen during adolescence around puberty.[20] As with the sleepiness of other sleep disorders, sleepiness or EDS of narcolepsy presents an increased propensity to fall asleep, nodding, or easily dozing in relaxed or sedentary situations or a need to exert extra effort to avoid sleeping in these situations.[21] Additionally, irresistible or overwhelming urges to sleep commonly occur from time to time during wakeful periods in patients with untreated narcolepsy. These so-called sleep attacks are not instantaneous lapses into sleep, as is often thought of by the general public,

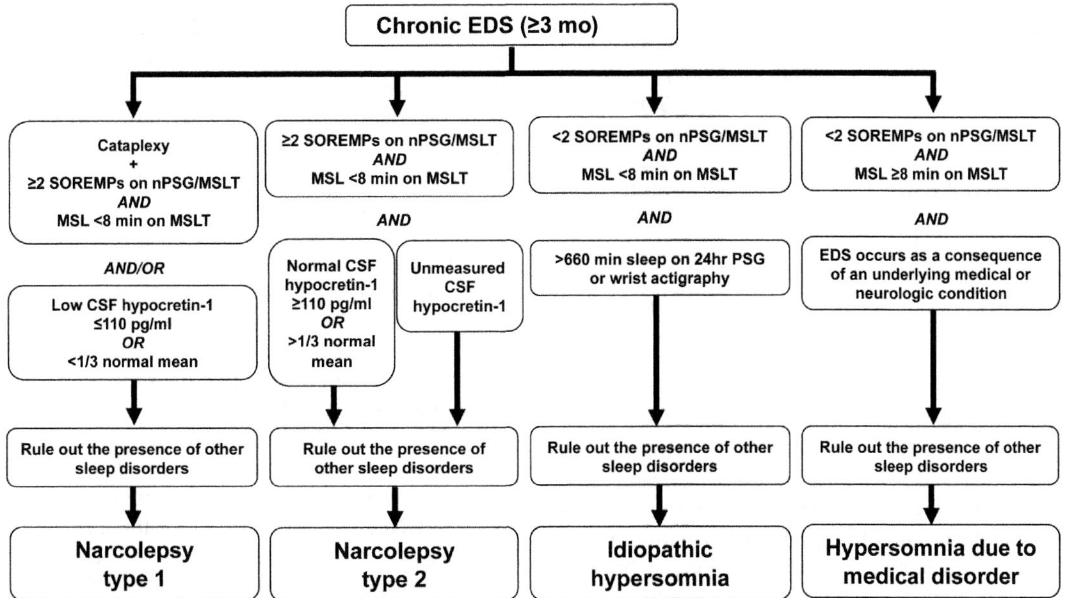

Fig. 1. Diagnostics of narcolepsy type 1, type 2, idiopathic hypersomnia, and hypersomnia due to the medical disorder. CSF, cerebrospinal fluid; EDS, excessive daytime sleepiness; MSL, mean sleep latency; MSLT, multiple sleep latency test; nPSG, nocturnal polysomnogram; SOREMP, sleep onset REM period.

but represent episodes of profound sleepiness experienced by those with marked sleep deprivation or other severe sleep disorders. This feeling is most often relieved by short naps (15–30 minutes), but in most cases, the refreshed sensation only lasts a short time after awaking. The refreshing value of short naps is of considerable diagnostic value for EDS associated with narcolepsy.

EDS can be objectively measured with the standardized multiple sleep latency test (MSLT), and the MSLT findings (mean sleep latency <8 minutes) were included in the diagnostic criteria of EDS associated with narcolepsy and other hypersomnias (see **Fig. 1**).[17] The maintenance of wakefulness test (MWT) was also developed to measure how alert patients are when they are set in a boring situation during the day.[22] Although MWT is not included in the diagnostic criteria of any hypersomnias, many researchers believe that MWT is more sensitive in evaluating effects of treatments, such as pharmacotherapy with wake-promoting compounds. One of the reasons for this is the floor effects seen with MSLT; when the EDS is severe, it is often difficult to detect the therapeutic effects (to sleep vs to stay awake with MWT) with the MSLT protocol. Therefore, MWT is often used to examine the therapeutic effects of wake-promoting compounds. There is not enough evidence, however, to set the cutoff value even when the MWT is used to measure the effectiveness of the treatment of diseases.[23,24]

In addition to EDS, patients with narcolepsy exhibit cataplexy and other abnormal manifestations of REM sleep, such as hypnagogic hallucinations and sleep paralysis.[25] Cataplexy, the sudden occurrence of muscle weakness in association with emotions, such as laughing, joking, or anger, has long been considered a pathognomonic symptom of the syndrome.[21,26,27] Cataplectic events usually last from a few seconds to 2 or 3 minutes but occasionally continue longer.[28] Patients are usually alert and oriented during the event despite their inability to respond. Positive emotions, such as laughter, more commonly trigger cataplexy than negative emotions; however, any strong emotion is a potential trigger.[29]

Hypnagogic or hypnopompic hallucinations may be visual, tactile, auditory, or multisensory events, usually brief but occasionally continuing for a few minutes, that occur at transitions from wakefulness to sleep (hypnagogic) or from sleep to wakefulness (hypnopompic).[21] Hallucinations may contain combined elements of dream sleep and consciousness and are often bizarre or disturbing to patients.

Sleep paralysis is the inability to move, lasting from a few seconds to a few minutes, during the transition from sleep to wakefulness or from wakefulness to sleep. Episodes of sleep paralysis may alarm patients, particularly those who experience the sensation of being unable to breathe. Although accessory respiratory muscles may not be active during these episodes, diaphragmatic activity continues, and air exchange remains adequate.

One of the most frequently associated symptoms is insomnia, best characterized as a difficulty to maintain nighttime sleep. Typically, patients with narcolepsy fall asleep easily, only to wake up after a short nap and are unable to return to sleep for another hour or so. Patients with narcolepsy do not usually sleep more than normal individuals over the 24-hour cycle[30–32] but frequently have disrupted nighttime sleep.[30–32] Frequently associated problems include periodic leg movements,[33,34] REM sleep behavior disorders, other parasomnias,[35,36] and obstructive sleep apnea.[34,37,38]

Other commonly reported symptoms include automatic behavior—absent-minded behavior or speech that is often nonsensical that the patient does not remember. Hypnagogic hallucinations, sleep paralysis, and automatic behavior are nonspecific to narcolepsy and occur in other sleep disorders (as well as in healthy individuals); however, these symptoms are far more common and occur with much greater frequency in narcolepsy.[39]

Hypocretin / Orexin Deficiency in Type 1 Narcolepsy

In most patients with cataplexy, a deficiency in the hypocretin (orexin) neuropeptide system is involved in the pathophysiology of human narcolepsy.[40] The observation that cerebrospinal fluid (CSF) hypocretin-1 (orexin-A) levels are decreased in patients with narcolepsy provides a new diagnostic tool and refines the nosologic considerations for narcolepsy.

Using a large sample of patients and controls, the authors determined that 110 pg/mL (30% of mean control values) was the most specific and sensitive cutoff value for diagnosing narcolepsy.[41] Most samples had undetectable levels (<40 pg/mL), and a few had detectable but very diminished levels. None of the patients with idiopathic hypersomnia, sleep apnea, restless legs syndrome, or insomnia had abnormal hypocretin levels. Because the specificity of the CSF finding is also high, low CSF hypocretin-1 levels were included in the *International Classifications of Sleep Disorder, Second Edition,* as a positive diagnosis for narcolepsy-cataplexy.[42] In the most recent revision of the *ICSD, ICSD-3,* published in 2014,[15] narcolepsy-cataplexy was renamed narcolepsy type 1, or hypocretin deficiency syndrome, whereas narcolepsy without cataplexy was renamed narcolepsy type 2 (hypocretin nondeficient) to emphasize the pathophysiologic basis of the diseases.

Immune Systems and Narcolepsy

It has been reported that a large majority of people with narcolepsy have tissue-type HLA DR2.[21,28] High-resolution typing revealed that narcolepsy has the closest association with HLA-DQB1*0602, which is found in 95% of patients with narcolepsy with cataplexy and 41% of patients with narcolepsy without cataplexy but only 18% to 35% of the general population.[21,43] The tight association between narcolepsy and antigen-presenting class II HLA type suggests that autoimmune processes may play a critical role in type 1 narcolepsy because many autoimmune diseases exhibit tight associations with class II HLA haplotypes. Type 1 narcolepsy cases could thus involve an autoimmune alteration of hypocretin-containing cells in the central nervous system (CNS), but the antigen for this pathologic process has not yet been identified. Dauvilliers and colleagues[44] reported an HLA-DQB1*0602-positive monozygotic twin pair discordant for narcolepsy and CSF hypocretin-1 (only the affected subject had a low hypocretin-1 level), suggesting that altered CSF hypocretin levels are state dependent and not trait dependent and likely an acquired deficit. In other words, the genetic background is likely not sufficient to develop an abnormality in the hypocretin system. This finding is also complementary to the autoimmune hypothesis.

Considerations for the Pathophysiology of Type 2 Narcolepsy

There are debates about the pathophysiology of narcolepsy with normal hypocretin levels (ie, type 2 narcolepsy). More than 90% of the patients with narcolepsy without cataplexy show normal CSF hypocretin levels, yet they show apparent REM sleep abnormalities (ie, sleep-onset REMs [SOREMs]). Furthermore, even if the strict criteria for narcolepsy-cataplexy are applied, up to 10% of patients with narcolepsy-cataplexy show normal CSF hypocretin levels. Considering that occurrence of cataplexy is tightly associated with hypocretin deficiency, impaired hypocretin neurotransmission is still likely involved in narcolepsy-cataplexy with normal CSF hypocretin levels. Conceptually, there are 2 possibilities to explain these mechanisms: (1) specific impairment of hypocretin receptor and their downstream pathway and (2) partial/localized loss of hypocretin ligand (yet normal CSF levels exhibited). A good example of the former is Hcrtr 2-mutated narcoleptic dogs; they exhibit normal CSF hypocretin-1 levels[45] while having full-blown narcolepsy. Thannickal and colleagues[46] reported 1 narcolepsy without cataplexy patient (HLA typing was unknown) who had an overall loss of 33% of hypocretin cells compared with normal, with maximal cell loss in the posterior hypothalamus. This result favors the second hypothesis, but studies with more cases are needed.

Treatment of Excessive Daytime Sleepiness Associated with Narcolepsy Types 1 and 2

Nonpharmacologic treatments (ie, behavioral modification, such as regular napping and work accommodations) are often helpful. In a survey by a patient group organization;[47–49] however, 94% of all patients reported using pharmacologic therapies, mostly stimulant medications.[50]

Sleepiness is usually treated using amphetamine-like CNS stimulants (ie, methylphenidate) or modafinil (ie, 2-[(diphenylmethyl)sulfinyl]acetamide) and its R-enantiomer, armodafinil, which are wake-promoting compounds unrelated to amphetamines (**Table 1**).[51] More recently, the American Academy of Sleep Medicine (AASM) recommended the use of sodium oxybate, a short-lasting sedative of unknown mechanisms, as first-line treatment of EDS and cataplexy. The most commonly used amphetamine-like compounds are methylphenidate, methamphetamine, D-amphetamine (all schedule II compounds), and mazindol (a schedule IV compound) (**Fig. 2**, see **Table 1**). The clinical use of stimulants in narcolepsy has often been the subject of standards of practice published by AASM.[52] Typically, a patient is started on a low dose, which is then increased progressively to obtain satisfactory results. Studies have shown that daytime sleepiness can be greatly improved subjectively, but sleep variables are never completely normalized by stimulant treatments.[53] Milder stimulants with low efficacy and potency, such as modafinil or armodafinil, are usually tried first (see **Fig. 1**). More effective amphetamine-like stimulants (methylphenidate, D-amphetamine, and methamphetamine) are then used if needed (see **Fig. 2**). Stimulant compounds are generally well tolerated in patients with narcolepsy. Minor adverse effects, such as headaches, irritability, nervousness, tremors, anorexia, palpitations, sweating, and gastric discomfort, are common. Cardiovascular impact, such as increased blood pressure, is possible, considering that sympathomimetic effects of these classes of compounds have been established in animals, although they have been remarkably difficult to document in human studies. Surprisingly, tolerance rarely occurs in this patient population and drug holidays are not recommended by the AASM.[52] Stimulant abuse is rare among patients with well-defined narcolepsy.[11–14] A compliance study has shown that approximately 50% of patients who receive stimulants reduce or withdraw stimulant medications by themselves.[54] Exceptionally, psychotic complications may be observed, most often when the medications are used at high doses and chronically disrupt nocturnal sleep.[55]

Modafinil/armodafinil

Modafinil (2-[(diphenylmethyl)sulfinyl]acetamide) is a chemically unique compound developed in France. Modafinil has been available in France since 1984 in compassionate mode and was officially approved in France in 1992. Modafinil (and its R-enantiomer) was approved in 1998 in the United States for the treatment of narcolepsy, shift-work disorder, and residual sleepiness in treated patients with sleep apnea syndrome.

Armodafinil, the R-enantiomer of racemic modafinil with a longer half-life, was also recently approved by the US Food and Drug Administration (FDA) for EDS associated with narcolepsy as well as for residual sleepiness in nasal continuous positive airway pressure-treating individuals and sleepiness in shift work sleep disorder. Importantly, the R-enantiomer of modafinil has a half-life of 10 to 15 hours, which is longer than that of the S-enantiomer of modafinil (3–4 hours).[56] The dual pharmacokinetic properties of the racemic mixture may explain why modafinil is often more potent when taken twice per day at the beginning of therapy, during the period of drug accumulation. In terms of plasma concentrations, armodafinil is higher than modafinil late in the day on a milligram-to-milligram basis.[57] That is the reason why modafinil is given twice a day at the beginning of therapy, and armodafinil is given once a day.

Several randomized trials have shown that modafinil is effective against EDS in narcolepsy compared with placebo.[58,59] Armodafinil improves the MWT compared with placebo among patients with narcolepsy.[60] Both modafinil and armodafinil are classified as schedule IV (defined as drugs with low potential for abuse and low risk of dependence) (see **Table 1**).[61]

The prevalence of side effects of modafinil/armodafinil is not high, and headache, nausea, dry mouth, and anorexia are known side effects.[62] Modafinil can cause a serious rash in children, although rarely.[63]

In clinical practice, modafinil is given once a day in the morning on an empty stomach in bed to maximize the effect of the drug. The starting dose is usually 200 mg, and the dose range can vary between 100 mg and 400 mg, as needed, depending on the effect.[64] If the maximum dose (400 mg/d) is not sufficient to treat EDS among

Table 1
Current pharmacologic treatment for excessive daytime sleepiness associated with narcolepsy

Compound	Scheduled Class[a]	Usual Daily Doses	Half-Life (h)	Side Effects/Notes
Modafinil	IV	100–400 mg	9–14[b]	No peripheral sympathomimetic action, headaches, nausea
Armodafinil	IV	100–250 mg	10–15[b]	Similar to those of modafinil
Mazindol	IV	2–8 mg	10–13	Reduce appetite or increase in blood pressure
Methylphenidate hydrochloride	II	10-60 mg	2–4	Same as amphetamines; less reduction in appetite or increase in blood pressure
Methamphetamine	II	10-40 mg	9–12	Irritability, mood changes, headaches, palpitations, tremors, excessive sweating, insomnia
D-Amphetamine sulfate	II	5-60 mg	10–28	Irritability, mood changes, headaches, palpitations, tremors, excessive sweating, insomnia
Pitolisant	na	17.8–35.6 mg	20	Headaches, nausea, anxiety, reducing the efficacy of hormonal contraceptives, prolongation of the QT Interval
Solriamfetol	IV	37.5–150 mg	7.1	Headaches, nausea, anxiety, decreased appetite, insomnia, increased blood pressure, increased heart rate, irritability, agitation
Sodium oxybate	III	4.5–9 g	0.5–1	Overdoses (a single dose of 60–100 mg/kg) induce dizziness, nausea, vomiting, confusion, agitation, epileptic seizures, hallucinations, coma with bradycardia, and respiratory depression; evidence of withdrawal syndrome

[a] All compounds in the list are scheduled and the class is listed.
[b] The half-life of the S-enantiomer of modafinil is short (approximately 3–4 h), so the half-life of racemic modafinil mostly reflects the R-enantiomer (armodafinil).

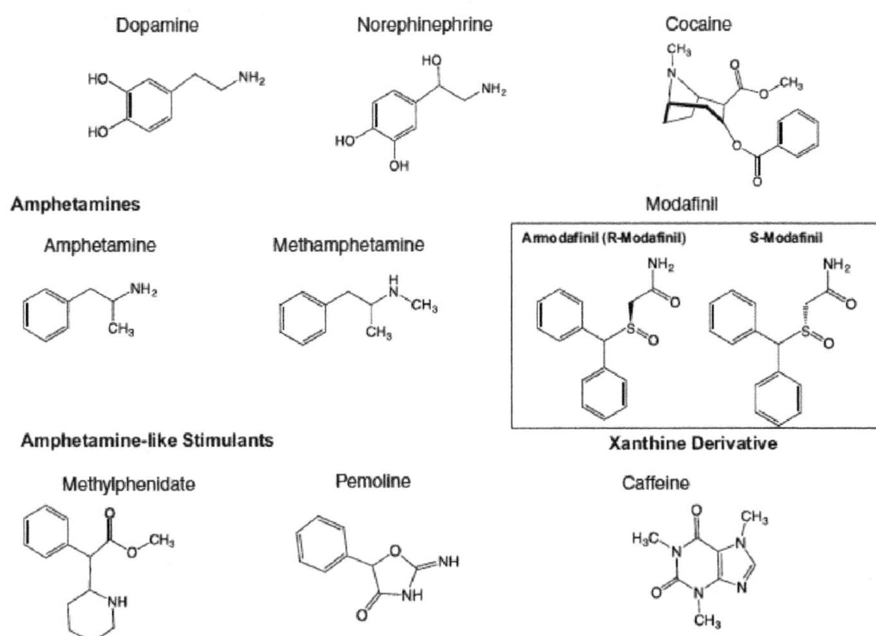

Fig. 2. The most commonly used amphetamine-like compounds.

patients with narcolepsy, then it is recommended to increase the dose up to 600 mg per day.

As discussed previously, armodafinil is usually given once a day in the early morning, and the dose range of armodafinil is 100 mg to 250 mg each morning.

The mechanism of action of modafinil/armodafinil is highly debated. There are few studies addressing the mode of action of armodafinil, and this review mostly discusses the action of racemic modafinil. Modafinil/armodafinil has not been shown to bind to or inhibit any receptors or enzymes of known neurotransmitters.[65,66] In vitro, modafinil/armodafinil binds to the dopamine transporter (DAT) and inhibits dopamine (DA) reuptake.[66,67] These binding inhibitory effects have been shown associated with increased extracellular DA levels in the striatum in rats and dog brains.[68,69]

The most striking finding was that DAT knockout mice were completely unresponsive to the wake-promoting effects of methamphetamine, GBR12909 (a selective DAT blocker), and modafinil. These results further confirm the critical role of DAT in mediating the wake-promoting effects of amphetamines and modafinil and that an intact DAT molecule is required for mediating the arousal effects of these compounds.[69] Qu and colleagues[70] further demonstrated that wake-promoting effects of modafinil were attenuated in D2 receptor knockout mice and were completely abolished in D2 receptor knockout mice with D1 antagonist, confirming the importance of dopaminergic neurotransmission for the modes of the action of modafinil.

Furthermore, a recent human PET study in 10 healthy humans with $[^{11}C]$ cocaine (DAT radioligand) and $[^{11}C]$ raclopride (D2/D3 radioligand sensitive to changes in endogenous DA) also demonstrated that modafinil (200 mg and 400 mg given orally) decreased $[^{11}C]$ cocaine binding potential in the caudate (53.8%), putamen (47.2%), and nucleus accumbens (39.3%).[71] In addition, modafinil also reduced the binding potential of $[^{11}C]$ raclopride in these structures, suggesting that the increases in extracellular DA were caused by DAT blockades.[71] These results are highly consistent with the results of the animal studies, discussed previously; modafinil's effects on alertness are entirely abolished in mice without the DAT protein[69] and in animals lacking D1 and D2 receptor functions.[70]

Methylphenidate and amphetamines

In 1935, amphetamine was used for the first time for the treatment of narcolepsy. Narcolepsy was possibly the first condition for which amphetamine was used clinically. It revolutionized therapy for the condition, even though it was not curative.

Methylphenidate, the piperazine derivative of amphetamine, was introduced for the treatment of narcolepsy in 1959 and both compounds share similar pharmacologic properties.[72] Phenylisopropylamine (amphetamine) has a simple chemical structure resembling endogenous catecholamines.

Amphetamine-like compounds, such as methylphenidate, pemoline, and fencamfamine, are structurally similar to amphetamines; all compounds include a benzene core with an ethylamine group side chain (phenethylamine derivatives). Methylphenidate is commonly used for the treatment of EDS in narcolepsy, and a racemic mixture of both the D-enantiomer and L-enantiomer is used, but D-methylphenidate mainly contributes to clinical effects, especially after oral administration.

Molecular targets mediating amphetamine-like stimulant effects are complex and vary depending on the specific analog/isomer and the dose administered. Amphetamine per se increases catecholamine (DA and norepinephrine (NE)) release and inhibits reuptake. These effects are mediated by specific catecholamine transporters (ie, DAT and NE transporter).[73] Amphetamine derivatives inhibit the uptake and enhance the release of DA, NE, or both by interacting with these molecules. These mechanisms, as well as the reverse transport (ie, exchange diffusion) and the blocking of the reuptake of DA/NE by amphetamine, all lead to an increase in NE and DA synaptic concentrations.[73]

Methylphenidate is now recommended for use as one of the second-line options. Because there are new medicines available, like sodium oxybate and modafinil/armodafinil, methylphenidate is used when patients do not respond to these new classes of drugs.

The mechanism of action of methylphenidate is similar to that of amphetamines and mainly increases the extracellular concentration of DA by blockage of the DAT and also, to a lesser degree, increases DA release.[74,75]

The side effects of methylphenidate are reduced appetite, nausea, headache, insomnia, and psychosis, which are similar to that of amphetamine.[74] It has been said that methylphenidate increases the risk of cardiovascular events in children and adults[76]; however, a large cohort, including more than 1 million children and young adults, has shown that the risk of the cardiovascular event is not strongly associated with attention deficit-hyperactivity disorder drugs, which is mainly methylphenidate.[77]

In clinical practice, methylphenidate is initially prescribed at 10 mg per day at first. The recommended maximum dose is up to 60 mg per day.

Sodium oxybate

Sodium oxybate, the sodium salt of g-hydroxybutyrate (GHB), taken in the evening and once again during the night, reduces daytime sleepiness, cataplectic attacks, and other manifestations of REM sleep.[78–82] GHB has been used in Canada and European countries for the treatment of narcolepsy-cataplexy. The administration of GHB was followed by a significant decrease in the number of stage shifts and awakenings, wakefulness after sleep onset, and percentage of sleep stage 1. Sleep efficiency and slow-wave sleep percentage increased REM latency decreased significantly.[83] Although improvement in sleepiness occurs relatively quickly, anticataplectic effects appear 1 week to 2 weeks after the initiation of the treatment. Due to its positive effects on mood and libido, its slow-wave sleep-enhancing properties, and a subsequent increase in growth hormone release, GHB is widely abused by athletes and other populations.[84,85] In addition, because of its euphorigenic, behavioral disinhibitive, and amnestic properties, coupled with simple administration (ie, high solubility, colorlessness, and tastelessness when mixed with a drink), the abuse/misuse of GHB as a recreational substance and as a date rape drug has risen sharply in recent years, leading to an increased number of overdoses and intoxications for which no specific antidote exists.[81,86] GHB was classified as a schedule I drug that currently has no accepted medical use for treatment in the United States. Recent large-scale, double-blind, placebo-controlled clinical trials in the United States, however, led to reestablish sodium oxybate (the sodium salt of GHB) as a first-line treatment of narcolepsy-cataplexy.[79–81,87] In the United States, sodium oxybate is the approved formula of GHB and is classified as a schedule III compound. The compound is especially useful in patients with severe insomnia and cataplexy who do not tolerate antidepressant medication well because of its side effects on sexual potency. Although improvement in sleepiness occurs quickly, anticataplectic effects appeared 1 week to 2 weeks after the initiation of the treatment. Sodium oxybate has demonstrated statistically significant improvements in both symptoms, EDS and cataplexy, either as a monotherapy or in combination with modafinil, in clinical trials.[88] According to the meta-analysis, sodium oxybate was superior to placebo in increasing MWT (5.18 minutes; 95% CI, 2.59–7.78) and reducing weekly sleep attacks (−9.65 times; 95% CI, −17.72–1.59).[89] From these wake-promoting effects (on the day after the intake of the compound at night), some researchers try to classify sodium oxybate as a CNS stimulant, but the mode of

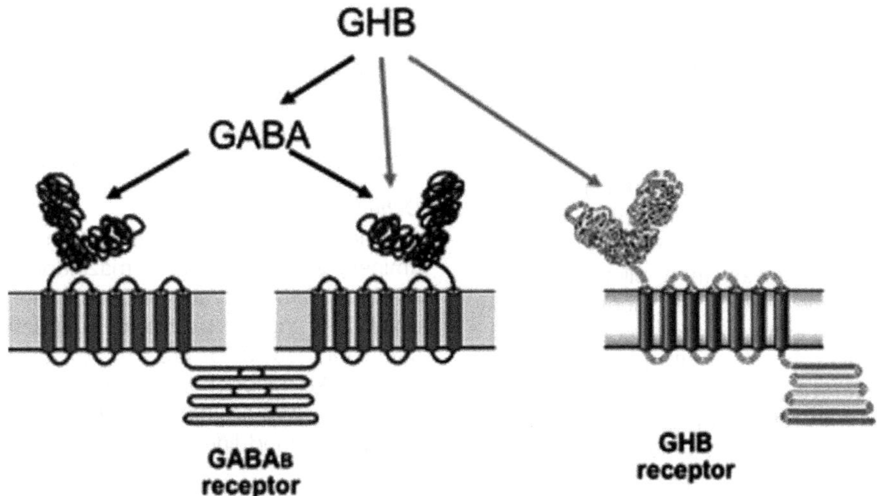

Fig. 3. GHB receptor.

action of wake-promoting effects of sodium oxybate is unknown. Patients first need to take liquid sodium oxybate before they go to bed, and then they need to take the second dose 2.5 hours to 4 hours after the first dose. This is because of the short half-life (0.5–1 hours in the body) and the short duration of action (2–4 hours) of sodium oxybate.[90] The recommended starting dose is 4.5 g a night divided into 2 equal doses of 2.25 g, which may be adjusted up to a maximum of 9 g per night in increments of 1.5 g per night with 1-week to 2- week intervals. The benefit was significant after 4 weeks, highest after 8 weeks, and maintained during long-term therapy.[91] The side effects of sodium oxybate are nausea, insomnia, headache, dizziness, vomiting, weight loss, psychiatric complications, and sleep apnea[92] (see **Table 1**).

Because of the abuse potency of the compound, the Risk Evaluation and Mitigation Strategies program operated by the US FDA mandates prescriber/patient education for safe use and registration to prescribe sodium oxybate.[93] There are also economic drawbacks to using sodium oxybate for the treatment of narcolepsy. The cost of sodium oxybate is expensive, at up to $143,604 per 1 year.[94] The patent will expire in 2024, and the cost of sodium oxybate is likely to be more economical after 2024.

The mechanism of how sodium oxybate works has not been fully understood and it may have multiple mechanisms of action in the brain. A series of experimental evidence suggests that sodium oxybate may work as an agonist on g- aminobutyric acid $(GABA)_b$ receptors.[95] Sodium oxybate is one of the precursors of GABA, and a portion of it may be converted to GABA and stimulate GABA receptors.[96] Several researchers also claimed that sodium oxybate has its own receptor (GHB receptor),[97] but functional roles of this receptor are still largely unknown (**Fig. 3**).

Despite these new findings, the physiological significance of the brain's GHB signaling pathway, especially for the therapeutic effects against EDS and cataplexy, is still unknown. One of the possible modes of action is mediating the regulation of activities of adrenergic locus coeruleus (LC) neurons. The activity of the LC is essential for the maintenance of muscle tone, and the LC ceases to fire during cataplectic attacks.[98] GHB may prevent a cataplectic attack by dampening the tone of LC neurons via the stimulation of inhibitory extrasynaptic GABA receptors in the LC, thus increasing the threshold for autoinhibition.[99] Worsening of periodic leg movements in patients with narcolepsy by sodium oxybate may suggest dopaminergic involvements in the drug action.

Pitolisant (H_3 antagonist/inverse agonist)

Histamine has long been implicated in the control of vigilance, and H_1 antagonists are strongly sedative. The downstream effects of hypocretins on the histaminergic system (hcrtr2 excitatory effects) are likely important in mediating the wake-promoting properties of hypocretin.[100] Although centrally injected histamine and histaminergic H_1 agonists promote wakefulness, systemic administrations of these compounds induce various unacceptable side effects via peripheral H_1 receptor stimulation. In contrast, the histaminergic H_3 receptors are regarded as inhibitory autoreceptors and are enriched in the CNS. H3 antagonists and inverse agonists enhance wakefulness in normal rats and cats[101] and in narcoleptic mice models.[102]

Histaminergic H3 antagonists might be useful as wake-promoting compounds for the treatment of EDS or as cognitive enhancers,[103] and several histaminergic H3 receptor antagonists/inverse agonists are currently being investigated. Pitolisant (previously known as BF2.649 and tiprolisant; Bioprojet, Wakix, Paris, France) was the first clinically used inverse agonist of the histamine H_3 autoreceptor and increases histamine release in the hypothalamus and cortex. In a pilot single-blind study of 22 patients with narcolepsy/cataplexy, pitolisant (40 mg in the morning) reduced EDS.[104] Recent double-blind phase III trials on 95 narcoleptic subjects in 32 sleep disorder centers in 5 European countries revealed that pitolisant (10 mg, 20 mg, or 40 mg) once a day was efficacious on the 2 major symptoms of narcolepsy, EDS and cataplexy, compared with placebo and was better tolerated compared with twice-a-day modafinil (100 mg, 200 mg, or 400 mg).[105] Pitolisant is currently available in the US and is not classified as a scheduled drug by the US Drug Enforcement Administration. The side effects are gastrointestinal pain, increased appetite, weight gain, headache, insomnia, and anxiety.[106] The initial dose of pitolisant is 8.9 mg, taken as a single dose in the morning. The maximum dose is up to 35.6 mg.

Solriamfetol (dopamine/norepinephrine reuptake inhibitor)

Solriamfetol is a dopamine/norepinephrine reuptake inhibitor and is approved for the treatment of adult patients with EDS associated with narcolepsy or obstructive sleep apnea[107] (US Food and Drug Administration, 2019). The starting dose for patients with narcolepsy is 75 mg per day, and that for patients with OSA is 37.5 mg once daily. It is taken in a single dose upon awakening. The efficacy of solriamfetol for the treatment of EDS in patients with narcolepsy has been reported in randomized controlled studies, which demonstrated on the Maintenance of Wakefulness Test and Epworth Sleepiness Scale.[108,109] The maximum dose is 150 mg once daily[107] (US Food and Drug Administration, 2019). The most common side effects include headaches, nausea, decreased appetite, anxiety, and problems sleeping such as insomnia. Solriamfetol may also cause serious side effects, including increased blood pressure, increased heart rate, irritability, and agitation.[107] Solriamfetol is a schedule IV drug in the United States.[110]

Combination strategy

Combination therapy of some stimulants is also recommended when the administration of a single type of stimulant is not effective against EDS in patients with narcolepsy.

The recommended combinations of stimulants are sodium oxybate + modafinil/armodafinil, pitolisant, or methylphenidate + sodium oxybate, and modafinil or methylphenidate + pitolisant.

Other stimulants

Amphetamine and dextroamphetamine (amphetamines, dose 5–60 mg/d), mazindol (a weak DA releaser with DA and NE reuptake inhibitor, dose 2–8 mg/d), pemoline (amphetamine-like stimulant, dose 37.5–112.5 mg/d), and bupropion (DA uptake inhibitor with wake-promotion, dose 150–300 mg/d) are occasionally used if the first-line and second-line medications turn out to be insufficient.

Pharmacotherapy for Rapid Eye Movement Sleep-Related Symptoms in Narcolepsy

The pharmacotherapy for REM sleep-related symptoms in narcolepsy is briefly discussed. Besides sodium oxybate, tricyclic antidepressants; serotonin-NE reuptake inhibitors such as milnacipran and selective serotonin reuptake inhibitors such as paroxetine and fluvoxamine are recommended for patients suffering from cataplexy, hypnagogic hallucinations, and sleep paralysis.[111] Side effects of these antidepressants include dry mouth, obesity, sexual dysfunction, type 2 diabetes, and suicidal tendencies.[112] Antidepressants suppress cataplexy, hypnagogic hallucinations, and sleep paralysis, and this effect seems due to suppression of REM sleep or prolongation of REM sleep latency.[21,113]

Idiopathic Hypersomnia

With the clear definition of narcolepsy (cataplexy and dissociated manifestations of REM sleep), it became apparent that some patients with hypersomnia suffer from a different disorder. In the late 1950s and early 1960s, Bedrich Roth[114] first described a syndrome characterized by EDS, prolonged sleep, and sleep drunkenness, and by the absence of sleep attacks, cataplexy, sleep paralysis, and hallucinations. The terms *independent sleep drunkenness* and *hypersomnia with sleep drunkenness* were initially suggested, but now this syndrome is categorized as idiopathic hypersomnia with and without long sleep time.[42]

In the absence of systematic studies, the prevalence of idiopathic hypersomnia is unknown. Nosologic uncertainty causes difficulty in determining the epidemiology of the disorder. Recent reports from large sleep centers reported the ratio of idiopathic hypersomnia to narcolepsy to be

1:10.[115] The age of onset of symptoms varies, but it is frequently between 10 and 30 years. The condition usually develops progressively over several weeks or months. Once established, symptoms are generally stable and long lasting, but spontaneous improvement in EDS may be observed in up to one-quarter of patients.[115]

The pathogenesis of idiopathic hypersomnia is unknown. Hypersomnia usually starts insidiously. Occasionally, EDS is first experienced after transient insomnia, abrupt changes in sleep-wake habits, overexertion, general anesthesia, viral illness, or mild head trauma.[115] Despite reports of an increase in HLA-DQ1, DQ11, DR5, Cw2, and DQ3 and decrease in Cw3, no consistent findings have emerged.[115]

The most recent attempts to understand the pathophysiology of idiopathic hypersomnia relate to the investigation of the potential role of the hypocretins. Most studies suggest, however, normal CSF levels of hypocretin-1 in idiopathic hypersomnia.[41,116]

Patients with idiopathic hypersomnia have less sleep paralysis (20% of patients with idiopathic hypersomnia) and sleep hallucinations (25%) than narcolepsy. Among patients with idiopathic hypersomnia, sleep drunkenness and long nocturnal sleep times without fragmentation are common, and the effects and duration of naps are unrefreshing and long compared with patients with narcolepsy.[15,117,118] Recently, the US FDA has approved an oral solution of calcium, magnesium, potassium, and sodium oxybate for the treatment of idiopathic hypersomnia in adults. In a clinical setting, modafinil is also used off-label to treat EDS in idiopathic hypersomnia, as in narcolepsy.[119,120] If EDS is irresistible and resistant to modafinil, methylphenidate and amphetamine-like compounds are also used. A recent article has shown that sodium oxybate improves the sleepiness of idiopathic patients as much as it improves sleepiness in narcolepsy type 1; however, sodium oxybate has strong side effects and dependency, as discussed prevously.[120,121]

Hypersomnia Due to a Medical Disorder

The prevalence of symptomatic narcolepsy (ie, narcolepsy due to a medical disorder) is likely small, and only approximately 120 such cases have been reported in the literature in the past 30 years.[122] The prevalence of symptomatic (ie, hypersomnia due to a medical disorder) hypersomnia, however, may be much higher. For example, several million subjects in the United States suffer from chronic brain injury; 75% of these patients have sleep problems and approximately half of them claim sleepiness.[123] Patients with hypersomnia due to a medical disorder have EDS caused by coexisting medical or neurologic disorders. Daytime sleepiness of this disorder may be similar to that of narcolepsy or idiopathic hypersomnia.[15,118] Common disorders are discussed later, and in any secondary hypersomnia, it is important to treat the underlying disease besides providing symptomatic therapies.

Post-traumatic Hypersomnia

According to a meta-analysis research, the prevalence of EDS among patients with post-traumatic brain injury is 27%.[124] CSF hypocretin-1 levels are low in most patients with moderate to severe traumatic brain injuries during their acute injury phase.[125] Regarding treatment, the effectiveness of modafinil is still under controversy. A randomized controlled trial (RCT) has shown that modafinil improves the Epworth Sleepiness Scale (ESS) score significantly compared with placebo at 6 treatment weeks.[126] Another RCT shows, however, that modafinil did not consistently improve the ESS score compared with the placebo at 10 treatment weeks.[127] Another RCT has demonstrated that armodafinil does not improve the ESS score compared with placebo at 12 treatment weeks.[128]

Hypersomnia Secondary to Parkinson's Disease

Like narcolepsy and idiopathic hypersomnia, daytime sleepiness is measured by ESS and MSLT. Among patients with Parkinson's disease, 20% to 50% are said to have EDS.[129–131]

The effect of modafinil on this disorder is still controversial. There are some studies that have shown that modafinil improves EDS in patients with Parkinson's disease,[132,133] whereas there are other that have shown that modafinil does not improve EDS in patients with Parkinson's disease.[133,134] An article has also shown that sodium oxybate can improve EDS in patients with Parkinson's disease.[135]

Common Stimulants in Daily Life

Caffeine is probably the most popular and widely consumed CNS stimulant in the world. Caffeine is digested from foods, drinks, and sometimes chocolate, coffee, energy drinks, soft drinks, and so forth. Caffeine is a xanthine derivative and acts as an adenosine A1 and adenosine A2A receptor agonist.[136] Adenosine content is increased in the basal forebrain after sleep deprivation. Adenosine has thus been proposed as a sleep-inducing substance accumulating in the brain during prolonged wakefulness.[137] Side effects of caffeine are often overlooked; however, sometimes they are crucial. A variety of side effects of caffeine is well known, which are headache, stomach upset, nervousness, and so forth. For the common side effects of caffeine in terms of sleep, caffeine typically prolongs sleep latency, reduces total sleep time and sleep efficiency, and worsens perceived sleep quality.[136] An average cup of coffee contains 50 mg to 150 mg of caffeine. Caffeine is also available over the counter (NoDoz, 200 mg caffeine [GlaxoSmithKline plc, Middlesex, United Kingdom]; Vivarin, 200 mg caffeine [Meda Consumer Healthcare Inc, NJ]). This suggests that the stimulant effects of caffeine tablets are not strong enough to manage pathologic sleepiness, but patients with narcolepsy often take caffeine before they are diagnosed. According to a recent review, moderate caffeine intake (400 mg/d) is not associated with adverse effects.[138] The average cup of ground roasted coffee contains 85 mg of caffeing, and instant coffee contains 60 mg of caffeing.[139] Drinking fewer than 5 cups of ground roasted coffee per day is better for health.

FUTURE TREATMENT OPTIONS

Hypocertin/Orexin-Based Treatments

Because a large majority of human patients with narcolepsy are hypocretin ligand deficient, hypocretin replacement therapy may be a new therapeutic option. This may be effective for both sleepiness (ie, fragmented sleep/wake pattern) and cataplexy. Animal experiments using ligand-deficient narcoleptic dogs suggest that stable and centrally active hypocretin analogs (possibly nonpeptide synthetic hypocretin ligands) need to be developed to be peripherally effective.[140,141] This is also substantiated by a mice study that found the normalization of sleep/wake patterns and behavioral arrest episodes (equivalent to cataplexy and REM sleep onset) in hypocretin-deficient mice knockout models supplemented by central administration of hypocretin-1.[142] In addition, orexin gene therapy (injection of adenoassociated viral vector coding for prepro-orexin plus a red fluorescence protein into the mediobasal hypothalamus) markedly improved the MWT in orexin/ataxin-3 narcoleptic mice.[143] These results demonstrate that cell transplantations and gene therapy may be developed in the future. One of the peptides does not cross the blood–brain barrier (BBB) well. Intranasal delivery is a noninvasive method of bypassing the BBB to deliver therapeutic agents to the brain and spinal cord. Developments of small molecule nonpeptide hypocretin receptor agonists are in progress and have shown effectiveness in mouse models.[144] Recently, orexin 2 receptor-selective agonists, TAK-925 and TAK-994, were discovered.[145,146] Both compounds are now progressing to clinical studies. Regarding TAK-925, the results of the Phase I study have been reported. Low-dose TAK-925 (44 mg), high-dose TAK-925 (112 mg), and modafinil (300 mg) significantly increased wakefulness compared to placebo, and high-dose TAK-925 was more effective than low-dose TAK-925 and modafinil.[147] The results show TAK-925 to be effective at promoting wakefulness. Unfortunately, both phase 2 studies of TAK-994 were stopped owing to participants having a significant liver function test elevation.167,168 Recent reports in both rhesus monkeys and humans show some effects using intranasal hypocretin-1 administration.[148,149] A recent double-blind, randomized, placebo-controlled crossover design study on 7 patients with narcolepsy/cataplexy and matched healthy controls showed that intranasal hypocretin-1 restores olfactory function in patients with narcolepsy/cataplexy.[148] However, no data exist concerning potential effects of daytime sleepiness and cataplexy at this time.

Immune-Based Treatments

Type 1 narcolepsy is currently thought to be an autoimmune disorder targeting hypothalamus hypocretin neurons. An autoimmune basis for the hypocretin cell loss in narcolepsy has been suspected due to its strong DQB1*0602 association and association with T-cell receptor polymorphisms.[150] Based on the autoimmune hypothesis of narcolepsy, immune-based therapy, such as steroids (in 1 patient), intravenous immunoglobulins, and plasmapheresis have been proposed, with some promising results in a few cases.[151,152] Recently, a case of narcolepsy with cataplexy with undetectable CSF hypocretin-1 level that completely reversed shortly after disease onset was reported.[151] Although needing replication in well-designed trials, these results suggest that immune-based therapy could become a new treatment option for patients with narcolepsy/cataplexy at disease onset.

Other Possible Treatments of Interest (Nonhypocretin-Based Treatments)

In addition to hypocretin replacement, preclinical and clinical trials for new classes of compounds are also in progress.

In 1983, Osamu Hayaishi[153] and his group claimed that prostaglandin (PG) D2 is an endogenous sleep substance, and a series of animal studies by his group reported that PGD2 or

PGD2 receptor (DP1) agonists promote sleep in animals (see Huang and colleagues[154]). The same research group also reported that PG DP1 potently promotes wakefulness. This suggests the possible use of PG DP1 antagonists as wake-promoting compounds. This may also be clinically important because it is reported that increased serum lipocalin-type PGD synthase (beta-trace) levels correlate with EDS associated with narcolepsy.[155] Wake-promoting effects of a DP1 antagonist, ONO-4127, were evaluated in a mouse model of narcolepsy (ie, orexin/ataxin-3 transgenic mice) and compared with effects of modafinil.[156] ONO-4127 perfused in the basal forebrain area potently promoted wakefulness in both wild-type and narcoleptic mice, and the wake-promoting effects of ONO-4127 at $2.93 \times 10{\sim}^{4}$ M approximately corresponded to those of modafinil at 100 mg/kg, orally; ONO-4127 reduced DREM (direct transitions from wake to REM sleep), an electro-encephalogram/ electromyogram assessment of behavioral cataplexy, in narcoleptic mice, suggesting that ONO-4127 is likely to have anticataplectic effects; DP1 antagonists may be a new class of compounds for the treatment of narcolepsy-cataplexy.

Another possible area that currently gathers less pharmaceutical interest is the use of thyrotropin-releasing hormone (TRH) direct or indirect agonists. TRH itself is a small peptide, which penetrates the BBB at very high doses. Small molecules with agonistic properties and increased BBB penetration (ie, CG3703, CG3509, orTA0910) have been developed, partially thanks to the small nature of the starting peptide.[157] TRH (at a high dose of several milligrams/kilograms) and TRH agonists increase alertness and have been shown to be wake promoting and anticataplectic in the narcoleptic canine model,[158,159] and these effects might be related to the excitatory effects of TRH on motoneurons.[160] Initial studies have demonstrated that TRH enhances DA and NE neurotransmission,[161,162] and these properties may partially contribute to the wake-promoting and anticataplectic effects of TRH. Recent studies have suggested that TRH may promote wakefulness by directly interacting with the thalamocortical network; TRH itself and TRH receptor type 2 are abundant in the reticular thalamic nucleus.[163] Local application of TRH in the thalamus abolishes spindle wave activity,[164] and in the slice preparations, TRH depolarized thalamocortical and reticular/ perigeniculate neurons by the inhibition of leak K+ conductance.[164]

Other pathways with possible applications in the development of novel stimulant medications include the adenosinergic system (more selective receptor antagonists than caffeine), the dopaminergic/adrenergic system (for example, DA/NE-reuptake inhibitors), the GABAergic system (for example, inverse benzodiazepine agonists), and the glutamatergic system (ampakines).[165]

SUMMARY

This article overviews pharmacotherapy of EDS associated with narcolepsy type 1, narcolepsy type 2, idiopathic hypersomnia, and hypersomnia due to a medical disorder.

Narcolepsy-cataplexy is most commonly caused by a loss of hypocretin-producing cells in the hypothalamus (ie, type 1 narcolepsy). Low CSF hypocretin-1 levels can be used to diagnose the condition. The disorder is tightly associated with HLA-DQB1*0602, suggesting that the cause in most patients may be the autoimmune destruction of these cells. Treatment of EDS includes the use of amphetamine-like CNS stimulants, modafinil, and its R-enantiomer armodafinil. Methylphenidate is the most commonly prescribed amphetamine-like stimulant in the United States, and this compound is efficacious and well tolerated by most patients with narcolepsy. Because of its safe and low side-effect profile, modafinil became the first-line treatment of choice for EDS associated with narcolepsy. These wake-promoting compounds, however, do not improve cataplexy and dissociated manifestations of REM sleep, so antidepressants (monoamine uptake inhibitors) are additionally used to treat these aspects. Sodium oxybate (a sodium salt of GHB, available in the United States), when given at night, improves EDS and cataplexy, Therefore, the number of US patients treated with sodium oxybate is increasing, and it has become the first-line treatment of narcolepsy. Combination therapy with some stimulants is also recommended when the administration of a single stimulant type is not effective against EDS in patients with narcolepsy. Recently, the US FDA has approved an oral solution of calcium, magnesium, potassium, and sodium oxybate for the treatment of idiopathic hypersomnia in adults. Treatments of EDS associated with symptomatic hypersomnia (ie, hypersomnias due to a medical disorder) are more complex because these conditions are heterogeneous, and hypocretin involvements are seen in some disease conditions but not in all. Specific brain structures that have been damaged and mechanisms involved in EDS are likely varied. Unresponsiveness to stimulant treatments may occur depending on the underlying pathophysiologic mechanism. In this regard, the development of new types of wake-promoting compounds would likely benefit these patients.

Emerging treatments undergoing investigation include TRH agonists, DP1 antagonists, hypocretin replacement/supplement therapies, and immunomodulation for prevention.

There are many potential approaches for narcolepsy; compounds and new therapies, such as hypocretin transplant or gene technology, are being developed.[166] The development of small molecular synthetic hypocretin receptor agonists, however, is likely the next step for this therapeutic option in humans, because hypocretin peptides themselves do not penetrate the brain effectively. Recently, orexin 2 receptor-selective agonists were discovered and are now progressing to clinical studies. If ligand replacement therapy is demonstrated as effective in hypocretin-deficient narcolepsy, hypocretin cell transplant or gene therapy technology may also be applicable in the near future. These therapies, however, are many years away, and the efficacy of exogenously administered hypocretin analogs (nonpeptide agonists) in humans should be established first.

To prevent hypoceretin neuronal loss (ie, narcolepsy type 1), immune-based treatments are promising, but the accumulation of many cases is needed to prove the efficacy of this approach.

CLINICS CARE POINTS

- Treatment of EDS includes the use of amphetamine-like CNS stimulants, modafinil, and its R-enantiomer armodafinil.
- Modafinil is the first-line treatment of choice for EDS associated with narcolepsy because of its safe and low side-effect profile.
- Antidepressants (monoamine uptake inhibitors) are used to treat cataplexy and dissociated manifestations of REM sleep.
- Sodium oxybate (a sodium salt of GHB, available in the United States), when given at night, improves EDS and cataplexy.

DISCLOSURE

The authors declare no conflicts of interest associated with this article.

REFERENCES

1. Arand D, Bonnet M, Hurwitz T, et al. The clinical use of the MSLT and MWT. Sleep 2005;28(1):123–44.
2. Pagnin D, de Queiroz V, Carvalho YT, et al. The relation between burnout and sleep disorders in medical students. Acad Psychiatry 2014;38(4):438–44.
3. Swanson LM, Arnedt JT, Rosekind MR, et al. Sleep disorders and work performance: findings from the 2008 National Sleep Foundation Sleep in America poll. J Sleep Res 2011;20(3):487–94.
4. Young TB. Epidemiology of daytime sleepiness: definitions, symptomatology, and prevalence. J Clin Psychiatry 2004;65(Suppl 16):12–6.
5. Wu S, Wang R, Ma X, et al. Excessive daytime sleepiness assessed by the Epworth Sleepiness Scale and its association with health related quality of life: a population-based study in China. BMC Public Health 2012;12:849.
6. Plante DT, Finn LA, Hagen EW, et al. Longitudinal associations of hypersomnolence and depression in the Wisconsin sleep cohort study. J Affect Disord 2017;207:197–202.
7. Roth T. Effects of excessive daytime sleepiness and fatigue on overall health and cognitive function. J Clin Psychiatry 2015;76(9):e1145.
8. Garbarino S, Durando P, Guglielmi O, et al. Sleep apnea, sleep debt and daytime sleepiness are independently associated with road accidents. A cross-sectional study on truck drivers. PLoS One 2016;11(11):e0166262.
9. Murray BJ. A practical approach to excessive day time sleepiness: a focused review. Can Respir J 2016;2016:4215938.
10. Doyle JB, Daniels LE. Symptomatic treatment for narcolepsy. J Am Med Assoc 1931;96(17):1370–2.
11. Akimoto H, Honda Y, Takahashi Y. Pharmacotherapy in narcolepsy. Dis Nerv Syst 1960;21:704–6.
12. Guilleminault C, Carskadon M, Dement WC. On the treatment of rapid eye movement narcolepsy. Arch Neurol 1974;30(1):90–3.
13. Parkes JD, Baraitser M, Marsden CD, et al. Natural history, symptoms and treatment of the narcoleptic syndrome. Acta Neurol Scand 1975;52(5):337–53.
14. Passouant P, Billiard M. [Narcolepsy]. Rev Prat 1976;26(27):1917–23.
15. ICSD-3. International classification of sleep disorders. 3rd edition. Rochester (MN): American Sleep Disorders Association; 2014. Medicine AAoS.
16. Arnulf I. Kleine-levin syndrome. Sleep Med Clin 2015;10(2):151–61.
17. Medicine AAoS. International classification of sleep disorders. 3rd edition. Daren (IL): American Academy of Sleep Medicine; 2014.
18. Hublin C, Kaprio J, Partinene M, et al. The prevalence of narcolepsy: an epidemiological study of the Finnish twin cohort. Ann Neurol 1994;35:709–16.
19. TashiroT, KanbayashiT, HishikawaY. An epidemiological study of narcolepsy in Japanese. Paper

pre sented at: The 4th International Symposium on Narcolepsy. Tokyo, Japan, June 16-17, 1994. p. 13.
20. Dauvilliers Y, Montplaisir J, Molinari N, et al. Age at onset of narcolepsy in two large populations of pa tients in France and Quebec. Neurology 2001; 57(11):2029–33.
21. Nishino S, Mignot E. Pharmacological aspects of human and canine narcolepsy. Prog Neurobiol 1997;52(1):27–78.
22. Pizza F, Contardi S, Mondini S, et al. Daytime sleepiness and driving performance in patients with obstructive sleep apnea: comparison of the MSLT, the MWT, and a simulated driving task. Sleep 2009;32(3):382–91.
23. Littner MR, Kushida C, Wise M, et al. Practice pa rameters for clinical use of the multiple sleep latency test and the maintenance of wakefulness test. Sleep 2005;28(1):113–21.
24. Sullivan SS, Kushida CA. Multiple sleep latency test and maintenance of wakefulness test. Chest 2008;134(4):854–61.
25. Scammell TE. Narcolepsy. N Engl J Med 2015; 373(27):2654–62.
26. Dauvilliers Y, Billiard M, Montplaisir J. Clinical aspects and pathophysiology of narcolepsy. Clin Neurophysiol 2003;114(11):2000–17.
27. Guilleminault C, Kryger MH, Roth T, et al. Narco lepsy syndrome. Principles and practice of sleep medicine. 2nd edition. Philadelphia: WB Saunders; 1994. p. 549–61.
28. Juji T, Satake M, Honda Y, et al. HLA antigens in Japanese patients with narcolepsy. All the patients were DR2 positive. Tissue Antigens 1984;24(5):316–9.
29. Gelb M, Guilleminault C, Kraemer H, et al. Stability of cataplexy over several months-information for the design of therapeutic trials. Sleep 1994;17(3): 265–73.
30. Hishikawa Y, Wakamatsu H, Furuya E, et al. Sleep satiation in narcoleptic patients. Electroencephalogr Clin Neurophysiol 1976;41:1–18.
31. Broughton R, Dunham W, Newman J, et al. Ambulatory 24 hour sleep-wake monitoring in narcolepsy-cataplexy compared to matched control. Electroencephalogr Clin Neurophysiol 1988; 70:473–81.
32. Montplaisir J, Billard M, Takahashi S, et al. Twenty-four-hour recording in REM-narcoleptics with special reference to nocturnal sleep disruption. Biol Psychiatry 1978;13(1):78–89.
33. Godbout R, Montplaisir J. Comparison of sleep pa rameters in narcoleptics with and without periodic movements of sleep. In: Koella WP, Ruther E, Schulz H, editors. Sleep '84. New York: Gustav Fischer Verlag; 1985. p. 380–2.
34. Mosko SS, Shampain DS, Sassin JF. Nocturnal REM latency and sleep disturbance in narcolepsy. Sleep 1984;7:115–25.
35. Mayer G, Pollmächer T, Meier-Ewert K, et al. Zur Einschatzung des Behinderungsgrades bei Narkolepsie. Gesundheitswesen 1993;55:337–42.
36. Schenck CH, Mahowald MW. Motor dyscontrol in narcolepsy: rapid-Eye-Movement (REM) sleep without atonia and REM sleep behavior disorder. Ann Neurol 1992;32(1):3–10.
37. Chokroverty S. Sleep apnea in narcolepsy. Sleep 1986;9(1):250–3.
38. Guilleminault C, Dement WC, Passouant P, editors. Narcolepsy. New York: Spectrum Publications; 1976. Advances in Sleep Research; No. 3.
39. Juji T, Matsuki K, Tokunaga K, et al. Narcolepsy and HLA in the Japanese. Ann N Y Acad Sci 1988;540:106–14.
40. Nishino S, Ripley B, Overeem S, et al. Hypocretin (orexin) deficiency in human narcolepsy. Lancet 2000;355(9197):39–40.
41. Mignot E, Lammers GJ, Ripley B, et al. The role of cerebrospinal fluid hypocretin measurement in the diagnosis of narcolepsy and other hypersomnias. Arch Neurol 2002;59(10):1553–62.
42. ICSD-2. ICSD-2-International classification of sleep disorders. In: Sateia MJ, editor. Diagnostic and cod ing manual. 2nd edition. Westchester (IL): American Academy of Sleep Medicine; 2005. p. 38–43.
43. Mignot E, Hayduk R, Black J, et al. HLA DQB1*0602 is associated with cataplexy in 509 narcoleptic patients. Sleep 1997;20(11):1012–20.
44. Dauvilliers Y, Maret S, Bassetti C, et al. A monozygotic twin pair discordant for narcolepsy and CSF hypocretin-1. Neurology 2004;62(11):2137–8.
45. Ripley B, Fujiki N, Okura M, et al. Hypocretin levels in sporadic and familial cases of canine narco lepsy. Neurobiol Dis 2001;8(3):525–34.
46. Thannickal TC, Nienhuis R, Siegel JM. Localized loss of hypocretin (orexin) cells in narcolepsy without cataplexy. Sleep 2009;32(8):993–8.
47. Garma L, Marchand F. Non-pharmacological approaches to the treatment of narcolepsy. Sleep 1994;17(8 Suppl):S97–102.
48. Roehrs T, Zorick F, Wittig R, et al. Alerting effects of naps in patients with narcolepsy. Sleep 1986;9(1): 194–9.
49. Rogers AE. Problems and coping strategies identified by narcoleptic patients. J Neurosurg Nurs 1984;16(6):326–34.
50. Morgenthaler TI, Kapur VK, Brown T, et al. Practice parameters for the treatment of narcolepsy and other hypersomnias of central origin. Sleep 2007; 30(12):1705–11.
51. Hirai N, Nishino S. Recent advances in the treat ment of narcolepsy. Curr Treat Options Neurol 2011;13(5):437–57.
52. Mitler MM, Aldrich MS, Koob GF, et al. Narcolepsy and its treatment with stimulants. ASDA standards of practice. Sleep 1994;17(4):352–71.

53. Mitler MM, Hajdukovic R. Relative efficacy of drugs for the treatment of sleepiness in narcolepsy. Sleep 1991;14(3):218–20.
54. Rogers AE, Aldrich MS, Berrios AM, et al. Compli ance with stimulant medications in patients with narcolepsy. Sleep 1997;20(1):28–33.
55. Auger RR, Goodman SH, Silber MH, et al. Risks of high-dose stimulants in the treatment of disorders of excessive somnolence: a case-control study. Sleep 2005;28(6):667–72.
56. Nishino S, Okuro M. Armodafinil for excessive day time sleepiness. Drugs Today (Barc) 2008;44(6): 395–414.
57. Darwish M, Kirby M, Hellriegel ET, et al. Armodafinil and modafinil have substantially different pharma cokinetic profiles despite having the same terminal half-lives: analysis of data from three randomized, single-dose, pharmacokinetic studies. Clin Drug Investig 2009;29(9):613–23.
58. Randomized trial of modafinil for the treatment of pathological somnolence in narcolepsy. US Moda finil in Narcolepsy Multicenter Study Group. Ann Neurol 1998;43(1):88–97.
59. Randomized trial of modafinil as a treatment for the excessive daytime somnolence of narcolepsy: US Modafinil in Narcolepsy Multicenter Study Group. Neurology 2000;54(5):1166–75.
60. Harsh JR, Hayduk R, Rosenberg R, et al. The effi cacy and safety of armodafinil as treatment for adults with excessive sleepiness associated with narcolepsy. Curr Med Res Opin 2006;22(4):761–74.
61. United States Department of Justice. Drug enforce ment administration. Drug scheduling. Available at: https://www.dea.gov/druginfo/ds.shtml. Accessed February 10, 2017.
62. Roth T, Schwartz JR, Hirshkowitz M, et al. Evalua tion of the safety of modafinil for treatment of excessive sleepiness. J Clin Sleep Med 2007; 3(6):595–602.
63. U.S. Food & Drug Administration. Drug safety. Medication guide. Available at: https://www.sec.gov/Archives/edgar/ data/873364/ 000110465907048203/a07-16834_ 1ex99d1.htm. Accessed February 11, 2017.
64. Schwartz JR, Feldman NT, Bogan RK, et al. Dosing regimen effects of modafinil for improving daytime wakefulness in patients with narcolepsy. Clin Neuropharmacol 2003;26(5):252–7.
65. Cephalon, Inc. FDA approval of NUVIGIL. Available at: https://www.sec.gov/Archives/edgar/data/873364/000110465907048203/a07-16834_ 1ex99d1.htm. Accessed February 11, 2017.
66. Mignot E, Nishino S, Guilleminault C, et al. Modafinil binds to the dopamine uptake carrier site with low affinity. Sleep 1994;17(5):436–7.
67. Nishino S, Mao J, Sampathkumaran R, et al. Increased dopaminergic transmission mediates the wake-promoting effects of CNS stimulants. Sleep Res Online 1998;1(1):49–61.
68. Dopheide MM, Morgan RE, Rodvelt KR, et al. Mod afinil evokes striatal [(3)H]dopamine release and alters the subjective properties of stimulants. Eur J Pharmacol 2007;568(1–3):112–23.
69. Wisor JP, Nishino S, Sora I, et al. Dopaminergic role in stimulant-induced wakefulness. J Neurosci 2001;21(5):1787–94.
70. Qu WM, Huang ZL, Xu XH, et al. Dopaminergic D1 and D2 receptors are essential for the arousal effect of modafinil. J Neurosci 2008;28(34):8462–9.
71. Volkow ND, Fowler JS, Logan J, et al. Effects of modafinil on dopamine and dopamine transporters in the male human brain: clinical implications. JAMA 2009;301(11):1148–54.
72. Yoss RE, Daly D. Treatment of narcolepsy with ritalin. Neurology 1959;9(3):171–3.
73. Kuczenski R, Segal DS. Neurochemistry of amphetamine, in psychopharmacology, toxicology and abuse. San Diego (CA): Academic Press; 1994. p. 81–113.
74. Leonard BE, McCartan D, White J, et al. Methylphenidate: a review of its neuropharmacological, neuropsychological and adverse clinical effects. Hum Psychopharmacol 2004;19(3):151–80.
75. Schenk JO. The functioning neuronal transporter for dopamine: kinetic mechanisms and effects of amphetamines, cocaine and methylphenidate. Prog Drug Res 2002;59:111–31.
76. Nissen SE. ADHD drugs and cardiovascular risk. N Engl J Med 2006;354(14):1445–8.
77. Cooper WO, Habel LA, Sox CM, et al. ADHD drugs and serious cardiovascular events in children and young adults. N Engl J Med 2011;365(20): 1896–904.
78. Broughton R, Mamelak M. The treatment of narcolepsy-cataplexy with nocturnal gamma-hydroxybutyrate. Can J Neurol Sci 1979;6(1):1–6.
79. Group USXMS. A randomized, double blind, placebo-controlled multicenter trial comparing the effects of three doses of orally administered sodium oxybate with placebo for the treatment of nar colepsy. Sleep 2002;25(1):42–9.
80. Group USXMS. A 12-month, open-label, multi- center extension trial of orally administered sodium oxybate for the treatment of narcolepsy. Sleep 2003;26(1):31–5.
81. Group USXMS. Sodium oxybate demonstrates long-term efficacy for the treatment of cataplexy in patients with narcolepsy. Sleep Med 2004;5(2):119–23.
82. Mamelak M, Scharf MB, Woods M. Treatment of narcolepsy with gamma-hydroxybutyrate. A review of clinical and sleep laboratory findings. Sleep 1986;9(1 Pt 2):285–9.
83. Plazzi G, Pizza F, Vandi S, et al. Impact of acute administration of sodium oxybate on nocturnal

sleep polysomnography and on multiple sleep la tency test in narcolepsy with cataplexy. Sleep Med 2014;15(9):1046–54.
84. Mack RB. Love potion number 8 1/2. Gamma- hydroxybutyrate poisoning. N C Med J 1993;54(5):232–3.
85. Wong CG, Gibson KM, Snead OC 3rd. From the street to the brain: neurobiology of the recreational drug gamma-hydroxybutyric acid. Trends Pharmacol Sci 2004;25(1):29–34.
86. Nicholson KL, Balster RL. GHB: a new and novel drug of abuse. Drug Alcohol Depend 2001;63(1): 1–22.
87. Black J, Houghton WC. Sodium oxybate improves excessive daytime sleepiness in narcolepsy. Sleep 2006;29(7):939–46.
88. Robinson DM, Keating GM. Sodium oxybate: a review of its use in the management of narcolepsy. CNS Drugs 2007;21(4):337–54.
89. Alshaikh MK, Tricco AC, Tashkandi M, et al. Sodium oxybate for narcolepsy with cataplexy: systematic review and meta-analysis. J Clin Sleep Med 2012; 8(4):451–8.
90. Thorpy MJ. Update on therapy for narcolepsy. Curr Treat Options Neurol 2015;17(5):347.
91. Palatini P, Tedeschi L, Frison G, et al. Dose-dependent absorption and elimination of gamma- hydroxybutyric acid in healthy volunteers. Eur J Clin Pharmacol 1993;45(4):353–6.
92. Wang YG, Swick TJ, Carter LP, et al. Safety over view of postmarketing and clinical experience of sodium oxybate (Xyrem): abuse, misuse, depen dence, and diversion. J Clin Sleep Med 2009; 5(4):365–71.
93. Administration tUSFaD. Available at: http://www.fda.gov/Drugs/DrugSafety/PostmarketDrugSafetyInformationforPatientsandProviders/ucm332408.htm. Accessed February 9, 2017.
94. Saini P, Rye DB. Hypersomnia: evaluation, treat ment, and social and economic aspects. Sleep Med Clin 2017;12(1):47–60.
95. Maitre M, Klein C, Mensah-Nyagan AG. Mecha nisms for the specific properties of gamma- hydroxybutyrate in brain. Med Res Rev 2016;36(3): 363–88.
96. Pardi D, Black J. g-hydroxybutyrate/sodium oxy bate. CNS drugs 2006;20(12):993–1018.
97. Andriamampandry C, Taleb O, Viry S, et al. Cloning and characterization of a rat brain receptor that binds the endogenous neuromodulator gamma- hydroxybutyrate (GHB). Faseb J 2003;17(12):1691–3.
98. Wu MF, Gulyani SA, Yau E, et al. Locus coeruleus neurons: cessation of activity during cataplexy. Neuroscience 1999;91(4):1389–99.
99. Szabadi E. GHB for cataplexy: possible mode of action. J Psychopharmacol 2015;29(6):744–9.
100. Nishino S, Ripley B, Mignot E, et al. CSF hypocretin-1 levels in schizophrenics and controls: relationship to sleep architecture. Psychiatry Res 2002;110(1):1–7.
101. Shiba T. Wake promoting effects of thioperamide, a histamine H3 antagonist in orexin/ataxin-3 narco leptic mice. Sleep 2004;27(Suppl):A241–2.
102. Parmentier R, Anaclet C, Guhennec C, et al. The brain H3-receptor as a novel therapeutic target for vigilance and sleep-wake disorders. Biochem Pharmacol 2007;73(8):1157–71.
103. Lin JS, Dauvilliers Y, Arnulf I, et al. An inverse agonist of the histamine H(3) receptor improves wakefulness in narcolepsy: studies in orexin-/- mice and patients. Neurobiol Dis 2008;30(1): 74–83.
104. Dauvilliers Y, Bassetti C, Lammers GJ, et al. Pitolisant versus placebo or modafinil in patients with narcolepsy: a double-blind, randomised trial. Lancet Neurol 2013;12(11):1068–75.
105. Sharif NA, To ZP, Whiting RL. Analogs of thyrotropin- releasing hormone (TRH): receptor affinities in brains, spinal cords, and pituitaries of different spe- cies. Neurochem Res 1991;16(2):95–103.
106. Leu-Semenescu S, Nittur N, Golmard JL, et al. Ef fects of pitolisant, a histamine H3 inverse agonist, in drug-resistant idiopathic and symptomatic hy persomnia: a chart review. Sleep Med 2014;15(6): 681–7.
107. U.S. Food and Drug Administration. SUNOSI (solriamfetol): Highlights of prescribing information. Available from: https://www.accessdata.fda.gov/drugsatfda_docs/label/2019/211230s000lbl.pdf. Cited July 1, 2022.
108. Bogan RK, Feldman N, Emsellem HA, et al. Effect of oral JZP-110 (ADX-N05) treatment on wakefulness and sleepiness in adults with narcolepsy. Sleep Med 2015;16:1102–8.
109. Ruoff C, Swick TJ, Doekel R, et al. Effect of oral JZP-110 (ADX-N05) on wakefulness and sleepiness in adults with narcolepsy: a phase 2b study. Sleep 2016;39:1379–87.
110. Gandhi KD, Mansukhani MP, Silber MH, et al. Excessive daytime sleepiness: a clinical review. Mayo Clin Proc 2021;96:1288–301.
111. Swick TJ. Treatment paradigms for cataplexy in narcolepsy: past, present, and future. Nat Sci Sleep 2015;7:159–69.
112. Santarsieri D, Schwartz TL. Antidepressant efficacy and side-effect burden: a quick guide for clini cians. Drugs Context 2015;4:212290.
113. Thase ME. Depression, sleep, and antidepres sants. J Clin Psychiatry 1998;59(Suppl 4):55–65.
114. Roth B. Narkolepsie und hypersomnie. Berlin: VEB Verlag Volk und Gesundheit; 1962.
115. Bassetti C, Aldrich MS. Idiopathic hypersomnia. A series of 42 patients. Brain 1997;120(Pt 8):1423–35.
116. Bassetti C, Gugger M, Bischof M, et al. The narcoleptic borderland: a multimodal diagnostic

approach including cerebrospinal fluid levels of hypocretin-1 (orexin A). Sleep Med 2003;4(1):7–12.
117. Vernet C, Leu-Semenescu S, Buzare MA, et al. Subjective symptoms in idiopathic hypersomnia: beyond excessive sleepiness. J Sleep Res 2010; 19(4):525–34.
118. International classification of sleep disorders: diag nostic and coding manual. 3rd edition. Westches ter (IL): American Academy of Sleep Medicine; 2014.
119. Mayer G, Benes H, Young P, et al. Modafinil in the treatment of idiopathic hypersomnia without long sleep time-a randomized, double-blind, placebo-controlled study. J Sleep Res 2015;24(1):74–81.
120. Billiard M, Sonka K. Idiopathic hypersomnia. Sleep Med Rev 2016;29:23–33.
121. Leu-Semenescu S, Louis P, Arnulf I. Benefits and risk of sodium oxybate in idiopathic hypersomnia versus narcolepsy type 1: a chart review. Sleep Med 2016;17:38–44.
122. Nishino S, Kanbayashi T. Symptomatic narcolepsy, cataplexy and hypersomnia, and their implications in the hypothalamic hypocretin/orexin system. Sleep Med Rev 2005;9(4):269–310.
123. Verma A, Anand V, Verma NP. Sleep disorders in chronic traumatic brain injury. J Clin Sleep Med 2007;3(4):357–62.
124. Mathias JL, Alvaro PK. Prevalence of sleep distur bances, disorders, and problems following trau matic brain injury: a meta-analysis. Sleep Med 2012;13(7):898–905.
125. Baumann CR, Stocker R, Imhof HG, et al. Hypocretin-1 (orexin A) deficiency in acute traumatic brain injury. Neurology 2005;65(1):147–9.
126. Kaiser PR, Valko PO, Werth E, et al. Modafinil ame liorates excessive daytime sleepiness after trau matic brain injury. Neurology 2010;75(20): 1780–5.
127. Jha A, Weintraub A, Allshouse A, et al. A randomized trial of modafinil for the treatment of fatigue and excessive daytime sleepiness in individuals with chronic traumatic brain injury. J Head Trauma Rehabil 2008;23(1):52–63.
128. Menn SJ, Yang R, Lankford A. Armodafinil for the treatment of excessive sleepiness associated with mild or moderate closed traumatic brain injury: a 12-week, randomized, double-blind study followed by a 12-month open-label extension. J Clin Sleep Med 2014;10(11):1181–91.
129. Braga-Neto P, da Silva-Junior FP, Sueli Monte F, et al. Snoring and excessive daytime sleepiness in Par kinson's disease. J Neurol Sci 2004;217(1): 41–5.
130. Gjerstad MD, Alves G, Wentzel-Larsen T, et al. Excessive daytime sleepiness in Parkinson disease: is it the drugs or the disease? Neurology 2006;67(5):853–8.
131. Verbaan D, van Rooden SM, Visser M, et al. Nighttime sleep problems and daytime sleepi- ness in Parkinson's disease. Mov Disord 2008;23(1):35–41.
132. Adler CH, Caviness JN, Hentz JG, et al. Randomized trial of modafinil for treating subjective daytime sleepiness in patients with Parkinson's disease. Mov Disord 2003;18(3):287–93.
133. Hogl B, Saletu M, Brandauer E, et al. Modafinil for the treatment of daytime sleepiness in Parkinson's disease: a double-blind, randomized, crossover, placebo-controlled polygraphic trial. Sleep 2002; 25(8):905–9.
134. Ondo WG, Fayle R, Atassi F, et al. Modafinil for daytime somnolence in Parkinson's disease: double blind, placebo controlled parallel trial. J Neurol Neurosurg Psychiatr 2005;76(12):1636–9.
135. Ondo WG, Perkins T, Swick T, et al. Sodium oxybate for excessive daytime sleepiness in Parkinson disease: an open-label polysomnographic study. Arch Neurol 2008;65(10):1337–40.
136. Fisone G, Borgkvist A, Usiello A. Caffeine as a psychomotor stimulant: mechanism of action. Cell Mol Life Sci 2004;61(7–8):857–72.
137. Porkka-Heiskanen T, Strecker RE, Thakkar M, et al. Adenosine: a mediator of the sleep-inducing effects of prolonged wakefulness. Science 1997; 276(5316):1265–8.
138. Nawrot P, Jordan S, Eastwood J, et al. Effects of caffeine on human health. Food Addit Contam 2003;20(1):1–30.
139. Barone JJ, Roberts HR. Caffeine consumption. Food Chem Toxicol 1996;34(1):119–29.
140. Mieda M, Willie JT, Hara J, et al. Orexin peptides prevent cataplexy and improve wakefulness in an orexin neuron-ablated model of narcolepsy in mice. Proc Natl Acad Sci U S A 2004;101(13): 4649–54.
141. Schatzberg SJ, Cutter-Schatzberg K, Nydam D, et al. The effect of hypocretin replacement therapy in a 3-year-old Weimaraner with narcolepsy. J Vet Intern Med 2004;18(4):586–8.
142. Kantor S, Mochizuki T, Janisiewicz AM, et al. Orexin neurons are necessary for the circadian control of REM sleep. Sleep 2009;32(9):1127–34.
143. Deadwyler SA, Porrino L, Siegel JM, et al. Systemic and nasal delivery of orexin-A (Hypocretin-1) re duces the effects of sleep deprivation on cognitive performance in nonhuman primates. J Neurosci 2007;27(52):14239–47.
144. Nagahara T, Saitoh T, Kutsumura N, et al. Design and synthesis of non-peptide, selective orexin receptor 2 agonists. J Med Chem 2015;58(20): 7931–7.
145. Kimura H, Ishikawa T, Suzuki M. A novel, orally available orexin 2 receptor-selective agonist, tak-994, ameliorates narcolepsy-like symptoms in narcolepsy mouse models. Sleep Med 2019;64:S199.

146. Yukitake H, fujimoto T, Ishikawa T, et al. TAK-925, an orexin 2 receptor-selective agonist, shows robust wake-promoting effects in mice. Pharmacol Biochem Behav 2019;187:172794.
147. Evans R, Hazel J, Faessel H, et al. Results of a phase 1, 4-period crossover, placebo-controlled, randomized, single dose study to evaluate the safety, tolerability, pharmacokinetics, and pharmacodynamics of TAK-925, a novel orexin 2 receptor agonist, in sleep-deprived healthy adults, utilizing modafinil as an active comparator. Sleep Med 2019;64:S106.
148. Baier PC, Hallschmid M, Seeck-Hirschner M, et al. Effects of intranasal hypocretin-1 (orexin A) on sleep in narcolepsy with cataplexy. Sleep Med 2011;12(10):941–6.
149. Mishima K, Fujiki N, Yoshida Y, et al. Hypocretin re ceptor expression in canine and murine narcolepsy models and in hypocretin-ligand deficient human narcolepsy. Sleep 2008;31(8):1119–26.
150. Kawashima M, Lin L, Tanaka S, et al. Anti-Tribbles homolog 2 (TRIB2) autoantibodies in narcolepsy are associated with recent onset of cataplexy. Sleep 2010;33(7):869–74.
151. Dauvilliers Y, Abril B, Mas E, et al. Normalization of hypocretin-1 in narcolepsy after intravenous immu noglobulin treatment. Neurology 2009;73(16):1333–4.
152. Dauvilliers Y, Carlander B, Rivier F, et al. Successful management of cataplexy with intravenous immunoglobulins at narcolepsy onset. Ann Neurol 2004;56(6):905–8.
153. Ueno R, Honda K, Inoue S, et al. Prostaglandin D2, a cerebral sleep-inducing substance in rats. Proc Natl Acad Sci U S A 1983;80(6):1735–7.
154. Huang ZL, Urade Y, Hayaishi O. Prostaglandins and adenosine in the regulation of sleep and wakefulness. Curr Opin Pharmacol 2007;7(1):33–8.
155. Jordan W, Tumani H, Cohrs S, et al. Narcolepsy increased L-PGDS (beta-trace) levels correlate with excessive daytime sleepiness but not with cat aplexy. J Neurol 2005;252:1372–8.
156. Sagawa Y, Sato M, Sakai N, et al. Wake-promoting effects of ONO-4127Na, a prostaglandin DP1 re ceptor antagonist, in hypocretin/orexin deficient narcoleptic mice. Neuropharmacology 2016;110(Part A):268–76.
157. Riehl J, Honda K, Kwan M, et al. Chronic oral administration of CG-3703, a thyrotropin releasing hormone analog, increases wake and decreases cataplexy in canine narcolepsy. Neuropsychopharmacology 2000;23(1):34–45.
158. Nicoll RA. Excitatory action of TRH on spinal motoneurones. Nature 1977;265(5591):242–3.
159. Nishino S, Arrigoni J, Shelton J, et al. Effects of thyrotropin-releasing hormone and its analogs on daytime sleepiness and cataplexy in canine narco lepsy. J Neurosci 1997;17(16):6401–8.
160. Sharp T, Bennett GW, Marsden CA. Thyrotrophin-releasing hormone analogues increase dopamine release from slices of rat brain. J Neurochem 1982;39(6):1763–6.
161. Heuer H, Schafer MK, O'Donnell D, et al. Expression of thyrotropin-releasing hormone receptor 2 (TRH-R2) in the central nervous system of rats. J Comp Neurol 2000;428(2):319–36.
162. Keller HH, Bartholini G, Pletscher A. Enhancement of cerebral noradrenaline turnover by thyrotropin-releasing hormone. Nature 1974;248(448):528–9.
163. Broberger C. Neurotransmitters switching the thal amus between sleep and arousal: functional ef fects and cellular mechanism. New Frontiers in Neuroscience Research. Showa University Interna tional Symposium for Life Science. 1st Annual Meeting Showa University Kamijo Hall. Tokyo, August 31, 2004.
164. Mignot E, Nishino S. Emerging therapies in narcolepsy-cataplexy. Sleep 2005;28(6):754–63.
165. Okura M, Riehl J, Mignot E, et al. Sulpiride, a D2/D3 blocker, reduces cataplexy but not REM sleep in canine narcolepsy. Neuropsychopharmacology 2000;23(5):528–38.
166. Nishino S, Mignot E. Narcolepsy and cataplexy. Handb Clin Neurol 2011;99:783–814.
167. Takeda Pharmaceutical Company Limited. Clinical Trial Summary October 2021 (Accessed 6 July 2022).
168. Takeda Pharmaceutical Company Limited. Takeda Provides Update on TAK-994 Clinical Program (Accessed 6 July 2022).

Brain Stimulation for Improving Sleep and Memory

Roneil G. Malkani, MD, MS[a,b,*], Phyllis C. Zee, MD, PhD[c]

KEYWORDS

- Slow wave sleep • Memory • Brain stimulation • Acoustic stimulation • Closed-loop stimulation
- Transcranial electric stimulation • Targeted memory reactivation
- Transcranial magnetic stimulation

KEY POINTS

- Transcranial electrical stimulation enhances sleep slow oscillations and can improve declarative memory, but its effects on memory have been inconsistent.
- Transcranial magnetic stimulation during sleep increases slow oscillations, and stimulation during wake improves memory, but the relationship between sleep and memory with this method has not been established.
- Acoustic stimulation in non-rapid eye movement sleep increases slow oscillations, spindles, and their phase coupling, all of which correlate with improvements in declarative memory.
- Targeted memory reactivation in sleep using verbal and nonverbal auditory cues consolidates specific recently encoded memories.
- Future research to determine optimal stimulation parameters and examine long-term safety and effects on cognition and performance is needed in healthy and clinical populations.

INTRODUCTION

Over the past few decades, the importance of sleep has become increasingly recognized for many physiologic functions, including cognition. Many studies have reported the deleterious effect of sleep loss or sleep disruption on cognitive performance. Beyond ensuring adequate sleep quality and duration, discovering methods to enhance sleep to augment its restorative effects is important to improve learning in many populations, such as the military, students, age-related cognitive decline, and cognitive disorders. In the past two decades, noninvasive sleep stimulation techniques have emerged, including transcranial electrical stimulation (TES), transcranial magnetic stimulation (TMS), acoustic stimulation, and targeted memory reactivation (TMR). This article reviews the role of sleep in memory consolidation, these neurostimulation techniques, and their effects on memory.

SLEEP PHYSIOLOGY AND MEMORY

Sleep Physiology

Non-rapid eye movement (NREM) sleep is characterized by cortical neuronal synchrony that increases with deeper stages of NREM sleep.

Sleep Med Clin 15 (2020) 101-115 https://doi.org/10.1016/j.jsmc.2019.11.002 1556-407X/20/

[a] Division of Sleep Medicine, Department of Neurology, Center for Circadian and Sleep Medicine, Northwestern University Feinberg School of Medicine, 710 North Lake Shore Drive, Suite 525, Chicago, IL 60611, USA; [b] Jesse Brown Veterans Affairs Medical Center, Chicago, IL 60612, USA; [c] Division of Sleep Medicine, Department of Neurology, Center for Circadian and Sleep Medicine, Northwestern University Feinberg School of Medicine, 710 North Lake Shore Drive, Suite 520, Chicago, IL 60611, USA

* Corresponding author. Division of Sleep Medicine, Department of Neurology, Center for Circadian and Sleep Medicine, Northwestern University Feinberg School of Medicine, 710 North Lake Shore Drive, Suite 525, Chicago, IL 60611.

E-mail address: R-malkani@northwestern.edu

Sleep Med Clin 17 (2022) 505–521
https://doi.org/10.1016/j.jsmc.2022.06.013
1556-407X/22/

During stage NREM 2 (N2) sleep, there is a prominence of K-complexes and sleep spindles. Sleep spindles are short bursts of oscillations in the 9-Hz to 15-Hz frequency range that are generated by the thalamic reticular neurons and synchronized by corticothalamic feedback. They are present throughout stages N2 and N3 but are more difficult to visualize during stage N3.[1] Sleep spindles can be divided into slow (10–12 Hz) and fast (13–15 Hz) spindles with differing topographic distribution and functional significance.[2]

The deepest stage of NREM sleep is stage N3, or slow-wave sleep (SWS), and is characterized by electroencephalogram (EEG) slow waves in the delta (0.5–4.5 Hz) frequency band. SWS is implicated in many physiologic functions, including cognitive function,[2] hormonal regulation,[1,3,4] immune function, energy saving, and clearance of β-amyloid and toxic metabolites from the brain.[1,5,6] Slow oscillations (SOs), in ~1-Hz frequency band, are generated by the thalamocortical system with potential influences from the locus coeruleus[7,8] SOs represent synchronous changes in membrane potential of large populations of cortical neurons in a bistable manner with an upstate and downstate. During the depolarized upstate of the SOs, there is sustained neuronal firing of neurons; during the hyperpolarized downstate, there is neuronal quiescence.[9] SOs originate in the medial prefrontal cortex and propagate posteriorly.[10,11] Stimulation of frontal cortex results in EEG slow waves and sleep,[12] and slow-wave activity (SWA; the quantification of power in the delta frequency band using power spectral analysis) is most prominent in the frontal areas.[13]

Rapid eye movement (REM) sleep is characterized by cortical desynchrony, REMs, and motor atonia that spares respiratory and extraocular muscles. This sleep stage is associated with dreams and seems to play a more important role in procedural and emotional memory.[14,15] Earlier research focused on REM sleep, but recent attention has shifted to SWS. This article focuses on the role of NREM sleep because it has been the target of most of the recent sleep stimulation research.

Learning and Memory

The ability to remember is critical to adapt behaviors in response to the environment. There are two general types of memory: declarative and nondeclarative memory. Declarative memory refers to remembering facts and events and relies on the hippocampus. Nondeclarative memory, or procedural memory, refers to unconscious memory of performing a task, such as playing a musical instrument, and depends on corticostriatal and corticocerebellar networks.[2] However, there is some overlap between the memory function of these areas. Memory involves three components: encoding, consolidation, and retrieval.[2] During encoding, memory traces are coded and stored in the hippocampus.[16] These memory traces are unstable and are susceptible to interference from other information. Consolidation is the process of stabilization of memories, in which encoded information is transferred from the hippocampus to the neocortex for long-term storage. This process can occur when awake, but sleep has a critical role in the transfer of memory and integrating information into existing networks.[2,17]

The Role of Sleep in Memory Consolidation

Two major mechanisms have been proposed to explain the role of sleep in memory consolidation: the synaptic homeostasis hypothesis (SHY) and the active system consolidation model. SHY proposes that synaptic strength increases during wake and decreases during sleep, particularly SWS.[18] Because of energy and space constraints, the increase in synaptic density and strength that accumulates while awake is downscaled during sleep.[18] In support of this, markers of synaptic efficacy have been shown to increase while awake and decrease during sleep; these changes are blocked by sleep loss.[19] Furthermore, measures of synaptic strength, such as axon–spine interface, decrease with sleep.[20] Moreover, sleep deprivation increases net synaptic strength and decreases long-term potential-like plasticity.[21] Although SHY explains synaptic downscaling, it does not explain how memories are stored for long-term use or how some memories are retained and others are forgotten.

The active system consolidation model proposes that memories are stored in the hippocampus during encoding while awake. During NREM sleep, memories in the hippocampus are replayed, resulting in transfer of the memory for storage in the neocortex.[22–24] When memories are stabilized in the neocortex, the hippocampus no longer retains the information and returns to a state ready to encode new information.[25] One important unanswered question in this model is how memories are tagged and selected for replay and consolidation.

The SHY and active system consolidation models are not mutually exclusive and may be complementary. These models together could explain how, during sleep, memory replay transfers memories for long-term storage, and synaptic downscaling normalizes synaptic strength, erasing memory traces in the hippocampus, preparing for more learning.

SWS and sleep spindles are of particular importance to the consolidation of declarative memories. SWS and spindles[26,27] are independently linked to memory consolidation.[2,28,29] Blocking spindles with electric current impairs memory consolidation.[30] Fast spindles seem to be more consistently linked to memory consolidation, although many studies have not differentiated fast from slow spindles.[2] Sharp-wave ripples (SWRs)[31] are 100-Hz to 300-Hz oscillations that originate in the hippocampus and occur in SWS. SWRs increase with learning,[2] and disruption of SWRs impairs memory retention.[30,32]

The current neurophysiologic model of NREM sleep's role in memory consolidation is the interplay between SOs, spindles, and SWRs during SWS. In particular, these waveforms are coordinated in a nested fashion, with spindles occurring during upstate of the SO and SWRs occurring the spindle troughs.[2] This coordination represents the cross talk between the hippocampus and neocortex that underlies transfer of memories from short-term to long-term storage. This phase coupling seems to occur in a top-down manner with SOs synchronizing thalamocortical spindle and hippocampal SWR generation.[33–36] This phase coupling between SOs, spindles, and SWRs seems to be important for consolidation.[37] Furthermore, increased duration of the SO upstate, which may improve phase locking, is associated with improved declarative memory.[38]

Effect of Aging on Sleep and Memory

Understanding the role of sleep in cognition may be especially important to age-related cognitive decline. After age 55 years, function starts to decline in several cognitive domains, including declarative memory.[39,40] This change parallels reductions in SWS duration.[41] Aging results in decreases in SO density, number, and amplitude and impaired SO propagation.[10,11,42] These changes in SO characteristics may be explained by cortical thinning in areas involved in the default mode network, including medial prefrontal cortex, insula, temporal, and parietal areas.[10] Furthermore, aging decreases the slope and frequency of the SO, indicating decreased neuronal synchrony.[11] There are also reductions in spontaneous K-complexes and sleep spindle number, density, and duration.[43] In addition, aging is associated with reduced phase coupling between SOs and spindles, which predicts poorer overnight memory retention.[34]

Alzheimer's disease (AD) is a neurodegenerative memory disorder associated with aging and that involves deterioration of short-term memory, especially declarative memory. Pathologically, the disease is characterized by extracellular β-amyloid plaques and intracellular tau protein neurofibrillary tangles.[44] As AD progresses, other cognitive domains deteriorate, and patients become unable to independently perform usual activities of daily living. Given that the proportion of elderly is increasing, the prevalence of AD, already at 46.8 million worldwide, is expected to increase to 131.5 million by 2050.[45] Because there is no available cure or disease-modifying therapy, it is imperative to further understand AD and identify risk factors and therapeutic targets for disease prevention and modification. In addition, earlier disease detection may be critical to intervening before significant neurodegeneration.

Sleep disruption has emerged as a potential key player in the pathogenesis of AD. Sleep disturbances are common in people with AD and even confer risk of developing AD.[46] Sleep is involved in regulation of interstitial β-amyloid peptide levels, which increase during wake and decrease during sleep.[47] During sleep deprivation, β-amyloid peptide levels continue to increase while awake; with pharmacologically induced sleep beyond the usual sleep duration, these levels decrease further.[47] This regulation may depend on the glymphatic system, which is responsible for clearance of toxic metabolites from the brain during sleep.[5,6] In addition, reduction in SWS increases levels of tau protein, and sleep fragmentation is associated with the development of tau protein neurofibrillary tangles.[48,49] In AD transgenic mice that have less SWA and early Aβ deposition, optogenetic stimulation to restore SWA reduces Aβ deposition,[50] and optogenetic stimulation to increase the frequency of slow waves increases Aβ deposition.[51]

Alterations in sleep macrostructure and microstructure can even be seen in people with amnestic mild cognitive impairment (aMCI), a precursor state to AD in which there is memory decline but functional independence is maintained.[52] People with aMCI have lower SWS duration, lower SWA, and lower fast spindle density and count.[29,53] Furthermore, sleep disturbances in people with aMCI are associated with decreased functional connectivity between the prefrontal cortex and temporoparietal junction.[54] Therefore, restoration of normal sleep function is a novel and exciting avenue that may improve cognitive function and even alter the pathophysiology of AD.

METHODS TO ENHANCE SLEEP AND THEIR EFFECTS ON MEMORY

Given the relationship between sleep and memory, there has been growing research in methods to improve memory by modulating sleep. Enhancing sleep for memory has important implications in adults (eg, military, aging, and neurodegenerative disease). Most approaches have targeted SOs and spindles. Enhancing SWS is advantageous because it can occur during daytime naps, making this easier to study and providing more opportunities for therapeutic intervention. The most commonly studied methods include electrical stimulation, magnetic stimulation, acoustic stimulation, and TMR.

Transcranial Electrical Stimulation

Transcranial application of electricity with direct current (DC) or alternating current (AC) can be used to stimulate brain oscillations. Such currents induce neuronal membrane depolarization or hyperpolarization, resulting in entrainment of brain oscillations.[55–57] DC is a unidirectional current that is constant; AC changes in direction, amplitude, frequency, and phase variance/coherence. TES can be used to enhance[58] or disrupt[59] oscillations, depending on how it is applied. The most common sleep application of TES is for the enhancement of SO, in which case the electrical current is applied at low frequency (typically 0.75 Hz). TES can also be applied at other frequencies (eg, 12 Hz) to stimulate sleep spindles.

Most studies using TES have examined the effects of slow-oscillatory transcranial DC stimulation (SO-tDCS) on brain oscillations. Marshall and colleagues[60] reported that frontal SO-tDCS applied during a nap in young healthy adults increased frontal SO and delta power. These data led to the landmark study in overnight sleep in healthy young adults that showed enhancement of SO, delta power, and slow sleep spindles.[58] Since then, there have been multiple studies using similar methodology of SO-tDCS during sleep in healthy young and older adults. Most studies show an increase in spectral power in the SO and delta frequency bands during stimulation-free intervals or immediately after stimulation,[58,60–62] although some studies did not.[63–65] Although one study showed an increase in SWS,[58] most studies have found no effect on sleep stages, during nap or overnight,[61–63,66,67] and one found decreased SWS overnight in older adults.[65] A recent study using transcranial AC stimulation (tACS) targeting limbic areas showed increased SWS and SO power.[68]

The effects of tDCS on sleep spindles have been much more varied. Some studies report an increase in fast[66,69] or slow[58] spindle density, whereas others report lower spindle counts[60] or fast spindle density.[67,70] Several other studies with tDCS have found no effect on spindles.[62–65] These discrepancies in spindle effects may be related to several factors, including the type of current, the difference in spindle frequency bands assessed, spindle detection methodologies, and inability to examine the EEG during the stimulation itself.

The effects of TES on cognitive function have also been inconsistent among studies. The initial studies using tDCS showed improvement in word-pair association task (WPT), a test of declarative memory that has been used in many studies and is sensitive to sleep effects.[58,60] However, the effect of tDCS on the WPT has been inconsistent, regardless of how the WPT was given (eg, train to criterion, feedback provided). The mixed results do not seem to depend on the age of population studied or whether the tDCS was applied during a nap or overnight sleep.[63] All studies using tDCS have shown no benefit to procedural memory tasks, consistent with the effect of SWS on declarative memory.[58,60,62–67,69] One study using tACS showed improvement in a motor sequent tapping task response time but not accuracy.[70]

Although TES has had varied effects in healthy people, there are data to suggest that it may be more effective in clinical populations. For example, because people with aMCI have less SWA, increasing SO may be of particular benefit. One recent study in this population showed that tDCS improved SO power, fast spindle power (12–15 Hz), phase coupling, and visual declarative memory. Furthermore, the memory enhancement correlated with a higher degree of phase coupling.[69] SO-tDCS also improved SO power and memory in children with attention-deficit/hyperactivity disorder[71] and reduced forgetting in adults with paranoid schizophrenia.[72] There are two studies using TES in patients with epilepsy. One study using SO-tDCS during wakefulness before a nap in patients with temporal lobe epilepsy found increased total sleep duration, improved declarative verbal memory, and less forgetting of visuospatial memory. Although slow spindle current generator density increased, particularly in frontal areas, fast and slow spindle counts remained unchanged.[73] In contrast, the other study showed that low-frequency tACS during NREM sleep in patients undergoing surgery for medication-refractory epilepsy did not entrain sleep spindles.[74] Each of these populations has had limited data and small sample sizes, and the effects need to be confirmed with additional and larger studies.

Several inherent limitations to TES may explain the discrepancies in these results. First, the dose of current may not be sufficient to stimulate the cortex to reliably increase SWA, because TES affects only the superficial layers of the brain.[60] Second, the parameters of stimulation may need to be individualized to optimize stimulation potential. Third, it remains unclear whether multiple nights of stimulation have lasting and cumulative effects. Fourth, the EEG can be examined only during stimulation-free intervals and after stimulation, not during stimulation, because the application of electrical current interferes with such measurement. In addition, the utility of TES in its present form requires a technician to apply stimulation, limiting at-home or clinical use.

TES is generally safe with no known serious adverse events. Headache, fatigue, tingling, itching, and burning are the most common side effects, with skin lesions occurring under the electrodes in some people with repeated use.[75] However, side effects of nightly long-term use are unknown.

Transcranial Magnetic Stimulation

TMS is a noninvasive neurostimulation technique that can be applied over specific brain areas without requiring physical contact. The magnetic field is generated by passing a strong electric current through a coil positioned over the head by the brain region of interest. The magnetic field stimulates or inhibits nearby neurons and can modulate connected subcortical and transcortical areas.[76] TMS affects cortical neural plasticity, such as long-term potentiation or long-term depression, and can have long-lasting effects than TES, depending on the type and frequency of stimulation. Factors that influence the effects of TMS include the coil shape and orientation, cortical geometry, and TMS type and frequency. TMS can be used as an exploratory tool to assess relationships between brain areas or as a diagnostic tool by assessing functional connectivity as a biomarker. TMS can also be used therapeutically in pain disorders and depression.

TMS can be delivered using different modalities. Single-pulse TMS delivers pulses at least 4 seconds apart to avoid summation of effects. Paired pulse-TMS delivers 2 pulses with varying interstimulation intervals (ISIs) to evaluate conduction times between different brain areas. Repetitive TMS (rTMS) delivers a train of stimuli with ISIs less than 2 seconds apart. rTMS seems to have long-lasting effects and it is the typical modality used therapeutically.[77]

Despite the wealth of data available on TMS effects on the brain, there are sparse data available for its effects on sleep. A few studies have shown that TMS can evoke high-amplitude SO. Massimini and colleagues[78] applied TMS repetitively in blocks of ~0.8 Hz with intertrial intervals of ~1 minute at different midline sites. During NREM sleep, each pulse of the train triggered a high-amplitude SO resembling endogenous SO, which spread to the rest of the brain. The triggered SO upstate was associated with an increase in spindle amplitude. This response was state-dependent, because TMS did not evoke SO in the awake state. This effect was also dose and site-dependent, with greater stimulation intensity and stimulation over the sensorimotor cortex eliciting the greatest responses.[78] Furthermore, TMS-elicited SOs are larger if the pulse was delivered at the endogenous SO upstate.[79] Single-pulse[80] and paired-pulse TMS[81] techniques also enhanced sleep SO. However, it is unclear whether these induced slow waves serve the same physiologic function as endogenous ones. Further research needs to determine whether increasing trains of SO decrease the need for spontaneous SO, thereby reducing the sleep homeostatic drive, and whether enhancing SO affects cognitive performance.[82]

Although TMS applied in the wake state does not elicit SO, it can increase SWA in subsequent sleep.[83] The increase in SWA was most pronounced where cortical EEG response was most potentiated. This finding was confirmed using a paired associated stimulation protocol, in which the TMS of the motor cortex pulse immediately followed stimulation of the contralateral median nerve. Varying the frequency of stimulation led to either long-term potentiation or depression. If long-term potentiation was seen, SWA was increased in that area during subsequent sleep; if long-term depression was seen, SWA was decreased.[84]

Although studies using TMS have examined either sleep or cognitive effects separately, not linking them together, TMS applied in the wake state improves cognitive performance. For example, single-pulse TMS over the right dorsolateral prefrontal cortex in young adults increases pattern recognition and reaction time.[85] rTMS at 5 Hz applied to the midline parietal region improves working memory compared with sham TMS (same set up procedure but no stimulation applied) in young adults.[86] Effects are also seen with sleep deprivation, during which rTMS seems to rescue cognitive impairment. Stimulation with rTMS at 5 Hz over the upper occipital region, but not the parietal region, improved working memory after 1 day[87] or 2 days[88] of sleep deprivation. However, rTMS does not improve cognitive performance when given after recovery sleep.[88] One potential mechanism by which TMS improves cognitive function is in facilitating transfer of memories, because it seems to increase functional connectivity between the hippocampus and the stimulated cortical networks.[89]

TMS also has a potential therapeutic role in AD-related cognitive function. Earlier studies showed that rTMS at 20 Hz over the left or right dorsolateral prefrontal cortex improves cognitive function in mild-to-moderate AD in a single session[90,91] or with repeated sessions over 4 weeks.[92] Combining cognitive training and several sessions of rTMS (20 Hz, 6 stimulation sites, 30 sessions) also improves cognitive function,[93–95] although an optimal control group was not used in these studies. Several small, randomized, sham-controlled trials have also shown benefits in AD (for a review, see Ref.[96]). None of these studies examined the effects of rTMS on sleep EEG, so it is unclear whether sleep effects played a role in the cognitive benefits. Although these studies targeted cortical areas closer to the surface, one study used a different coil to stimulate deeper in the brain, specifically the medial prefrontal cortex, and showed improved cognitive performance in a small group of patients with moderate-to-severe AD.[97] Although this study did not examine effects on sleep, given the role of the medial prefrontal cortex in SWS generation, it is possible that benefits could have been mediated through enhancing sleep.

TMS seems to be safe overall. The most common adverse events reported are headache and fatigue.[98] There are several contraindications to TMS. Ferromagnetic or metallic materials cannot touch the coil. Because seizures have been reported with TMS, although a rare, history of seizures or conditions or medications that lower the seizure threshold are a contraindication. The risk of TMS in pregnancy, heart conditions, and cerebral stimulators is unknown.[77] The major limitations with the use of TMS to enhance sleep are related to the interface. TMS requires a trained technician to use. TMS also requires the patient keep the head still, so positioning for stimulation during sleep can be challenging, particularly if considering stimulation throughout the night. Ear plugs and masking sounds need to be used to prevent sleep disruption from the noise from TMS. Furthermore, duration of stimulation is limited because of potential overheating of the coil.[79,82]

Acoustic Stimulation

Another window into the brain to enhance sleep is acoustic stimulation. Sounds provoke a K-complex response, which may be associated with reactive SO.[99] Sound stimuli in sleep activate lemniscal and non-lemniscal pathways through the brainstem to the cortex.[100] The lemniscal pathway projects via the medial geniculate body of the thalamus to the primary auditory cortex. The non-lemniscal pathway projects through two parallel pathways to the medial geniculate body and then to the associative cortex. One of the non-lemniscal pathways travels through the locus coeruleus, a wake-promoting nucleus. Activation of the other non-lemniscal pathway results in widespread neuronal depolarization of the cortex. If the sound does not significantly activate the locus coeruleus and result in an arousal, then a K-complex without an arousal results in fast and efficient synchrony and promotes enhancement of the SO.[100] Stimulation does not depend on the side of stimulation, because even unilateral stimulation leads to increased SO in both hemispheres.[101] Nearly all studies on acoustic stimulation have used pink noise (one of the basic types of noise in nature), which comprises a wide range of sound frequencies in a 1/f distribution (ie, lower frequencies provide greater contribution).[102] An advantage of acoustic stimulation is the feasibility and practicality of using an automated system and the ability to develop a device for home use.

Most of the studies using acoustic stimulation have focused on enhancing SO, which is discussed later. However, sleep spindles can also be enhanced with acoustic stimulation. Recently, it was shown that oscillating white noise at 12 Hz or 14 Hz can boost slow and fast spindle density, respectively. Although the sounds also increased SO density, the spindle enhancement did not depend on the increase in SO.[103]

There are two general types of acoustic stimulation for SO enhancement: open-loop and closed-loop stimulation. Open-loop stimulation consists of delivery of sounds during SWS with the intent to evoke an SO. Sounds are delivered without respect to a particular phase of endogenous SO. Stimulation with trains of 15 to 20 clicks of pink noise at a frequency of 0.8 to 2 Hz during NREM sleep increased SWA throughout the night.[104] One recent study with open-loop low-frequency stimulation with three tones in a sequence also increased SO but decreased fast and slow spindle power and did not improve declarative memory.[105] Similarly, open-loop stimulation of 0.8 Hz increased SO power but did not improve vigilance.[106] In contrast with open-loop stimulation, closed-loop stimulation bases the timing of the sequence of tones to a targeted phase of endogenous SO to enhance them. This methodology involves monitoring the EEG in real time to identify

SOs in SWS and deliver the sounds on a specific phase of the SO. Most recent studies of acoustic stimulation using a form of closed-loop stimulation are based on the seminal work from Ngo and colleagues[107] in young adults. In this study, an algorithm for online detection of SO identified the negative half-wave of the SO and then delivered two clicks of pink noise. The first click occurred about 0.5 seconds after the negative peak of the SO to target the SO upstate. This delay was based on the interval between the negative peak and positive peak measured on the adaptation night. The second click occurred at a fixed interval of 1.075 seconds after the first. This method enhanced the amplitude of SO and fast and slow spindle power without increasing overall SWA across the night or changing sleep stage duration or distribution. The increase in SO power occurred predominantly in the frontal leads, much like the natural topographic distribution of SO power in humans. Furthermore, stimulation increased performance on the declarative memory task (WPT); this improvement correlated with increase in fast spindle power.

Timing of stimuli seems to matter for SO enhancement. Randomly timed stimulation did not increase SO power but increased fast spindle power.[108] Similar to findings from Ngo and colleagues,[109] other studies have replicated the finding that stimulation in the upstate rather than downstate of the SO increases SO amplitude.[109] This can change with age; in young adults, playing the sound anywhere on the upstate enhanced the SO, but in older adults, the range of phases on the upstate is narrower.[110] In contrast, delivery of the sounds during the negative peak of the SO enhanced neither SWA nor memory.[107] A mechanistic study using high-density EEG found that stimulation during the SO upstate enhanced cortical involvement and promoted propagation of smaller amplitude slow waves. Conversely, stimulation during the SO downstate disrupted such propagation, disengaging cortical networks. Such findings increased the possibility of not only SO enhancement but SO disruption, which could be useful clinically if such disruption is desired (eg, seizure prevention in epilepsy patients).[110]

Length of trains of stimuli may not be critical for SO enhancement. Because two-click stimulation increased SWA, it was plausible that increasing train length of stimuli would increase SWA further. However, stimulating continuously in the presence of SO to drive SO did not improve SWA any better that the two-click paradigm.[111] There has not been a direct comparison between shorter trains (eg, two-click vs five-click).

Similar protocols assessing 1-tone or 2-tone trains of stimulation also enhanced SWA.[112–114] A 1-tone stimulation method increased SWA and spindle power and improved declarative memory with WPT but not procedural memory.[112] This study also found that spindle activity increased at the peak of SO.[112]

An interesting point about acoustic stimulation of SO is that it seems to alter brain oscillations during stimulation but preserves the overall sleep architecture and spectral power. Most studies found no significant change in sleep stage duration or proportion[107,108,111–113,115–119] or in overall SWA.[107,116,117,119,120]Only one showed increase in SWA in young adults.[115] However, slow-wave energy—an accumulation of SWA during NREM stages N2 and N3 in the first four sleep cycles—seems to increase.[119,121] With the phase-locked loop (PLL) method, there is an increase in SO power during trains of stimulation but a decrease between trains, suggesting a reorganization of SO. The changes between the trains of stimulation and the intertrain interval were particularly associated with change in declarative memory performance[116,117] and autonomic function,[120] indicating that the reorganization of SO may be critical for memory consolidation.

Another emerging form of closed-loop stimulation is PLL stimulation. This method uses an automated algorithm that phase locks to the EEG and tracks SO in real time with the intent of delivering the sounds at the SO upstate (**Fig. 1**).[117,122] The potential advantage is that delivery of the sounds after the first tone in the block is most likely to be at the upstate. Other forms of closed-loop stimulation delivered the sound a fixed interval after the initial tone of the train, but delivery of subsequent tones on the upstate may be not precise because the frequency of SO can vary. The PLL phase targeting is precise,[116–118,122] and the PLL method enhances SO and increases fast spindle activity in young adults during a nap.[118] In older adults, it increases SO power and spindle density and amplitude during overnight sleep (**Fig. 2**)[117] and is associated with better performance on the WPT.

Several studies have indicated a high interindividual response to stimulation, such that some people respond to stimulation, although others do not. There are varying degrees of response to SO enhancement, and several studies have some subjects who did not have SO enhancement with acoustic stimulation.[116,117,119,121,123] Using correlational analyses or dividing participants into responders and nonresponders, these studies found that SO enhancement predicts cognitive response to the WPT and tests of executive cognitive function.[116,117,119,123] It will be important to

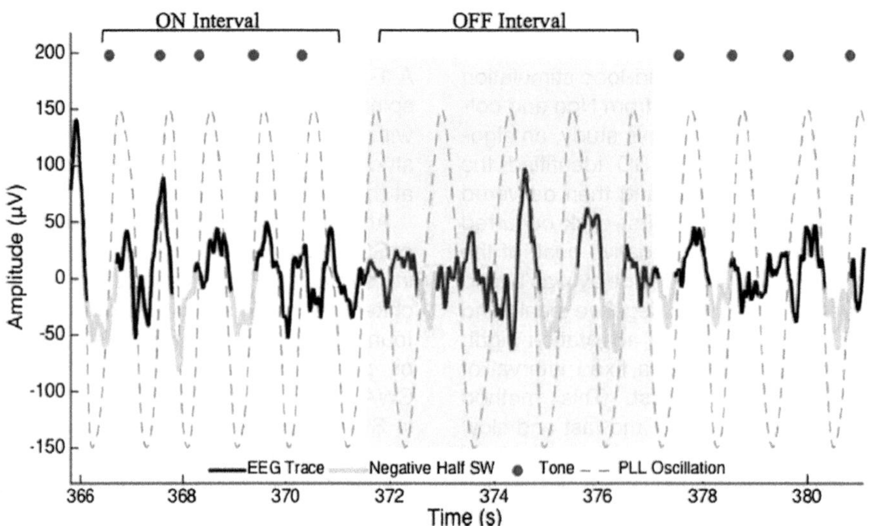

Fig. 1. A sample of electroencephalographs data (*solid black line*) with concurrent PLL acoustic stimulation. The PLL (*dashed gray line*) oscillates with variable frequency to match the endogenous SOs. During trains of stimulation (ON intervals), the tone of pink noise (*red dots*) is played just before the peak of the positive upstate for five PLL oscillations. During periods between trains (OFF intervals), no tones are given for five PLL oscillations. (*Adapted from* Papalambros NA, Santostasi G, Malkani RG, et al. Acoustic Enhancement of Sleep Slow Oscillations and Concomitant Memory Improvement in Older Adults. *Front Hum Neurosci.* 2017;11(March):1.)

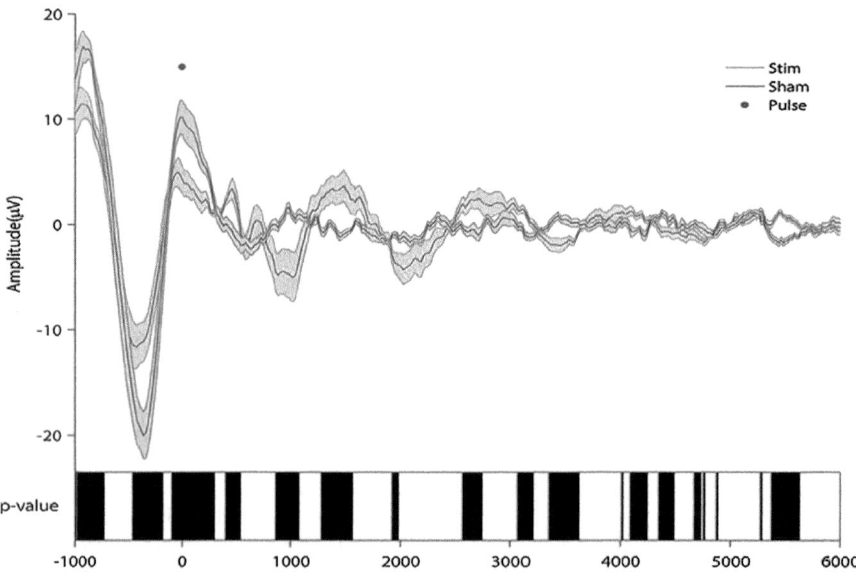

Fig. 2. A grand average event-related potential using PLL acoustic stimulation in older adults. The EEG of trains of stimulation (ON intervals with stimulation [Stim]) and trains of sham stimulation (ON intervals with sham) are aligned to the first tone (*purple dot*). In the sham condition, the timing of tone delivery is marked but no tones are given. Stimulation (*red line*) results in increased SO amplitude compared with sham (*blue line*). Because frequency of the PLL varies within each train, the remaining tones of each train are not shown. The black bars below indicate statistical significance ($P<.05$) between conditions. (*Adapted from* Papalambros NA, Santostasi G, Malkani RG, et al. Acoustic Enhancement of Sleep Slow Oscillations and Concomitant Memory Improvement in Older Adults. Front Hum Neurosci. 2017;11(March):1-14; with permission.)

determine the predictors of SO response to tailor the intervention.

Still, not all studies have shown improvement in cognitive performance. Although the most consistent improvement across studies has been with the semantically related WPT, one study replicating the initial closed-loop stimulation method did not find improvement in the WPT in young adults.[124] Furthermore, performance with semantically unrelated word pairs did not improve with closed-loop stimulation.[125]

Acoustic stimulation may also have effects beyond memory. In particular, stimulation seems to affect immune function,[113] reduce cortisol levels,[113,120] increase parasympathetic tone during sleep, and decrease sympathetic tone in the morning after stimulation.[120]

The ability of acoustic stimulation to enhance SWA persists even after multiple nights of stimulation. One recent study used a commercially available acoustic stimulation device for at-home use.[114] The validation study showed an increase in SO amplitude using a 2-tone PLL method to deliver pink noise via bone conduction through the mastoid in healthy young adults. SO amplitude enhancement was similar on the first and the tenth consecutive night of stimulation. Therefore, the brain does not seem to adapt to stimulation in a way that would limit long-term effects on SO.[114] Another protocol assessing stimulation of multiple nights used a different portable system that has an automated detection system to deliver a tone to the SO upstate followed by stimulation at 1-s intervals during NREM sleep.[115] Over a 5-night period, compared with sham, patients younger than 40 years had SWA enhancement even after the fifth night of stimulation; however, those more than 40 year old did not have SWA enhancement. The lack of effect seen in those more than 40 year old may be influenced by the sensitivity of SWS detection, which was much lower in this group compared with the younger group, or the method of stimulation,[115] because the PLL method did enhance SWA in older adults.[117] Two recent studies using closed-loop auditory stimulation over two nights in young-middle aged adults found improvements in alertness and vigilance.[119,121] One did not observe overall effects on executive cognitive function, but those who responded to the SO stimulation had improvements in verbal fluency and working memory.[119]

Many of these studies assessed stimulation in young adults. Given that SWA declines with aging[41,42] and reductions in SWA relate to declarative memory performance in older adults,[29,42] SWA enhancement in middle-aged and older adults may be a feasible way to mitigate age-related decline in declarative memory. Only two studies have examined acoustic stimulation in middle-aged people. In one study, acoustic stimulation enhanced SO amplitude in young to middle-aged people (mean age 40.8 years). The longitudinal analysis showed enhancement after 10 nights in those with mean age 45.4 years[114] but did not separately report young versus middle-aged adults. In contrast, another study showed no enhancement in those more than 40 years of age.[115] These differences may be caused by differences in either SO detection or sound delivery methods. However, the PLL method with trains of five clicks with a refractory period of about 5 to 6 seconds showed enhancement of SWA and fast spindle power and improvement in WPT performance in older adults.[117]

Therefore, acoustic stimulation has potential to improve sleep quality and memory in older adults.

Because people with aMCI have reduced SWA,[29] enhancing SO with acoustic stimulation may be a feasible method to mitigate cognitive dysfunction in aMCI. The PLL method of acoustic stimulation enhances SO in people with aMCI.[116] The degree of enhancement correlates with improvement in WPT performance, showing that even people with cognitive impairment retain adequate brain plasticity and integrity such that SO enhancement can improve memory. However, this effect was examined in a small sample and over only one night of stimulation, and it is unclear whether these potential benefits will be seen after multiple nights of stimulation.[116]

Although acoustic stimulation enhances SWA and sleep-sensitive declarative memory performance, there are several unanswered questions on optimal stimulation parameters.[100] First, the optimal timing of stimulation needs to be determined. Stimulation of the downstate of the SO does not seem to enhance SO.[107] However, it is unclear how precisely and accurately the sound stimulus needs to be delivered at the upstate of the SO to best enhance SWA. Because the closed-loop and PLL systems deliver sounds differently, one system may be more effective than the other at enhancing SWA, but this remains to be determined. Second, the optimal sound to enhance SWA is unclear. Most studies used pink noise in 50-ms pulses. Some used a ramping on and off with the pulse, whereas others did not. Other pulse durations or frequency distributions may also be effective, but studies are lacking. Third, the optimal volume for stimulation needs to be determined. Some studies have used a fixed volume, whereas others used an adaptive volume to deliver sounds, but it is unclear whether one method is more effective that the other and what the optimal volume adjustment method is. Fourth, entrainment of SOs may vary based on number of stimuli delivered in a train of SOs. Although one study did not show any benefit with continuous stimulation,[111] another showed that cumulative SWA increased with continuous stimulation.[115] However, continuous stimulation may lead to habituation, so intermittent stimulation across the night, as most studies have done with short trains of stimuli, may be more effective. Fifth, different populations may need different parameters. For example, older adults may need different sleep stage and SO detection parameters to start stimulation and may need more precise timing or different sound, volume, or train length to optimally improve SWA.[109,126]

Acoustic stimulation has some limitations. First, only sleep-sensitive tasks such as the WPT have shown improvements. Effects on other tasks of declarative memory and long-term effects have yet to be shown. Second, long-term effects on cognitive performance have not yet been shown, and it is unclear whether repeated sessions will continue to benefit cognition. No adverse events from acoustic stimulation have yet been reported.

Targeted Memory Reactivation

Both TES and acoustic stimulation enhance SWA and perhaps spindles to nonspecifically enhance declarative memory, but recent strategies have emerged to enhance specific memories. Because recently encoded memories are replayed during sleep-mediated consolidation, it may be possible to selectively replay specific memories to enhance their consolidation. TMR uses a sensory cue paired with information during encoding, and the cue is replayed during sleep to reactivate the associated memory and promote its consolidation.

Reactivation using cues is hippocampal-dependent. Replaying during sleep an odor cue associated with recently encoded information increases hippocampal activity during sleep[127] and improves hippocampal-dependent declarative memories but not hippocampal-independent procedural memories.[127] Furthermore, people with greater hippocampal volume have greater response to TMR, and people with bilateral hippocampal sclerosis do not respond to TMR.[128] Interestingly, TMR using odors can be applied locally based on a recent experiment pairing words to the left or right visual field and associated with an order to the right or left nostril, respectively. Replay of the memory in NREM using an odor cue improved memories processed in the ipsilateral hemisphere (eg, right nostril cue and right hemisphere processing left visual field information).[129]

Several types of cues have been used (odor, nonverbal auditory, and verbal cues) and can improve memory. Odor cues are less likely to cause an arousal during sleep than an auditory cue, and TMR with odor cues can strengthen hippocampal-dependent memory.[127]

Several studies have used nonverbal cues to reactivate and strengthen memories.[130–133] Replaying a melody during a nap enhances the recall and performance of playing that melody correctly.[134] This enhancement is accomplished by pairing a sound with information to be encoded. These studies then replay half of the sounds and examine which memories were better consolidated. Most studies tested memory with the picture-location task, a test of declarative memory, in which the patient learns the location of various objects (eg, cat) while a sound is played (eg, a meow). On the recall test, the patient reports the location of the presented object.[131–133,135,136] TMR reduces forgetting of cued items across several studies when done during a nap or overnight sleep.[131–133,135] TMR with nonverbal sounds can also alter proprioceptive and body ownership memory as tested using a rubber hand[137] and increased spatial accuracy of a throwing task.[138,139]

TMR using verbal cues also reduces forgetting on the WPT.[136] This finding does not seem to be caused only by the sound but also by the word. Changing the verbal cue from a male to female voice alters the sound but not the meaning of the word cue. This change effectively reduced forgetting in cued and non-cued memories. These data indicate that word memories are stored in an episodic form (with speaker detail) and abstract, speaker-independent form.[136,140]

TMR can also rescue memories that may have been forgotten. When value or importance is given to information during encoding, higher value information is consolidated more effectively. When sounds associated with object location of low-value items are played, low-value memories are also consolidated similarly to high-value memories.

Emotional memory may also be altered by TMR. Groch and colleagues[141] tested healthy adolescents and young adults on positive and negative memories. Subjects were shown ambiguous pictures and then either a positive or negative word, and half the positive and negative words were replayed in sleep. Not only was recall better for cued items but also cueing with positive words led to more positive interpretations, and cueing negative words led to less positive interpretations of new pictures.[141] Reactivation of emotional memories if replayed in REM sleep but not SWS reduced subjective arousal responses.[142]

Recent data have shown that the timing of TMR may be important to improve memory. The time of TMR relative to encoding has different effects on memory. If TMR is done soon after encoding, TMR with sounds improves object location memory. However, if TMR is delayed (hours later), then TMR weakens the memory.[132] In addition, the timing relative to the phase of SO may be critical. When cues were delivered between the peak of the upstate and the trough of the downstate of the SO, TMR led to less forgetting than if the cue was delivered in the other phase half.[133] The difference in timing relative to what has been tested in acoustic stimulation may be caused by the time needed to reach the auditory cortex and additional auditory processing needed to reactivate memories.[133]

There are several unanswered questions regarding the use of TMR.[130] First, the underlying neural mechanisms still need to be elucidated, including how cues activate certain memories and which neural pathways are involved. Second, the fidelity of the memory replayed is also unclear, including whether replayed memories are always exact or some memories are distorted. It is also unclear whether memories can be distorted. Third, the effects of repeated TMR are also largely unknown, including whether the effects are cumulative and enduring and whether the effects are generalizable across the lifespan. Recently, unsupervised TMR over three nights to improve language learning showed benefits but only after the third night. However, those who reported general sleep disturbance did not benefit, and those whose reported sleep disruption from the TMR sounds performed worse.[143] Fourth, TMR has potential to be used therapeutically, and clinical application needs to be tested. TMR has specific advantages compared with other techniques because of its targeted nature. For example, given the effects on positive and negative bias, TMR can potentially address unpleasant memories in people with post-traumatic stress disorder or help treat undesired habits. Answers to these important questions will be critical to better understand the role of memory replay in sleep and to develop clinical tools to enhance memory.

TMR also has several inherent limitations. First, TMR requires a learning program with built-in cues, and learned information is likely specific to that learning program. Second, there are limits to the number of cues that can be replayed during the finite amount of SWS. Third, although TMR improves cued memories, this enhancement may be at the expense of non-cued memories, indicating a consolidation bias.[144] Although there are no known adverse events from TMR, further data are needed to confirm the tolerability of TMR.

SUMMARY

Sleep's role in memory consolidation represents a critical avenue to improve the quality and effectiveness of sleep and memory. Multiple techniques have emerged to enhance sleep to improve declarative memory. Although TES increases SOs between stimulation periods or after stimulation, the effects on spindles and memory are inconsistent in healthy people. Furthermore, the utility of TES is limited because it requires a trained technician to apply the electrodes. TMS can elicit and enhance SWA locally and globally and improves cognitive function, but it is unclear whether its effects on memory are linked to sleep. Although the TMS interface limits its potential therapeutic utility to enhance SO during sleep, stimulation when awake may have potential benefits on sleep-related memory consolidation, but this requires further examination. Acoustic stimulation during sleep has been shown to enhance SOs and spindle activity and the phase relationship between the two. Furthermore, acoustic stimulation more consistently improves declarative memory and seems to have benefits in clinical populations. A significant advantage of acoustic stimulation is that it is easily adaptable for home use, and devices for auditory stimulation are already developed. TMR enhances selected information using associated cues and has particular relevance when specific information needs to be consolidated preferentially. A unique feature of TMR is that in addition to improving declarative memory, it may also rescue forgotten memories with the potential to alter emotional memories. Several unanswered questions need to be addressed for each of these techniques, including safety, long-term effects, and optimal parameters for a given person and therapeutic utility. Also, other techniques such as vestibular stimulation and vibrational stimulation to enhance sleep and memory are under study.[145,146] Future development of neurostimulation systems for therapeutic applications is promising for age-related cognitive disorders as well as sleep disorders.

CLINICS CARE POINTS

- Given sleep's role in memory consolidation, it is important to optimize sleep for cognitive health.
- Aging is associated with declines in sleep and memory, and sleep disruption appers to be a

key player in development of dementias such as Alzheimer's disease.

- Brain stimulation techniques have potential to leverage effects on sleep to improve memory but need to be further studied to determine clinical utility.
- Acoustic stimulation, in particular, has potential to be adapted for home use but further research is needed to determine long-term effects.

ACKNOWLEDGMENTS

This article was supported in part by the Northwestern University Feinberg School of Medicine Center for Circadian and Sleep Medicine. This material is also the result of work supported with resources and the use of facilities at the Jesse Brown VA Medical Center, Chicago, Illinois. The views expressed in this article are those of the authors and do not necessarily reflect the position or policy of the Department of Veterans Affairs or the United States government.

DISCLOSURE

R.G. Malkani has nothing to disclose. Dr P.C. Zee is an inventor on a patent application for the PLL technique of acoustic stimulation that has been filed by Northwestern University with the United States Patent and Trademark Office (US Patent Application Number 15/517,458). Dr P.C. Zee also serves on the Philips scientific advisory board.

REFERENCES

1. Léger D, Debellemaniere E, Rabat A, et al. Slow-wave sleep: from the cell to the clinic. Sleep Med Rev 2018;41:113–32.
2. Rasch B, Born J. About sleep's role in memory. Physiol Rev 2013;93(2):681–766.
3. Tasali E, Leproult R, Ehrmann DA, et al. Slow-wave sleep and the risk of type 2 diabetes in humans. Proc Natl Acad Sci U S A 2008;105(3):1044–9.
4. Van Cauter E, Spiegel K, Tasali E, et al. Metabolic consequences of sleep and sleep loss. Sleep Med 2008;9(suppl 1):S23–8.
5. Xie L, Kang H, Xu Q, et al. Sleep drives metabolite clearance from the adult brain. Science 2013;342(6156):373–7.
6. Roh JH, Huang Y, Bero AW, et al. Disruption of the sleep-wake cycle and diurnal fluctuation of amyloid-ß in mice with Alzheimer's disease pathology. Sci Transl Med 2012;4(150):150ra122.
7. Amzica F, Steriade M. Cellular substrates and laminar profile of sleep K-complex. Neuroscience 1997;82(3):671–86.
8. Durán E, Yang M, Neves R, et al. Modulation of prefrontal cortex slow oscillations by phasic activation of the locus coeruleus. Neuroscience 2021;453:268–79.
9. Amzica F, Steriade M. Electrophysiological correlates of sleep delta waves. Electroencephalogr Clin Neurophysiol 1998;107:69–83.
10. Dube J, Lafortune M, Bedetti C, et al. Cortical thin- ning explains changes in sleep slow waves during adulthood. J Neurosci 2015;35(20):7795–807.
11. Carrier J, Viens I, Poirier G, et al. Sleep slow wave changes during the middle years of life. Eur J Neu Rosci 2011;33(4):758–66.
12. Sterman MB, Clemente CD. Forebrain inhibitory mechanisms: sleep patterns induced by basal forebrain stimulation in the behaving cat. Exp Neu- Rol 1962;6(2):103–17.
13. Massimini M, Huber R, Ferrarelli F, et al. The sleep slow oscillation as a traveling wave. J Neurosci 2004;24(31):6862–70.
14. Plihal W, Born J. Effects of early and late nocturnal sleep on declarative and procedural memory. J Cogn Neurosci 1997;9(4):534–47.
15. Groch S, Zinke K, Wilhelm I, et al. Dissociating the contributions of slow-wave sleep and rapid eye movement sleep to emotional item and source memory. Neurobiol Learn Mem 2015;122:122–30.
16. Frankland PW, Bontempi B. The organization of recent and remote memories. Nat Rev Neurosci 2005;6(2):119–30.
17. Sutherland GR, McNaughton B. Memory trace reactivation in hippocampal and neocortical neuronal ensembles. Curr Opin Neurobiol 2000;10(2):180–6.
18. Tononi G, Cirelli C. Sleep and the price of plasticity: from synaptic and cellular homeostasis to memory consolidation and integration. Neuron 2014;81(1):12–34.
19. Cirelli C. Sleep, synaptic homeostasis and neuronal firing rates. Curr Opin Neurobiol 2017;44:72–9.
20. De Vivo L, Bellesi M, Marshall W, et al. Ultrastructural evidence for synaptic scaling across the wake/sleep cycle. Science 2017;355(6324):507–10.
21. Kuhn M, Wolf E, Maier JG, et al. Sleep recalibrates homeostatic and associative synaptic plasticity in the human cortex. Nat Commun 2016;7:12455.
22. Born J, Wilhelm I. System consolidation of memory during sleep. Psychol Res 2012;76(2):192–203.
23. Diekelmann S, Born J. The memory function of sleep. Nat Rev Neurosci 2010;11(2):114–26.

24. Buzsaki G. Memory consolidation during sleep: a neurophysiological perspective. J Sleep Res 1998;7(S1):17–23.
25. Van Der Werf YD, Altena E, Schoonheim MM, et al. Sleep benefits subsequent hippocampal func tion- ing. Nat Neurosci 2009;12(2):122–3.
26. Gais S, Molle M, Helms K, et al. Learning-dependent increases in sleep spindle density. J Neurosci 2002;22(15):6830–4.
27. Schabus M, Gruber G, Parapatics S, et al. Sleep spindles and their significance for declarative memory consolidation. Sleep 2004;27(8): 1479–85.
28. Chauvette S, Seigneur J, Timofeev I. Sleep oscillations in the thalamocortical system induce long-term neuronal plasticity. Neuron 2012;75(6): 1105–13.
29. Westerberg CE, Mander BA, Florczak SM, et al. Concurrent impairments in sleep and memory in amnestic mild cognitive impairment. J Int Neuro-Psychol Soc 2012;18(3):490–500.
30. Girardeau G, Benchenane K, Wiener SI, et al. Selective suppression of hippocampal ripples impairs spatial memory. Nat Neurosci 2009;12(10): 1222–3.
31. Buzsaki G, Horvath Z, Urioste R, et al. High-frequency network oscillation in the hippocampus. Science 1992;256(5059):1025–7.
32. Ego-Stengel V, Wilson MA. Disruption of ripple-associated hippocampal activity during rest impairs spatial learning in the rat. Hippocampus 2010;20(1):1–10.
33. Klinzing JG, Molle M, Weber F, et al. Spindle activity phase-locked to sleep slow oscillations. Neuroimage 2016;134:607–16.
34. Helfrich RF, Mander BA, Jagust WJ, et al. Old brains come uncoupled in sleep: slow wave- spindle synchrony, brain atrophy, and forgetting. Neuron 2018;97(1):221–30.
35. Steriade M, McCormick DA, Sejnowski TJ. Thalamocortical oscillations in the sleeping and aroused brain. Science 1993;262(5134):679–85.
36. Steriade M, Contreras D, Amzica F. Synchronized sleep oscillations and their paroxysmal develop ments. Trends Neurosci 1994;17(5): 199–208.
37. Maingret N, Girardeau G, Todorova R, et al. Hippocampo-cortical coupling mediates memory consol idation during sleep. Nat Neurosci 2016;19(7): 959–64.
38. Heib DPJ, Hoedlmoser K, Anderer P, et al. Slow oscillation amplitudes and up-state lengths relate to memory improvement. PLoS One 2013;8(12): e82049.
39. Hedden T, Gabrieli JDE. Insights into the ageing mind: a view from cognitive neuroscience. Nat Rev Neurosci 2004;5(2):87–96.
40. Schaie KW. Intellectual development in adulthood: the Seattle longitudinal study. Cambridge (En gland): Cambridge University Press; 1996.
41. Ohayon MM, Carskadon MA, Guilleminault C, et al. Meta-analysis of quantitative sleep parameters from childhood to old age in healthy individuals: developing normative sleep values across the hu- man lifespan. Sleep 2004;27(7): 1255–73.
42. Mander BA, Rao V, Lu B, et al. Prefrontal atrophy, disrupted NREM slow waves and impaired hippocampal-dependent memory in aging. Nat Neurosci 2013;16(3):357–64.
43. Crowley K, Trinder J, Kim Y, et al. The effects of normal aging on sleep spindle and K-complex pro duction. Clin Neurophysiol 2002;113(10): 1615–22.
44. Masters CL, Simms G, Weinman NA, et al. Amyloid plaque core protein in Alzheimer disease and Down syndrome. Proc Natl Acad Sci U S A 1985; 82:4245–9.
45. Prince M, Wimo A, Guerchet M, et al. World Alz heimer Report 2015: the global impact of dementia: an analysis, of prevalence, incidence, cost, and trends. London: Alzheimer's Disease International; 2015.
46. Shi L, Chen S-J, Ma M-Y, et al. Sleep disturbances increase the risk of dementia: a systematic review and meta-analysis. Sleep Med Rev 2017. https://doi.org/10.1016/j.smrv.2017.06.010.
47. Kang J-E, Lim MM, Bateman RJ, et al. Amyloid-beta dynamics are regulated by orexin and the sleep-wake cycle. Science 2009;326(5955): 1005–7.
48. Liguori C, Romigi A, Nuccetelli M, et al. Orexinergic system dysregulation, sleep impairment, and cognitive decline in Alzheimer disease. JAMA Neu rol 2014;71(12):1498–505.
49. Lim ASP, Yu L, Kowgier M, et al. Modification of the relationship of the apolipoprotein E e4 allele to the risk of Alzheimer disease and neurofibrillary tangle density by sleep. JAMA Neurol 2013;70(12): 1544–51.
50. Kastanenka KV, Hou SS, Shakerdge N, et al. Optogenetic restoration of disrupted slow oscillations halts amyloid deposition and restores calcium homeostasis in an animal model of Alzheimer's disease. PLoS One 2017;12: e0170275.
51. Kastanenka KV, Calvo-Rodriguez M, Hou SS, et al. Frequency-dependent exacerbation of Alzheimer's disease neuropathophysiology. Sci Rep 2019;9: 8964.
52. Petersen RC. Mild cognitive impairment as a clin ical entity. J Intern Med 2004;256(7):183–94.
53. Gorgoni M, Lauri G, Truglia I, et al. Parietal fast sleep spindle density decrease in Alzheimer's

dis- ease and amnesic mild cognitive impairment. Neu- Ral Plast 2016;2016:8376108.
54. McKinnon AC, Duffy SL, Cross NE, et al. Functional connectivity in the default mode network is reduced in association with nocturnal awakening in mild cognitive impairment. J Alzheimers Dis 2017;56(4):1373–84.
55. Herrmann CS, Rach S, Neuling T, et al. Transcra- nial alternating current stimulation: a review of the underlying mechanisms and modulation of cognitive processes. Front Hum Neurosci 2013; 7:279.
56. Antal A, Herrmann CS. Transcranial alternating cur rent and random noise stimulation: possible mech anisms. Neural Plast 2016;3616807. https://doi.org/10.1155/2016/3616807.
57. Jackson MP, Rahman A, Lafon B, et al. Animal models of transcranial direct current stimulation: methods and mechanisms. Clin Neurophysiol 2016;127(11):3425–54.
58. Marshall L, Helgadottir H, Molle M, et al. Boosting slow oscillations during sleep potentiates memory. Nature 2006;444(7119):610–3.
59. Garside P, Arizpe J, Lau CI, et al. Cross-hemispheric alternating current stimulation during a nap disrupts slow wave activity and associated memory consoli dation. Brain Stimul 2015;8(3): 520–7.
60. Marshall L, Molle M, Hallschmid M, et al. Transcranial direct current stimulation during sleep improves declarative memory. J Neurosci 2004; 24(44):9985–92.
61. Ladenbauer J, Kulzow N, Passmann S, et al. Brain stimulation during an afternoon nap boosts slow oscillatory activity and memory consolidation in older adults. Neuroimage 2016;142: 311–23.
62. Paßmann S, Kulzow N, Ladenbauer J, et al. Boost ing slow oscillatory activity using tDCS during early nocturnal slow wave sleep does not improve memory consolidation in healthy older adults. Brain Stimul 2016;9(5):730–9.
63. Bueno-Lopez A, Eggert T, Dorn H, et al. Slow oscil latory transcranial direct current stimulation (so-tDCS) during slow wave sleep has no effects on declarative memory in healthy young subjects. Brain Stimul 2019;12(4):948–739.
64. Sahlem GL, Badran BW, Halford JJ, et al. Oscil lating square wave transcranial direct current stim- ulation (tDCS) delivered during slow wave sleep does not improve declarative memory more than sham: a randomized sham controlled crossover study. Brain Stimul 2015; 8(3):528–34.
65. Eggert T, Dorn H, Sauter C, et al. No effects of slow oscillatory transcranial direct current stimulation (tDCS) on sleep-dependent memory consolidation in healthy elderly subjects. Brain Stimul 2013;6: 938–45.
66. Koo PC, Molle M, Marshall L. Efficacy of slow oscillatory-transcranial direct current stimulation on EEG and memory contribution of an inter- individual factor. Eur J Neurosci 2018;47(7): 812–23.
67. Westerberg CE, Florczak SM, Weintraub S, et al. Memory improvement via slow-oscillatory stimulation during sleep in older adults. Neurobiol Aging 2015;36(9):2577–86.
68. Hathaway E, Morgan K, Carson M, et al. Transcranial Electrical Stimulation targeting limbic cortex increases the duration of human deep sleep. Sleep Med 2021;81:350–7. https://doi.org/10.1016/j.sleep.2021.03.001.
69. Ladenbauer J, Ladenbauer J, Kulzow N, et al. Pro moting sleep oscillations and their functional coupling by transcranial stimulation enhances memory consolidation in mild cognitive impair ment. J Neurosci 2017;37(30):7111–24.
70. Lustenberger C, Boyle MR, Alagapan S, et al. Feedback-controlled transcranial alternating cur rent stimulation reveals a functional role of sleep spindles in motor memory consolidation. Curr Biol 2016;26(16):2127–36.
71. Prehn-Kristensen A, Munz M, Goder R, et al. Trans cranial oscillatory direct current stimulation during sleep improves declarative memory consolidation in children with attention-deficit/hyperactivity disor der to a level comparable to healthy controls. Brain Stimul 2014;7(6):793–9.
72. Goder R, Baier PC, Beith B, et al. Effects of trans cranial direct current stimulation during sleep on memory performance in patients with schizo phrenia. Schizophr Res 2013;144:153–4.
73. Del Felice A, Magalini A, Masiero S. Slow-oscillatory transcranial direct current stimulation modulates memory in temporal lobe epilepsy by altering sleep spindle generators: a possible reha- bilitation tool. Brain Stimul 2015;8(3): 567–73.
74. Lafon B, Henin S, Huang Y, et al. Low frequency transcranial electrical stimulation does not entrain sleep rhythms measured by human intracranial re- cordings. Nat Commun 2017;8(1):1199.
75. Antal A, Alekseichuk I, Bikson M, et al. Low inten sity transcranial electric stimulation: safety, ethical, legal regulatory and application guidelines. Clin Neurophysiol 2017;128(9):1774–809.
76. Luber B, McClintock SM, Lisanby SH. Applications of transcranial magnetic stimulation and magnetic seizure therapy in the study and treatment of disor ders related to cerebral aging. Dialogues Clin Neu Rosci 2013;15:87–98.
77. Babiloni AH, De Beaumont L, Lavigne GJ. Transcranial magnetic stimulation: potential use in

obstructive sleep apnea and sleep bruxism. Sleep Med Clin 2018;13(4):571–82.

78. Massimini M, Ferrarelli F, Esser SK, et al. Triggering sleep slow waves by transcranial magnetic stimula tion. Proc Natl Acad Sci U S A 2007;104(20): 8496–501.
79. Bergmann TO, Molle M, Schmidt MA, et al. EEG-guided transcranial magnetic stimulation reveals rapid shifts in motor cortical excitability during the human sleep slow oscillation. J Neurosci 2012; 32(1):243–53.
80. Manganotti P, Formaggio E, Del Felice A, et al. Time-frequency analysis of short-lasting modulation of EEG induced by TMS during wake, sleep deprivation and sleep. Front Hum Neurosci 2013; 7:767.
81. Stamm M, Aru J, Rutiku R, et al. Occipital long- interval paired pulse TMS leads to slow wave components in NREM sleep. Conscious Cogn 2015; 35:78–87.
82. Massimini M, Tononi G, Huber R. Slow waves, syn aptic plasticity and information processing: in sights from transcranial magnetic stimulation and high-density EEG experiments. Eur J Neurosci 2009;29(9):1761–70.
83. Huber R, Esser SK, Ferrarelli F, et al. TMS-induced cortical potentiation during wakefulness locally in creases slow wave activity during sleep. PLoS One 2007;2(3):e276.
84. Huber R, Maatta S, Esser SK, et al. Measures of cortical plasticity after transcranial paired associa tive stimulation predict changes in electroencepha logram slow-wave activity during subsequent sleep. J Neurosci 2008;28(31):7911–8.
85. Bashir S, Al-Hussain F, Hamza A, et al. Role of single low pulse intensity of transcranial magnetic stimulation over the frontal cortex for cognitive function. Front Hum Neurosci 2020;1–6. https://doi.org/10.3389/fnhum.2020.00205.
86. Luber B, Kinnunen LH, Rakitin BC, et al. Facilitation of performance in a working memory task with rTMS stimulation of the precuneus: frequency- and time-dependent effects. Brain Res 2007; 1128(1):120–9.
87. Martinez-Cancino DP, Azpiroz-Leehan J, Jimenez-Angeles L, et al. Effects of high frequency rTMS on sleep deprivation: a pilot study. Conf Proc IEEE Eng Med Biol Soc 2016;2016:5937–40.
88. Luber B, Stanford AD, Bulow P, et al. Remediation of sleep-deprivation-induced working memory impairment with fMRI-guided transcranial magnetic stimulation. Cereb Cortex 2008;18: 2077–85.
89. Wang JX, Rogers LM, Gross EZ, et al. Memory enhancement: targeted enhancement of cortical-hippocampal brain networks and associative mem- ory. Science 2014;345(6200):1054–7.
90. Cotelli M, Manenti R, Cappa SF, et al. Effect of transcranial magnetic stimulation on action naming in patients with Alzheimer disease. Arch Neurol 2006;63(11):1602–4.
91. Cotelli M, Manenti R, Cappa SF, et al. Transcranial magnetic stimulation improves naming in Alzheimer disease patients at different stages of cognitive decline. Eur J Neurol 2008;15(12): 1286–92.
92. Cotelli M, Calabria M, Manenti R, et al. Improved language performance in Alzheimer disease following brain stimulation. J Neurol Neurosurg Psychiatry 2011;82(7):794–7.
93. Bentwich J, Dobronevsky E, Aichenbaum S, et al. Beneficial effect of repetitive transcranial magnetic stimulation combined with cognitive training for the treatment of Alzheimer's disease: a proof of concept study. J Neural Transm 2011;118(3): 463–71.
94. Rabey JM, Dobronevsky E. Repetitive transcranial magnetic stimulation (rTMS) combined with cognitive training is a safe and effective modality for the treatment of Alzheimer's disease: clinical experience. J Neural Transm 2016;123(12):1449–55.
95. Lee J, Choi BH, Oh E, et al. Treatment of Alzheimer's disease with repetitive transcranial magnetic stimulation combined with cognitive training: a prospective, randomized, double-blind, placebo-controlled study. J Clin Neurol 2016;12(1): 57–64.
96. Buss SS, Fried PJ, Pascual-Leone A. Therapeutic noninvasive brain stimulation in Alzheimer's dis ease and related dementias. Curr Opin Neurol 2019;32(2):292–304.
97. Avirame K, Stehberg J, Todder D. Benefits of deep transcranial magnetic stimulation in Alzheimer disease case series. J ECT 2016;32(2): 127–33.
98. Chang C-H, Lane H-Y, Lin C-H. Brain stimulation in Alzheimer's disease. Front Psychiatry 2018;9:201.
99. Halasz P. The K-complex as a special reactive sleep slow wave A theoretical update. Sleep Med Rev 2016;29:34–40.
100. Bellesi M, Riedner BA, Garcia-Molina GN, et al. Enhancement of sleep slow waves: underlying mechanisms and practical consequences. Front Syst Neurosci 2014;8:208.
101. Simor P, Steinbach E, Nagy T, et al. Lateralized rhythmic acoustic stimulation during daytime NREM sleep enhances slow waves. Sleep 2018; 41(12):zsy176.
102. Zhou J, Liu D, Li X, et al. Pink noise: effect on complexity synchronization of brain activity and sleep consolidation. J Theor Biol 2012;306:68–72.
103. Antony JW, Paller KA. Using oscillating sounds to manipulate sleep spindles. Sleep 2017;40(3): zsw068.

104. Tononi G, Riedner BA, Hulse BK, et al. Enhancing sleep slow waves with natural stimuli. Medicamundi 2010;54(2):82–8.
105. Weigenand A, Molle M, Werner F, et al. Timing matters: open-loop stimulation does not improve overnight consolidation of word pairs in humans. Eur J Neurosci 2016;44(6):2357–68.
106. Schade MM, Mathew GM, Roberts DM, et al. Enhancing slow oscillations and increasing N3 sleep proportion with supervised, non-phase-locked pink noise and other non-standard auditory stimulation during NREM sleep. Nat Sci Sleep 2020;(12):411–29. https://doi.org/10.2147/NSS.S243204.
107. Ngo HVV, Martinetz T, Born J, et al. Auditory closed-loop stimulation of the sleep slow oscillation enhances memory. Neuron 2013;78(3):545–53.
108. Ngo HVV, Claussen JC, Born J, et al. Induction of slow oscillations by rhythmic acoustic stimulation. J Sleep Res 2013;22(1):22–31.
109. Navarrete M, Schneider J, Ngo HVV, Valderrama M, Casson AJ, Lewis PA. Examining the optimal timing for closed-loop auditory stimulation of slow-wave sleep in young and older adults. Sleep 2020;43(6):zsz315. https://doi.org/10.1093/sleep/zsz315.
110. Sousouri G, Krugliakova E, Skorucak J, et al. Neuromodulation by means of phase-locked auditory stimulation affects key marker of excitability and connectivity during sleep. Sleep 2021;zsab204. https://doi.org/10.1093/sleep/zsab204.
111. Ngo H-VV, Miedema A, Faude I, et al. Driving sleep slow oscillations by auditory closed-loop stimulation-A self-limiting process. J Neurosci 2015;35(17):6630–8.
112. Leminen MM, Virkkala J, Saure E, et al. Enhanced memory consolidation via automatic sound stimulation during non-REM sleep. Sleep 2017;40(3):zsx003.
113. Besedovsky L, Ngo HVV, Dimitrov S, et al. Auditory closed-loop stimulation of EEG slow oscillations strengthens sleep and signs of its immune- supportive function. Nat Commun 2017;8(1):1984.
114. Debellemaniere E, Chambon S, Pinaud C, et al. Performance of an ambulatory dry-EEG Device for auditory closed-loop stimulation of sleep slow oscillations in the home environment. Front Hum Neurosci 2018;12:88.
115. Garcia-Molina G, Tsoneva T, Jasko J, et al. Closed-loop system to enhance slow-wave activity. J Neural Eng 2018;15(6):066018.
116. Papalambros NA, Weintraub S, Chen T, et al. Acoustic enhancement of sleep slow oscillations in mild cognitive impairment. Ann Clin Transl Neurol 2019;6(7):1191–201.
117. Papalambros NA, Santostasi G, Malkani RG, et al. Acoustic enhancement of sleep slow oscillations and concomitant memory improvement in older adults. Front Hum Neurosci 2017;11:1–14.
118. Ong JL, Lo JC, Chee NIYN, et al. Effects of phase-locked acoustic stimulation during a nap on EEG spectra and declarative memory consolidation. Sleep Med 2016;20:88–97.
119. Diep C, Ftouni S, Manousakis JE, et al. Acoustic slow wave sleep enhancement via a novel, automated device improves executive function in middle-aged men. Sleep 2020;43:zsz197. https://doi.org/10.1093/sleep/zsz197.
120. Grimaldi D, Papalambros NA, Reid KJ, et al. Strengthening sleep-autonomic interaction via acoustic enhancement of slow oscillations. Sleep 2019;42(5):zsz036.
121. Diep C, Garcia-Molina G, Jasko J, et al. Acoustic enhancement of slow wave sleep on consecutive nights improves alertness and attention in chronically short sleepers. Sleep Med 2021;81:69–79. https://doi.org/10.1016/j.sleep.2021.01.044.
122. Santostasi G, Malkani R, Riedner B, et al. Phase-locked loop for precisely timed acoustic stimulation during sleep. J Neurosci Methods 2016;259:101–14.
123. Ong JL, Patanaik A, Chee NIYN, et al. Auditory stimulation of sleep slow oscillations modulates subsequent memory encoding through altered hippocampal function. Sleep 2018;41(5):1–11. https://doi.org/10.1093/sleep/zsy031.
124. Henin S, Borges H, Shankar A, et al. Closed-loop acoustic stimulation enhances sleep oscillations but not memory performance. eNeuro 2019;6(6). https://doi.org/10.1523/ENEURO.0306-19.2019.ENEURO.0306-19.
125. Harrington MO, Ngo HVV, Cairney SA. No benefit of auditory closed-loop stimulation on memory for semantically-incongruent associations. Neurobiol Learn Mem 2021;183:107482. https://doi.org/10.1016/j.nlm.2021.107482.
126. Salfi F, D'Atri A, Tempesta D, et al. Boosting slow oscillations during sleep to improve memory function in elderly people: a review of the literature. Brain Sci 2020;10(5):300. https://doi.org/10.3390/brainsci10050300.
127. Rasch B, Buchel C, Gais S, et al. Odor cues during slow-wave sleep prompt declarative memory consolidation. Science 2007;315(5817):1426–2114.
128. Fuentemilla L, Miro J, Ripolles P, et al. Hippocampus-dependent strengthening of targeted memories via reactivation during sleep in humans. Curr Biol 2013;23(18):1769–75.
129. Bar E, Marmelshtein A, Arzi A, et al. Local targeted memory reactivation in human sleep. Curr Biol 2020;30(8):1435–46. https://doi.org/10.1016/j.cub.2020.01.091.

130. Oudiette D, Paller KA. Upgrading the sleeping brain with targeted memory reactivation. Trends Cogn Sci 2013;17(3):142–9.
131. Rudoy JD, Voss JL, Westerberg CE, et al. Strengthening individual memories by reactivat- ing them during sleep. Science 2009;326(5956):1079.
132. Oyarzun JP, Moris J, Luque D, et al. Targeted memory reactivation during sleep adaptively promotes the strengthening or weakening of overlapping memories. J Neurosci 2017;37(32):7748–58.
133. Batterink LJ, Creery JD, Paller KA. Phase of spontaneous slow oscillations during sleep influences memory-related processing of auditory cues. J Neurosci 2016;36(4):1401–9.
134. Antony JW, Gobel EW, O'Hare JK, et al. Cued memory reactivation during sleep influences skill learning. Nat Neurosci 2012;15(8):1114–6.
135. Oudiette D, Antony JW, Creery JD, et al. The role of memory reactivation during wakefulness and sleep in determining which memories endure. J Neurosci 2013;33(15):6672–8.
136. Cairney SA, Sobczak JM, Lindsay S, et al. Mecha nisms of memory retrieval in slow-wave sleep. Sleep 2017;40(9):zsx114.
137. Honma M, Plass J, Brang D, et al. Sleeping on the rubber-hand illusion: memory reactivation during sleep facilitates multisensory recalibration. Neurosci Conscious 2016;2016(1):niw020.
138. Johnson BP, Scharf SM, Verceles AC, et al. Sensorimotor performance is improved by targeted memory reactivation during a daytime nap in healthy older adults. Neurosci Lett 2020;731:134973. https://doi.org/10.1016/j.neulet.2020.134973.
139. Johnson BP, Scharf SM, Verceles AC, et al. Use of targeted memory reactivation enhances skill performance during a nap and enhances declarative memory during wake in healthy young adults. J Sleep Res 2019;28(5):1–8. https://doi.org/10.1111/jsr.12832.
140. Goldinger SD. Words and voices: episodic traces in spoken word identification and recognition memory. J Exp Psychol Learn Mem Cogn 1996;22(5):1166–83.
141. Groch S, McMakin D, Guggenbuhl P, et al. Memory cueing during sleep modifies the interpretation of ambiguous scenes in adolescents and adults. Dev Cogn Neurosci 2016;17:10–8.
142. Hutchison IC, Pezzoli S, Tsimpanouli M-E, et al. Targeted memory reactivation in REM but not SWS selectively reduces arousal responses. doi: 10.1038/s42003-021-01854-3
143. Göldi M, Rasch B. Effects of targeted memory reactivation during sleep at home depend on sleep disturbances and habituation. Npj Sci Learn 2019;4(1):5. https://doi.org/10.1038/s41539-019-0044-2.
144. Batterink LJ, Paller KA. Sleep-based memory processing facilitates grammatical generalization: evidence from targeted memory reactivation. Brain Lang 2017;167:83–93.
145. Kumar Goothy SS, McKeown J. Modulation of sleep using electrical vestibular nerve stimulation prior to sleep onset: a pilot study. J Basic Clin Physiol Pharmacol 2021;32(2):19–23. https://doi.org/10.1515/jbcpp-2020-0019.
146. Choi SH, Kwon H Bin, Jin HW, et al. Weak closed-loop vibrational stimulation improves the depth of slow-wave sleep and declarative memory consolidation. Sleep 2021;44(6):zsaa285. https://doi.org/10.1093/sleep/zsaa285.

Hypnotic Discontinuation in Chronic Insomnia

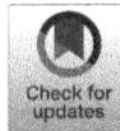

Jonathan P. Hintze, MD[a], Jack D. Edinger, PhD[b,*]

KEYWORDS

• Deprescribing • Discontinuation • Hypnotic • Benzodiazepines • Insomnia • Sleep disorder

KEY POINTS

- Patients with chronic insomnia are commonly prescribed hypnotic medications but discontinuation of these medications is difficult to achieve.
- A gradual taper is preferred over abrupt cessation to avoid rebound insomnia and withdrawal symptoms.
- Written information provided to the patient about medication discontinuation may be helpful.
- Cognitive behavioral therapy or behavioral therapies alone can improve hypnotic discontinuation outcomes.
- There is limited evidence for adjunct medications to assist in hypnotic cessation for insomnia.

INTRODUCTION

Insomnia disorder is common in adults and children. The estimated prevalence ranges from 9% to 15% in the general population, with higher prevalence in certain subpopulations.[1–6] Hypnotic medications are those that tend to produce sleep and are frequently used to treat insomnia.[7] Commonly used hypnotics in adults include benzodiazepines (BZDs), BZD receptor agonists (BzRAs), antihistamines, antidepressants, melatonin receptor agonists, orexin receptor antagonists, and antipsychotics. Although there are currently no medications for pediatric insomnia approved by the US Food and Drug Administration, commonly used medications include antihistamines, alpha agonists, antidepressants, BZDs, BzRAs, and antipsychotics.[8,9] The long-term health consequences of using hypnotics are not well described, and current guidelines recommend medication tapering and discontinuation when possible.[10] However, hypnotic discontinuation is difficult and often unsuccessful.[11] This article discusses strategies to discontinue hypnotics and evidence supporting their use.

HYPNOTIC TAPER STRATEGIES

Abrupt Hypnotic Cessation

Rapid drug cessation is an option for many medications. However, rebound insomnia and withdrawal symptoms may accompany abrupt hypnotic discontinuation. Rebound insomnia is generally defined as insomnia that is worse relative to baseline. This was first described with the discontinuation of triazolam[12] and has since been reported with several other BZDs[13,14]; sedating antidepressants, including amitriptyline[15] and trazodone[16]; and BzRAs, although with conflicting reports.[14,17–19] Additionally, withdrawal symptoms, largely defined as the emergence of previously absent symptoms, are frequently reported with abrupt discontinuation of BZDs.[20] Consequently, tapering hypnotics is generally preferred to abrupt cessation.

Tapering Hypnotics

Reported tapering strategies vary widely, with no consensus on the optimal tapering protocol. A frequently described approach is a dose reduction of 25% every 1 to 2 weeks until discontinued

Sleep Med Clin 13 (2018) 263-270 https://doi.org/10.1016/j.jsmc.2018.02.008. 1556-407X/18/© 2018 Elsevier Inc.

[a] Intermountain Healthcare Services, Inc, 652 S Medical Centre Drive, Suite 310, St George, UT 84790-7266, USA; [b] Department of Medicine, National Jewish Health, 1400 Jackson Street, Denver, CO 80206, USA
* Corresponding author.
E-mail address: edingerj@njhealth.org

Sleep Med Clin 17 (2022) 523–530
https://doi.org/10.1016/j.jsmc.2022.06.014
1556-407X/22/© 2022 Elsevier Inc. All rights reserved.

completely.[21–25] Complete discontinuation rates ranged from 24% to 61% in these studies but there is variability in the frequency of office visits and the follow-up period in these reports. Withdrawal symptoms were commonly reported. A slightly slower wean was used by Lopez-Peig and colleagues.[26] Subjects all took BZDs and were instructed to reduce their dose by 25% every 2 to 4 weeks. At the end of the taper period, 80.4% had successfully discontinued their BZD, and 64% remained BZD-free at 12 months. Another study weaned subjects from various BZDs by 10% to 25% every 2 to 3 weeks, with an approximately 40% hypnotic abstinence rate maintained at 36 months, without significant sleep dissatisfaction compared with a control group.[27] Drake[28] weaned subjects from temazepam by cutting doses roughly in half every 2 weeks, from 10 to 5 to 2 mg. Of the subjects, 59% successfully completed the taper, with 52% remaining hypnotic-free at follow-up 12 to 35 weeks later. Lemoine and colleagues[29] reported a similar taper with 2 BzRAs, zopiclone and zolpidem. In that study, subjects were weaned from zolpidem 10 to 5 mg for a week, followed by a placebo. Similarly, subjects were weaned from zopiclone 7.5 to 3.75 mg for a week, followed by a placebo. This regimen was associated with significantly higher withdrawal symptoms than the control group that was not weaned. In contrast, Raju and Meagher[30] used a more flexible taper protocol, in which subjects were able to control the rate of withdrawal. Given control over the weaning pace, some subjects rapidly discontinued hypnotic use (19 of 68), whereas others preferred a prolonged, yet complete, taper (13 of 68). The remainder did not completely discontinue medication use. To the authors' knowledge, there are no studies specifically comparing the success of different taper strategies. However, a clinical trial is currently underway that will compare different taper strategies among hypnotic-dependent subjects.[31]

Many practitioners find it helpful to switch from a short-acting to a long-acting BZD before initiating a taper.[27,32] This is done by switching to an equivalent dose of a long-acting BZD, commonly diazepam (**Table 1**). It is notable that a Cochrane Review published in 2006 noted higher dropout rates when tapering short half-life compounds compared with long-acting BZDs.[33] However, there was no difference in withdrawal symptoms between the groups, so switching from a short-acting to a long-acting BZD before a gradual taper was not supported. The authors are unaware of any studies specifically comparing the practice of switching to a long-acting BZD before gradual withdrawal versus a gradual withdrawal directly from a short-acting BZD.

ADJUNCT THERAPIES

Regardless of the taper strategy, several adjunct therapies have been studied to assist in hypnotic discontinuation. These include various degrees of patient education, psychological therapies, and medications.

Written Patient Education

There is some evidence that simply providing written information to patients can lead to hypnotic discontinuation. In 1 study, chronic BZD users were randomized to receive either routine care or advice during a single consultation supplemented by a self-help booklet.[34] The intervention resulted in a significant reduction in BDZ prescriptions compared with routine care alone (18% vs 5%). Several other studies used a letter sent to BZD users encouraging BZD reduction, with complete BZD cessation rates ranging from 14% to 27%[23,24,35–37]

Psychological Therapies

Many studies have used psychological therapies to aid in medication discontinuation. A brief description of the different types of therapy is provided in **Table 2**.

Sleep Hygiene Education

Sleep hygiene education is routinely provided to patients with insomnia. However, there is insufficient evidence to recommend sleep hygiene as a stand-alone therapy regardless of the presence or absence of hypnotic use.[38] Additionally, the authors are unaware of any studies that used sleep hygiene alone as an intervention to assist in hypnotic discontinuation.

Relaxation Therapy

Relaxation therapy is a technique used to reduce muscular tension and intrusive thought processes interfering with sleep and involves tensing and relaxing major muscle groups. Giblin and Clift[39] studied the effects of relaxation therapy on hypnotic discontinuation in 20 subjects. Notably, their intervention also included a discussion about sleep and insomnia, hypnotics and their effects on sleep, and general advice about problem-solving and optimism. There was a significant decrease in the number of subjects who resumed nightly hypnotic use at 12 weeks in the treatment group (2 of 10) compared with the control group (8 of 10), without any significant difference

Table 1
Approximate equivalent doses of benzodiazepines to 5 mg diazepam

BZD	Equivalent Dose (mg)
Alprazolam	0.25–0.5
Bromazepam	3–6
Lorazepam	0.5–1
Nitrazepam	5
Oxazepam	15
Temazepam	10
Triazolam	0.25

between the groups in reported sleep onset latency and overall sleep quality.

Lichstein and Johnson[40] used relaxation therapy for hypnotic cessation, resulting in a substantial reduction (47%) in sleep medication use. Lichstein and colleagues[41] assessed the usefulness of progressive relaxation techniques in addition to a standard drug withdrawal program in a randomized trial. All subjects had a 79% reduction in hypnotic consumption, without any significant difference between the groups. However, those assigned to the relaxation group had fewer withdrawal symptoms, greater sleep efficiency, and higher reported quality of sleep.

Stimulus Control Therapy

Stimulus control therapy is a method pioneered by Bootzin[42] and is used to reestablish the association between the bed and sleep. Patients are encouraged to remove themselves from the bed when unable to fall asleep, and only go to bed when sleepy rather than at a designated bedtime. They are also encouraged to keep a strict rise time and to avoid napping. A study of 7 long-term hypnotic users found that most (6 of 7) were able to reduce or stop their medication when stimulus control therapy was used.[43] Riedel and colleagues[44] randomized 21 subjects to either a medication withdrawal program, or the withdrawal program and stimulus control therapy. Both groups had significant reductions in the amount of sleep medication use but the stimulus control group also had significant improvements in total sleep time, sleep efficiency, sleep quality, and daytime sleepiness. Several other studies included stimulus control therapy as part of their intervention (see later discussion).

Sleep Restriction Therapy

Sleep restriction therapy is used to curtail the amount of time spent awake in bed. This is done by determining the amount of sleep a patient is regularly getting and limiting the total allowable time in bed to the same amount. For example, if a patient is currently spending 10 hours in bed per night but only sleeps 6 hours, then the amount of time in bed per night would be limited to 6 to 6.5 hours, depending on the specific sleep restriction protocol used.

Although sleep restriction is a well-established therapy for insomnia in general,[45] Taylor and colleagues[46] performed the only known study examining the effectiveness of sleep restriction in the setting of hypnotic discontinuation. Forty-six subjects were assigned to either sleep hygiene education or sleep restriction with medication withdrawal. In the sleep restriction group, 52.6% completely discontinued hypnotic medication use, compared with 15.4% in the sleep hygiene group. Additionally, there was improvement in sleep-onset latency and sleep efficiency, which was maintained through a 12-month follow-up period.

Cognitive Behavioral Therapy

Cognitive therapy is the method of challenging a patient's current beliefs about sleep that contribute to insomnia. Cognitive behavioral therapy (CBT) combines behavioral therapy (eg, relaxation, stimulus control, sleep restriction) with cognitive therapy to form a multicomponent and omnibus intervention. Therefore, CBT is a combination therapy with variation depending on the specific methods used. CBT has long been used for insomnia and an early study demonstrated its usefulness in hypnotic discontinuation.[47] Several subsequent studies have been performed.

Many studies specifically evaluated BZD cessation. Baillargeon and colleagues[48] studied 65 subjects with chronic insomnia taking BZDs nightly, randomizing subjects to a gradual supervised taper alone or combined with 8 weeks of CBT. At treatment completion, more subjects had complete drug cessation in the combined group (77%) compared with the taper-alone group (38%), with similar results at a 12-month follow-up (70% vs 24%). Although several other studies reported no improvement in BZD discontinuation rates with CBT,[23,49,50] other measures of sleep quality were generally improved. Morin and colleagues[25] considered the differential effects of supervised BZD withdrawal and CBT in their randomized trial. Seventy-six subjects underwent supervised withdrawal, CBT, or both. Although all groups had a significant reduction in quantity (90%) and frequency (80%) of BZD use, the combined treatment group was the most successful at achieving complete drug cessation (85%), with

Table 2
Psychological therapies for insomnia

Therapy	Description
Sleep hygiene education	Guidelines about practices and habits that support or interfere with sleep (eg, obtaining regular exercise, avoid electronics before bed)
Relaxation therapy	Techniques used to reduce muscular tension and intrusive thought processes interfering with sleep
Stimulus control therapy	Reinforcing the association of the bed with sleep by getting out of bed when unable to fall asleep, only going to bed when sleepy, keeping a strict rise time, and avoiding napping
Sleep restriction therapy	Reducing the amount of time spent in bed to match actual sleep time, with periodic adjustments as necessary
Cognitive therapy	A method of challenging false beliefs about sleep that contribute to insomnia
Cognitive behavioral therapy	Combining cognitive therapy with another behavioral treatment (eg, sleep restriction or stimulus control)
Self-efficacy enhancement	Improving perceived coping capabilities by providing positive vicarious experiences, discussing obstacles from prior failed attempts, and social persuasion

supervised withdrawal and CBT alone producing less-successful results (48% and 54%, respectively). Interestingly, the subjects in both groups that received CBT reported greater improvement in subjective sleep quality when compared with the group who only had supervised drug withdrawal. When a 24-month follow-up was conducted, 42.6% of subjects had resumed BZDs, with greater relapse in the CBT-alone group (69.2%) when compared with the combined (33.3%) and supervised withdrawal (30.8%) groups.

BzRAs have also been studied. Zavesicka and colleagues[51] reported 15 zolpidem-dependent subjects who were successfully weaned while receiving CBT, with associated improved sleep efficiency and decreased wakefulness after sleep onset. An 8-week hypnotic taper program, including 53 subjects taking either BZDs or BzRAs, found that those randomized to receive CBT had improved sleep efficiency and decreased total wake time when compared with the control group.[52] However, both groups successfully reduced hypnotic use, with no significant additional reduction in the CBT group. In contrast, Morgan and colleagues[53] found that CBT greatly reduced hypnotic drug use while improving sleep efficiency and reducing sleep onset latency in a cohort of 209 chronic hypnotic users. Lichstein and colleagues[54] further validated the usefulness of CBT in hypnotic-dependent insomnia patients using BZDs, BzRAs, or sedating antidepressants by randomizing subjects to CBT with drug withdrawal, placebo biofeedback with drug withdrawal, or drug withdrawal alone. There were no significant differences between groups in medication reduction, which decreased by 84% posttreatment and 66% at a 12-month follow-up. However, only the CBT group had significant improvement in sleep onset latency and subjective sleep measures.

Self-Efficacy Enhancement

In some analyses of factors leading to success in hypnotic cessation, an individual's perceived self-efficacy has been positively correlated with medication cessation.[50,55] To further pursue the effect of self-efficacy on patient outcomes, Yang and colleagues[56] randomized 48 long-term hypnotic users (BZDs or BzRAs) to a standard drug taper alone or a self-efficacy educational program followed by the same drug taper. Those in the treatment group had a higher percentage of dose reduction than those in the taper-alone group, suggesting that self-efficacy can be learned and can improve hypnotic cessation outcomes.

Pharmacologic Therapies

Several studies have evaluated the usefulness of medications to assist in BZD discontinuation, although generally in the setting of anxiety or other psychological disorders. These have included ondansetron,[57] imipramine,[58,59] buspirone,[58–60] paroxetine,[61] carbamazepine,[62] pregabalin,[63] progesterone,[64] antihistamines,[65] and propranolol.[66] Only a few have examined the usefulness of medications to assist in BZDs cessation specifically for insomnia. There have also been some reports of other supplements to aid in hypnotic discontinuation.

Zopiclone

Withdrawal symptoms and rebound insomnia have been shown to be less severe with BzRAs compared with some BZDs.[18] Therefore, some investigators have proposed using a BzRA as a bridge to BZD discontinuation. Pat-Horenczyk and colleagues[67] studied 24 subjects taking flunitrazepam for insomnia. All underwent a 5-week withdrawal protocol and were followed with nightly actigraphy and serial polysomnograms during the withdrawal period. One group was transitioned to zopiclone and then weaned off, whereas the other was weaned off flunitrazepam directly. Both objective (polysomnogram and actigraphy) and subjective (sleep diaries) measures were improved in the zopiclone group compared with the flunitrazepam group. Similar positive findings were found in other reports.[68–70] Two studies indicated that abrupt medication substitution yielded better results than gradual substitution.[68,70]

Melatonin

Some have postulated that melatonin therapy could aid in the discontinuation of hypnotics. In a large retrospective study of prolonged-release melatonin, 31% discontinued hypnotic use (BZDs or BzRAs) after the melatonin was started.[71] Several randomized trials have also considered the usefulness of melatonin in hypnotic discontinuation, specifically BZDs. Although 2 of these trials showed some effectiveness,[72,73] most found that melatonin did not enhance BZD discontinuation.[74–78] A meta-analysis also concluded that melatonin supplementation did not affect rates of BZD discontinuation.[79]

Valerian

The evidence for the use of the herbal supplement valerian in insomnia to date has been inconclusive.[80] However, Poyares and colleagues[81] reported some positive outcomes with the use of valerian in BZD discontinuation. Subjects treated with valerian had better subjective sleep quality than the placebo group, with decreased wakefulness after sleep onset at a 2-week polysomnogram, although with a longer sleep onset latency.

SUMMARY

Discontinuation of hypnotic medications is often challenging. The current evidence suggests that a gradual taper is preferred over abrupt discontinuation owing to both rebound insomnia and withdrawal symptoms. However, an ideal taper schedule has not been well established. A clinical trial is currently underway in an effort to improve understanding of the ideal wean schedule.[31] In addition to tapering hypnotics, providing patients with educational handouts may provide some benefit. Psychological therapies are also beneficial, with the most evidence supporting CBT in conjunction with a hypnotic taper. Some patients taking BZD hypnotics may benefit from bridging drug cessation with a BzRA. In those cases, an immediate switch to a BzRA was more beneficial than a gradual switch. Other medical therapies have not uniformly demonstrated benefit. Moreover, because most of the evidence for hypnotic discontinuation was done with BZDs, it is not clear that a similar approach can be made with sedating antidepressants, antihistamines, or other hypnotics. Furthermore, the discontinuation of hypnotics in the pediatric population is based only on the adult literature. Further research is needed to better establish optimal hypnotic discontinuation guidelines for both adults and children.

CLINICS CARE POINTS

- Taper hypnotics gradually rather than abruptly discontinuing them in patients on long-term hypnotic therapy for chronic insomnia to avoid rebound insomnia and withdrawal symptoms.
- Use cognitive behavioral therapy and provide educational materials to aid patients during the hypnotic tapering period.

DISCLOSURE

J.P. Hintze has no potential conflicts of interest or funding sources. J.D. Edinger conflicts of interest or funding: grant support from Merck, Philips, Respironics, Inc.

REFERENCES

1. Ohayon MM. Epidemiology of insomnia: what we know and what we still need to learn. Sleep Med Rev 2002;6(2):97–111.
2. Calhoun SL, Fernandez-Mendoza J, Vgontzas AN, et al. Prevalence of insomnia symptoms in a general population sample of young children and preadolescents: gender effects. Sleep Med 2014;15(1):91–5.
3. Chung KF, Yeung WF, Ho FY, et al. Cross-cultural and comparative epidemiology of insomnia: the Diagnostic and Statistical Manual (DSM), Interna tional Classification of Diseases (ICD) and International Classification of sleep disorders (ICSD). Sleep Med 2015;16(4):477–82.
4. Kronholm E, Partonen T, Härmä M, et al. Prevalence of insomnia-related symptoms continues to increase in the Finnish working-age population. J Sleep Res 2016;25(4):454–7.
5. Seow LS, Subramaniam M, Abdin E, et al. Sleep disturbance among people with major depressive disorders (MDD) in Singapore. J Ment Health 2016;25(6):492–9.
6. Kim KW, Kang SH, Yoon IY, et al. Prevalence and clinical characteristics of insomnia and its subtypes in the Korean elderly. Arch Gerontol Geriatr 2017;68: 68–75.
7. Walsh JK. Pharmacologic management of insomnia. J Clin Psychiatry 2004;65(Suppl 16):41–5.
8. Owens JA, Rosen CL, Mindell JA. Medication use in the treatment of pediatric insomnia: results of a sur vey of community-based pediatricians. Pediatrics 2003;111(5 Pt 1):e628–35.
9. Nguyen M, Tharani S, Rahmani M, et al. A review of the use of Clonidine as a sleep aid in the child and adolescent population. Clin Pediatr (Phila) 2014; 53(3):211–6.
10. Schutte-Rodin S, Broch L, Buysse D, et al. Clinical guideline for the evaluation and management of chronic insomnia in adults. J Clin Sleep Med 2008; 4(5):487–504.
11. Ostini R, Jackson C, Hegney D, et al. How is medi cation prescribing ceased? A systematic review. Med Care 2011;49(1):24–36.
12. Kales A, Scharf MB, Kales JD. Rebound insomnia: a new clinical syndrome. Science 1978;201(4360): 1039–41.
13. Roehrs T. Rebound insomnia: its determinants and significance. Am J Med 1990;88(3A):39S–42S.
14. Soldatos CR, Dikeos DG, Whitehead A. Tolerance and rebound insomnia with rapidly eliminated hypnotics: a meta-analysis of sleep laboratory studies. Int Clin Psychopharmacol 1999;14(5):287–303.
15. Staner L, Kerkhofs M, Detroux D, et al. Acute, subchronic and withdrawal sleep EEG changes during treatment with paroxetine and amitriptyline: a double-blind randomized trial in major depression. Sleep 1995;18(6):470–7.
16. Montgomery I, Oswald I, Morgan K, et al. Trazodone enhances sleep in subjective quality but not in objective duration. Br J Clin Pharmacol 1983;16(2): 139–44.
17. Monti JM, Attali P, Monti D, et al. Zolpidem and rebound insomnia-a double-blind, controlled polysomnographic study in chronic insomniac patients. Pharmacopsychiatry 1994;27(4):166–75.
18. Silvestri R, Ferrillo F, Murri L, et al. Rebound insomnia after abrupt discontinuation of hypnotic treatment: double-blind randomized comparison of zolpidem versus triazolam. Hum Psychopharmacol 1996;11(3):225–33.
19. Voshaar RC, van Balkom AJ, Zitman FG. Zolpidem is not superior to temazepam with respect to rebound insomnia: a controlled study. Eur Neuropsychopharmacol 2004;14(4):301–6.
20. Rickels K, Schweizer E, Case WG, et al. Long-term therapeutic use of benzodiazepines. I. Effects of abrupt discontinuation. Arch Gen Psychiatry 1990; 47(10):899–907.
21. Hopkins DR, Sethi KB, Mucklow JC. Benzodiazepine withdrawal in general practice. J R Coll Gen Pract 1982;32(245):758–62.
22. Murphy SM, Tyrer P. A double-blind comparison of the effects of gradual withdrawal of lorazepam, diaz epam and bromazepam in benzodiazepine depen dence. Br J Psychiatry 1991;158:511–6.
23. Voshaar RC, Gorgels WJ, Mol AJ, et al. Tapering off long-term benzodiazepine use with or without group cognitive-behavioural therapy: three-condition, randomised controlled trial. Br J Psychia Try 2003; 182:498–504.
24. Gorgels WJ, Oude Voshaar RC, Mol AJ, et al. Discontinuation of long-term benzodiazepine use by sending a letter to users in family practice: a pro spective controlled intervention study. Drug Alcohol Depend 2005;78(1):49–56.
25. Morin CM, Bastien CH, Guay B, et al. Randomized clinical trial of supervised tapering and cognitive-behavior therapy to facilitate benzodiazepine discontinuation in older adults with chronic insomnia. Am J Psychiatry 2004;161:332–42.
26. Lopez-Peig C, Mundet X, Casabella B, et al. Analysis of benzodiazepine withdrawal program managed by primary care nurses in Spain. BMC Res Notes 2012;5:684.
27. Vicens C, Sempere E, Bejarano F, et al. Efficacy of two interventions on the discontinuation of benzodi azepines in long-term users: 36-month follow-up of a cluster randomised trial in primary care. Br J Gen Pract 2016;66(643):e85–91.
28. Drake J. Temazepam 'Planpak': a multicentre gen eral practice trial in planned benzodiazepine hyp

notic withdrawal. Curr Med Res Opin 1991;12(6): 390–3.
29. Lemoine P, Allain H, Janus C, et al. Gradual withdrawal of zopiclone (7.5 mg) and zolpidem (10 mg) in insomniacs treated for at least 3 months. Eur Psychiatry 1995;10(Suppl 3):161s–5s.
30. Raju B, Meagher D. Patient-controlled benzodiazepine dose reduction in a community mental health service. Ir J Psychol Med 2005;22:42–5.
31. ClinicalTrials. gov. The role of tapering pace and selected traits on hypnotic discontinuation. Bethesda (MD): National Library of Medicine (US); 2016. Identifier NCT02831894, Available at: https://clinicaltrials.gov/ct2/show/NCT02831894. Accessed August 17, 2017.
32. Lader M, Tylee A, Donoghue J. Withdrawing benzodiazepines in primary care. CNS Drugs 2009;23(1): 19–34.
33. Denis C, Fatséas M, Lavie E, et al. Pharmacological in-terventions for benzodiazepine mono-dependence management in outpatient settings. Cochrane Data-base Syst Rev 2006;3:CD005194.
34. Bashir K, King M, Ashworth M. Controlled evaluation of brief intervention by general practitioners to reduce chronic use of benzodiazepines. Br J Gen Pract 1994;44(386):408–12.
35. Cormack MA, Sweeney KG, Hughes-Jones H, et al. Evaluation of an easy, cost-effective strategy for cut ting benzodiazepine use in general practice. Br J Gen Pract 1994;44(378):5–8.
36. Stewart R, Niessen WJ, Broer J, et al. General Prac titioners reduced benzodiazepine prescriptions in an intervention study: a multilevel application. J Clin Epidemiol 2007;60(10):1076–84.
37. Tannenbaum C, Martin P, Tamblyn R, et al. Reduc tion of inappropriate benzodiazepine prescriptions among older adults through direct patient educa tion: the EMPOWER cluster randomized trial. JAMA Intern Med 2014;174(6):890–8.
38. Morgenthaler T, Kramer M, Alessi C, et al. Amer ican Academy of Sleep Medicine. Practice param eters for the psychological and behavioral treatment of insomnia: an update. An american academy of sleep medicine report. Sleep 2006;29(11):1415–9.
39. Giblin MJ, Clift AD. Sleep without drugs. J R Coll Gen Pract 1983;33(255):628–33.
40. Lichstein KL, Johnson RS. Relaxation for insomnia and hypnotic medication use in older women. Psychol Aging 1993;8(1):103–11.
41. Lichstein KL, Peterson BA, Riedel BW, et al. Relaxa tion to assist sleep medication withdrawal. Behav Modif 1999;23(3):379–402.
42. Bootzin RR. Stimulus control treatment for insomnia. Am Psychol Ass Proc 1972;7:395–6.
43. Baillargeon L, Demers M, Ladouceur R. Stimulus-control: nonpharmacologic treatment for insomnia. Can Fam Physician 1998;44:73–9.
44. Riedel B, Lichstein K, Peterson BA, et al. A comparison of the efficacy of stimulus control for medicated and nonmedicated insomniacs. Behav Modif 1998;22(1):3–28.
45. Morin CM, Bootzin RR, Buysse DJ, et al. Psychological and behavioral treatment of insomnia: update of the recent evidence (1998-2004). Sleep 2006; 29(11):1398–414.
46. Taylor DJ, Schmidt-Nowara W, Jessop CA, et al. Sleep restriction therapy and hypnotic withdrawal versus sleep hygiene education in hypnotic using patients with insomnia. J Clin Sleep Med 2010; 6(2):169–75.
47. Morin CM, Colecchi CA, Ling WD, et al. Cognitive behavior therapy to facilitate benzodiazepine discontinuation among hypnotic-dependent patients with insomnia. Behav Ther 1995;26(4):733–45.
48. Baillargeon L, Landreville P, Verreault R, et al. Discontinuation of benzodiazepines among older insomniac adults treated with cognitive-behavioural therapy combined with gradual tapering: a random-ized trial. CMAJ 2003;169(10):1015–20.
49. Vorma H, Naukkarinen H, Sarna S, et al. Treatment of out-patients with complicated benzodiazepine dependence: comparison of two approaches. Addiction 2002;97(7):851–9.
50. O'Connor K, Marchand A, Brousseau L, et al. Cognitive-behavioural, pharmacological and psychosocial predictors of outcome during tapered discontinua tion of benzodiazepine. Clin Psychol Psychother 2008;15(1):1–14.
51. Zavesicka L, Brunovsky M, Matousek M, et al. Discontinuation of hypnotics during cognitive behavioural therapy for insomnia. BMC psychiatry 2008;8(1):80.
52. Belleville G, Guay C, Guay B, et al. Hypnotic taper with or without self-help of insomnia: a randomized clinical trial. J Consult Clin Psychol 2007;75: 325–35.
53. Morgan K, Dixon S, Mathers N, et al. Psychological treatment for insomnia in the management of long-term hypnotic drug use: a pragmatic randomised controlled trial. Br J Gen Pract 2003;53(497):923–8.
54. Lichstein KL, Nau SD, Wilson NM, et al. Psycholog ical treatment of hypnotic-dependent insomnia in a primarily older adult sample. Behav Res Ther 2013;51(12):787–96.
55. Bélanger L, Morin CM, Bastien C, et al. Self-efficacy and compliance with benzodiazepine taper in older adults with chronic insomnia. Health Psychol 2005; 24(3):281–7.
56. Yang CM, Tseng CH, Lai YS, et al. Self-efficacy enhancement can facilitate hypnotic tapering in pa tients with primary insomnia. Sleep Biol Rhythms 2015;13(3):242–51.
57. Romach MK, Kaplan HL, Busto UE, et al. A controlled trial of ondansetron, a 5-HT3 antago-

nist, in benzodiazepine discontinuation. J Clin Psychopharmacol 1998;18(2):121–31.
58. Rickels K, DeMartinis N, García-España F, et al. Imipramine and buspirone in treatment of patients with generalized anxiety disorder who are discontinuing long-term benzodiazepine therapy. Am J Psy-Chiatry 2000;157(12):1973–9.
59. Rynn M, García-España F, Greenblatt DJ, et al. Imip ramine and buspirone in patients with panic disorder who are discontinuing long-term benzodiazepine therapy. J Clin Psychopharmacol 2003;23(5):505–8.
60. Ashton CH, Rawlins MD, Tyrer SP. A double-blind placebo-controlled study of buspirone in diazepam withdrawal in chronic benzodiazepine users. Br J Psychiatry 1990;157:232–8.
61. Nakao M, Takeuchi T, Nomura K, et al. Clinical appli cation of paroxetine for tapering benzodiazepine use in non-major-depressive outpatients visiting an internal medicine clinic. Psychiatry Clin Neurosci 2006;60(5):605–10.
62. Schweizer E, Rickels K, Case WG, et al. Carbamazepine treatment in patients discontinuing long-term benzodiazepine therapy. Effects on withdrawal severity and outcome. Arch Gen Psychiatry 1991; 48(5):448–52.
63. Bobes J, Rubio G, Terán A, et al. Pregabalin for the discontinuation of long-term benzodiazepines use: an assessment of its effectiveness in daily clinical practice. Eur Psychiatry 2012;27(4):301–7.
64. Schweizer E, Case WG, Garcia-Espana F, et al. Pro gesterone co-administration in patients discontinu ing long-term benzodiazepine therapy: effects on withdrawal severity and taper outcome. Psychopharmacology (Berl) 1995;117(4):424–9.
65. Gilhooly TC, Webster MG, Poole NW, et al. What happens when doctors stop prescribing temazepam? Use of alternative therapies. Br J Gen Pract 1998;48(434):1601–2.
66. Hallström C, Crouch G, Robson M, et al. The treat ment of tranquilizer dependence by propranolol. Postgrad Med J 1988;64(Suppl 2):40–4.
67. Pat-Horenczyk R, Hacohen D, Herer P, et al. The ef fects of substituting zopiclone in withdrawal from chronic use of benzodiazepine hypnotics. Psycho-Pharmacol (Berl) 1998;140(4):450–7.
68. Shapiro CM, MacFarlane JG, MacLean AW. Allevi ating sleep-related discontinuance symptoms associated with benzodiazepine withdrawal: a new approach. J Psychosom Res 1993;37(Suppl 1): 55–7.
69. Shapiro C, Sherman D, Peck D. Withdrawal from benzodiazepines by initially switching to zopiclone. Eur Psychiatry 1995;10(Suppl 3). 145s-51s.
70. Lemoine P, Ohayon MM. Is hypnotic withdrawal facilitated by the transitory use of a substitute drug? Prog Neuropsychopharmacol Biol Psychiatry 1997; 21(1):111–24.
71. Kunz D, Bineau S, Maman K, et al. Benzodiazepine discontinuation with prolonged-release melatonin: hints from a German longitudinal prescription data base. Expert Opin Pharmacother 2012;13(1):9–16.
72. Garfinkel D, Zisapel N, Wainstein J, et al. Facilitation of benzodiazepine discontinuation by melatonin: a new clinical approach. Arch Intern Med 1999; 159(20):2456–60.
73. Garzón C, Guerrero JM, Aramburu O, et al. Effect of melatonin administration on sleep, behavioral disor ders and hypnotic drug discontinuation in the elderly: a randomized, double-blind, placebo-controlled study. Aging Clin Exp Res 2009;21(1): 38–42.
74. Cardinali DP, Gvozdenovich E, Kaplan MR, et al. A double blind-placebo controlled study on melatonin efficacy to reduce anxiolytic benzodiaze pine use in the elderly. Neuroendocrinol Lett 2002;23: 55–60.
75. Peles E, Hetzroni T, Bar-Hamburger R, et al. Mela tonin for perceived sleep disturbances associated with benzodiazepine withdrawal among patients in methadone maintenance treatment: a double-blind randomized clinical trial. Addiction 2007;102(12): 1947–53.
76. Vissers FH, Knipschild PG, Crebolder HF. Is mela tonin helpful in stopping the long-term use of hyp notics? A discontinuation trial. Pharm World Sci 2007;29(6):641–6.
77. Lähteenmäki R, Puustinen J, Vahlberg T, et al. Mela tonin for sedative withdrawal in older patients with primary insomnia: a randomized double-blind placebo-controlled trial. Br J Clin Pharmacol 2014; 77(6):975–85.
78. Baandrup L, Lindschou J, Winkel P, et al. Prolonged-release melatonin versus placebo for benzodiaze pine discontinuation in patients with schizophrenia or bipolar disorder: a randomised, placebo-controlled, blinded trial. World J Biol Psychiatry 2016;17(7):514–24.
79. Wright A, Diebold J, Otal J, et al. The effect of melatonin on benzodiazepine discontinuation and sleep quality in adults attempting to dis- continue benzodiazepines: a systematic review and meta-analysis. Drugs Aging 2015;32(12):1009–18.
80. Fernández-San-Martín MI, Masa-Font R, Palacios-Soler L, et al. Effectiveness of Valerian on insomnia: a meta-analysis of randomized placebo-controlled trials. Sleep Med 2010;11(6):505–11.
81. Poyares DR, Guilleminault C, Ohayon MM, et al. Can valerian improve the sleep of insomniacs af- ter benzodiazepine withdrawal? Prog Neuropsy- Chopharmacol Biol Psychiatry 2002;26(3):539–45.

Sleep-Related Drug Therapy in Special Conditions: Children

Nicholas-Tiberio Economou, MD, PhD[a,b], Luigi Ferini-Strambi, MD, PhD[c], Paschalis Steiropoulos, MD, PhD, FCCP[d,*]

KEYWORDS

• Pediatric obstructive sleep apnea • Pediatric insomnia • Pediatric narcolepsy
• Pediatric parasomnias • Pediatric restless legs syndrome

KEY POINTS

- Early detection of sleep disorders in childhood is of great importance in order to proceed to treatment and prevent neurodevelopmental, neurocognitive, and other consequences.
- Insomnia and parasomnias in children present with various complaints, depending on the child's age, and are treated pharmacologically only after nonpharmacologic treatment has failed.
- Sleep apnea in children can be managed with nonpharmacologic, pharmacologic, or surgical treatment, based on specific indications and severity.
- Narcolepsy in children is frequently addressed with stimulants; however, behavioral and lifestyle modifications are still important.
- Restless legs syndrome in children can be treated with pharmacologic and nonpharmacologic options. Iron and ferritin levels should always be evaluated.

INTRODUCTION

There is a continuously growing body of evidence pointing out the importance of detecting and consequently assessing sleep disorders in children, resulting from the bimodal association between sleep and neurodevelopment, cognition, and behavior. Thus, poor sleep quality and/or quantity, especially in the presence of sleep disorders, is related to neurodevelopmental and neurocognitive deficits; reduced learning and social skills; and difficulties in adaptation, behavior, and emotion.[1,2]

Numerous reasons can be found to emphasize the importance of focusing on pediatric sleep medicine and on pediatric sleep pharmacotherapy. First, symptoms of sleep disorders in children are not only different compared with those of adults but also heterogeneous among children of different age. Obstructive sleep apnea (OSA) in children, for example, is related neither to body mass index nor to male sex, in contrast with adults. Moreover, the cardinal daytime symptom of OSA in adults is excessive daytime sleepiness (EDS), whereas children are more often characterized by attention or behavior disorders (such as irritability, overactivity, and inattentiveness), instead of full-blown sleepiness.[3–5] Furthermore, there is variance in clinical manifestation according to

Sleep Med Clin 13 (2018) 251-262 https://doi.org/10.1016/j.jsmc.2018.02.007. 1556-407X/18/
Conflicts of Interest: All authors declare no conflict of interest related to this publication.
[a] Sleep Unit, Department of Psychiatry, University of Athens, 74 Vas Sofias Avenue, Athens 11528, Greece; [b] Enypnion Sleep-Epilepsy Center, Bioclinic Hospital Athens, 15 M. Geroulanou Street, Athens 11524, Greece; [c] Division of Neuroscience, University Vita-Salute San Raffaele, Via Stamira d'Ancona 20, Milan 20127, Italy; [d] Department of Pulmonology, Medical School, Democritus University of Thrace, University Campus, Dragana, Alexandroupolis 68100, Greece
* Corresponding author.
E-mail address: pstirop@med.duth.gr

Sleep Med Clin 17 (2022) 531–542
https://doi.org/10.1016/j.jsmc.2022.06.015
1556-407X/22/

age. For example, during the first years of life, insomnia (sleep-onset difficulty or frequent awakenings during the night), parasomnia, and sleep-disordered breathing are the most prevalent sleep disorders. Later, among school-aged children and mostly among teenagers, suboptimal sleep hygiene, sleep deprivation, delayed sleep phase syndrome, and other circadian disorders are the most prominent abnormalities.[1,6] Another issue, which makes sleep disorder assessment in children even more complicated, is the overall lack of training in pediatric sleep medicine worldwide. Thus, hesitancy of use or improper prescription of drugs (erroneous choice, underdosing, or overdosing) is observed. Moreover, there is also a lack of evidence-based guidelines and of officially approved pediatric sleep pharmacotherapy.[6,7] For example, pediatric insomnia is often treated in an empiric way with clonidine, a drug that is not used and approved for insomnia in adults.[8,9]

This article summarizes the current therapeutic management of sleep disorders in children, bearing in mind the absence of evidence-based guidelines on this topic.

Management of Insomnia in Children

Insomnia is defined as a difficulty to fall asleep, or difficulty in maintaining sleep (nocturnal awakenings), or as waking up earlier than desired. The last phenomenon is related to daytime functioning.[10]

In children, insomnia has mainly behavioral features (commonly called behavioral insomnias of childhood [BIC]) and is classified in 2 main categories: sleep-onset association disorder (SOAD) and limit-setting sleep disorder, whereas there is a third subtype, which represents a mixture of the 2 types of behavioral insomnia.[11,12] SOAD occurs when a child needs special settings or objects (ie, a pacifier) in order to get to sleep or to return to sleep once awakened. In the BIC limit-setting type, delayed sleep onset is observed with or without awakenings and is caused by inappropriate limit setting by parents, with the child refusing to go to bed or asking repeatedly for attention (eg, for a beverage or to use the bathroom).[12] As age advances, other types of insomnia may occur. Adolescents may have insomnia caused by poor sleep hygiene, delayed sleep phase syndrome, or by psychophysiologic conditioning. It is very common among adolescents to adopt bad sleep habits (ie, use of electronic devices in bed; having huge variation in sleep–wake schedule between weekdays and weekends; consuming considerable amounts of alcohol, caffeine [energy drinks], or stimulating substances), or going to bed late at night and consequently waking up late in the morning. In addition, psychophysiologic insomnia is defined as hypervigilance and learned sleep-preventing associations. Therefore, there is an overall preoccupation regarding sleep in adolescents (going to sleep, falling asleep, time spent asleep, possible presence of nonrefreshing sleep, and consequent daytime fatigue, sleepiness, and low performance).[12–15]

The prevalence of insomnia in children is variable because of different classification criteria and its variation with age. It is thought that insomnia prevalence is up to 30% when referring to infants, toddlers, and preschoolers, whereas it is reduced to approximately 15% in later ages.[12,16] The causes of pediatric insomnia are also age related. In infants and toddlers, except for SOAD, medical issues are mostly involved (food allergies, gastroesophageal reflux, colic, chronic, or acute infectious diseases). In preschoolers, nightmares, fear, parental separation, and anxiety may be more likely to be the insomnia aggravating factors. In addition, in adolescents, bad sleep hygiene practices, other sleep disorders such as circadian burdens (delayed sleep–wake phase disorder) or sleep-related movement disorders, in combination with psychiatric comorbidities (attention-deficit/hyperactivity disorder, depression, anxiety), are the main insomnia triggering factors.[12,17–19]

PHARMACOLOGIC TREATMENT

As previously mentioned, guidelines are lacking, such as US Food and Drug Administration (FDA) approvals/indications regarding pediatric sleep pharmacotherapy. Moreover, relevant literature is scarce. Pharmacotherapy in pediatric insomnia should be introduced if conservative measures, such as sleep hygiene and behavioral therapies, are not sufficient or efficacious.[20,21] Before opting for drug therapy in insomnia, as recommended for adults, comorbidities (medical, psychiatric, and other sleep disorders; that is, restless legs syndrome [RLS]) should be thoroughly assessed.

Melatonin

Melatonin has been mostly used in the treatment of insomnia in the context of autism spectrum disorder and in (Attention Deficit Hyperactivity Disorder (ADHD), whereas it has also been shown beneficial in other developmental disorders, such as Angelman syndrome and fragile X syndrome. Melatonin is a sleep-promoting hormone, produced in the pineal gland, with a peak secretion between 2 AM and 4 AM. It has an impact on sleep-onset latency and frequency of awakenings.

The effective dose is 0.05 mg/kg taken 1 to 2 hours before bedtime, although it has also been proposed that melatonin should be taken 9 to 10 hours after the child wakes up.[22,23] Melatonin has a safe pharmacokinetic profile, with mild and rare side effects (mostly sedation). Moreover, melatonin does not interfere with antiepileptic drugs, it does not affect the developmental process, and it is not linked with addiction.[24–26]

Antihistaminergic Drugs

Antihistaminergic drugs (ie, diphenhydramine, promethazine, hydroxyzine) are widely used in the treatment of insomnia. Histamine is one of the main wake-promoting neurotransmitters. Antihistaminergic drugs act via blocking histamine H1 receptors, which results in a sleep-promoting effect (shown by reduced sleep-onset latency and less awakenings) but can cause sedation. Sedation, which may last until the next morning, together with dizziness, is the major side effect of these drugs. Anticholinergic side effects may also be present (dry mouth, blurred vision, constipation, urinary retention, tachycardia). Moreover, tolerance develops with habitual use.[27–29] The duration of the hypnotic effect lasts approximately 4 to 6 hours (peak circulation level is reached 2 hours after ingestion), and recommended dose is 0.5 to 20 mg/kg and 1 mg/kg for diphenhydramine and hydroxyzine, respectively.[12,28,29]

Alpha-Adrenergic Receptor Agonists (α-Agonists)

Alpha-adrenergic receptor agonists (α-agonists; basically clonidine and guanfacine) may promote sleep via a pathophysiologic mechanism that is still unclear.[30] They act as central α2-agonists with onset of action less than 1 hour after ingestion, with peak blood levels 2 to 4 hours later.[8] The off-label daily recommended dose for clonidine starts from 0.05 mg and goes up to 0.1 mg and 0.5 up to 4 mg for guanafacine.[8,30] Common side effects may be hypotension, bradycardia, and anticholinergic effects, whereas rapid discontinuation of clonidine can lead to tachycardia, hypertension, and shortness of breath. Other common indications for these α-agonists are ADHD and ADHD-related sleep problems. Clonidine is also used to treat posttraumatic stress disorder and nightmares.[30–32]

Benzodiazepines Hypnotics

Benzodiazepines hypnotics (eg, estazolam, triazolam), which act on gamma-aminobutyric acid (GABA) receptors, although commonly used for insomnia in adults, are much less prescribed in children (with the exception of clonazepam, which is extremely often used, especially in sleep motor-phenomena and is discussed later). Thus, the trend is to substitute typical hypnagogic benzodiazepines with other drugs (ie, nonbenzodiazepine receptor agonists [nBZRAs]) because of a better pharmacologic profile (they do not induce muscle relaxation, hence avoiding the aggravation of possible comorbid sleep apnea).[24,33] As far as the effect of the benzodiazepines on sleep architecture is concerned, they reduce sleep latency and slow wave sleep (SWS), whereas, in contrast, they increase sleep stage 2 and the amplitude and total number of sleep spindles.

Nonbenzodiazepine Receptor Agonists

nBZRAs (zolpidem, zaleplon) have no indication in children; further, their use in children aged less than 12 years is contraindicated. Nevertheless, because of their few side effects, they are used as off-label hypnotic drugs at doses of 5 mg or 0.25 mg/kg (for zolpidem) at bedtime.[24,27] Zolpidem and zaleplon have half-lives of 1.5 to 2.4 hours and 1 hour, respectively, explaining their different clinical impacts: zolpidem is indicated for sleep-onset insomnia and sometimes for maintenance insomnia, whereas zaleplon only for sleep-onset insomnia.

Antidepressants

Antidepressants (trazodone, mirtazapine) and tricyclic antidepressants (ie, imipramine, amitriptyline, doxepin) are commonly used in adult insomnia but not as much in pediatric insomnia. Trazodone is a 5-HT2 receptor antagonist that blocks histamine receptors and is the most commonly prescribed insomnia drug for children with mood and anxiety disorders.[34] Its dosage is up to 50 mg/d. Tricyclic antidepressants are typically used to treat nonrapid eye movement (NREM) parasomnias because of their suppressive effect on SWS. In cases of insomnia, they are usually indicated for maintenance insomnia but have considerable side effects (sedation, anticholinergic activity, and so forth). In pediatric insomnia, amitriptyline is used at a starting dose of 5 mg at bedtime (maximum 50 mg), whereas imipramine is used at a dose of 0.5 mg/kg.[7,24]

L-5-Hydroxytryptophan

L-5-Hydroxytryptophan is a serotonin precursor and a precursor of melatonin as well. It has some use in parasomnia (1–2 mg/kg at bedtime) because of an overall stabilizing impact on sleep. It may also be used for insomnia given its safe drug profile.[27]

Chloral Hydrate

Chloral hydrate (CH) was used frequently as a hypnotic agent for both adults and children. It results in drowsiness and sedation within 1 hour after ingestion, whereas its half-life is 8 to 12 hours for toddlers and 3 to 4 hours more for neonates and infants. Dose regimen is 25 to 50 mg/kg. CH interferes with respiratory and cardiovascular function (respiratory suppression and cardiovascular instability if overdosed).[35]

NONPHARMACOLOGIC TREATMENT

As stated previously, insomnia treatment should be started with a nonpharmacologic approach that encompasses sleep hygiene routines and behavioral strategy. In short, sleep hygiene rules are the following: (1) maintenance of consistent sleep schedules (bedtime and wake-up time), (2) avoidance of caffeine (and other wake-promoting substances such as tea and chocolate), (3) regular physical activity (preferably until afternoon), and (4) sleep-promoting nocturnal atmosphere (relaxing activities at evening before sleep, appropriate sleep environment [bedroom]).

In adults, the behavioral approach targets the elimination of negative associations/thoughts about sleep, which lead to insomnia. This approach has been proved to be efficacious in children as well, and should be started after the age of 6 months. Relaxation techniques, sleep restriction, and stimulus control can be applied in children, and in the pediatric setting, they are called planned bedtime and programmed awakening. Moreover, extinction and gradual extinction (which consist of ignoring, totally or partially respectively, the child's agitated nocturnal behavior) are further behavior techniques used in children.[21,36]

Management of Obstructive Sleep Apnea in Children

Obstructive sleep apnea syndrome (OSAS) can occur at any age in children, and its prevalence is estimated between 2% and 5%.[37] The choice of treatment is made on an individual basis and depends on the following factors: child's age, polysomnographic pattern, comorbidities, and complications related to OSAS.[38] Surgical treatment, including tonsillectomy and adenoidectomy, is the first choice of treatment in children with adenotonsillar hypertrophy and OSAS. However, nasal continuous positive airway pressure (nCPAP) application remains a viable option for children not eligible for surgery, or in cases of residual disease.[39] Pharmacologic interventions for the treatment of OSAS in pediatric populations are very limited.

Pharmacologic Treatment

Intranasal corticosteroids have been suggested as treatment of children with mild OSAS, to whom adenotonsillectomy is contraindicated or for mild postoperative OSAS.[38] Brouillette and colleagues[40] examined the effect of nasal corticosteroids on the frequency of mixed and obstructive apneas and hypopneas in 25 children with OSAS. More specifically, nasal fluticasone propionate was administered in 13 children versus 12 children receiving placebo, for a period of 6 weeks. The mixed obstructive apnea/hypopnea index (AHI) decreased in the treatment group and increased in children receiving placebo (from 10.7 $\pm$ 2.6 to 5.8 $\pm$ 2.2/h in the fluticasone group and from 10.9 $\pm$ 2.3 to 13.1 $\pm$ 3.6/h in the placebo group; $P = .04$). The rates of oxyhemoglobin desaturation and arousals significantly improved in the fluticasone group compared with controls, whereas there were no changes in tonsillar size, adenoidal size, or symptom score. In another randomized placebo-controlled trial, intranasal mometasone furoate and placebo were administered, respectively, in 24 and 26 children with mild OSAS, for a total period of 4 months. The obstructive AHI decreased in the treatment group (from 2.7 $\pm$ 0.2/h to 1.7 $\pm$ 0.3/h) but increased in the placebo group (from 2.5 $\pm$ 0.2/h to 2.9 $\pm$ 0.6/h; $P = .039$).[41] In the same study, oxygen desaturation index also significantly decreased in the study group compared with controls (-0.6 ± 0.5/h vs 0.7 ± 0.4/h, respectively; $P = .037$). In conclusion, intranasal corticosteroids can reduce the severity of the syndrome in children with mild OSAS. However, data on the minimum duration of therapy for sustained benefit are still lacking.

Leukotriene modifiers have also been studied in pediatric OSAS. In a double-blind, randomized, placebo-controlled trial, Kheirandish-Gozal and colleagues[42] showed a decrease in AHI in the montelukast-treated children, compared with children receiving placebo (from 9.2 $\pm$ 4.1/h to 4.2 $\pm$ 2.8/h and from 8.2 $\pm$ 5.0/h to 8.7 $\pm$ 4.9/h, respectively; $P<.0001$).[42] Similar results were observed in another double-blind, placebo-controlled study by Goldbart and colleagues.[43] In another study with children with OSAS, 12 weeks of treatment with montelukast, after tonsillectomy and/or adenoidectomy, significantly improved AHI, nadir oxyhemoglobin saturation, and OSAS symptoms ($P<.001$).[44] In summary, leukotriene modifiers represent a valid option in the therapeutic approach of pediatric OSAS. In addition, as a complementary therapy, montelukast can improve sleep disturbances in children with OSAS after adenotonsillectomy. However, further research is necessary in order to better establish which pediatric patients with OSAS are most likely to benefit from montelukast therapy.

Recently, the combination of a leukotriene receptor antagonist with intranasal corticosteroids was evaluated in children with OSAS. A total of 183 children with OSAS were divided in 3 groups: group A received oral montelukast, group B received a nasal spray of mometasone furoate, and group C received a combination of montelukast plus mometasone furoate. After 12 weeks of treatment, OSAS symptoms such as snoring ($P<.01$), buccal respiration ($P<.05$), restless sleep ($P<.05$), hyperhidrosis ($P<.05$), and apnea ($P<.01$) improved in all groups compared with before treatment.[45] In addition, AHI decreased ($P<.05$) and minimum oxyhemoglobin saturation increased ($P<.05$) in all groups, whereas the adenoidal/nasopharyngeal ratio, assessed radiographically, decreased ($P<.05$).[45] Compared with the other groups, children belonging to group C showed shorter response duration regarding snoring, apnea, and restless sleep ($P<.05$).[45] The total effective rate was higher in group C than in A and B ($P<.05$).[45] Kheirandish and colleagues[46] studied children with residual OSAS after tonsillectomy and adenoidectomy who received treatment with montelukast and intranasal budesonide for a period of 12 weeks. Compared with children not receiving any therapy, the treatment group showed a significant improvement in AHI (0.3 ± 0.3/h; $P<.001$), nadir oxyhemoglobin saturation ($92.5 \pm 3.0\%$; $P<.01$), and arousal index (0.8 ± 0.7/h; $P<.001$).[46]

Several studies evaluated the role of antibiotic treatment in pediatric OSAS. Antibiotics act by reducing the size of the tonsils and adenoids in some children, thus temporarily alleviating OSAS symptoms. In a prospective randomized trial comparing azithromycin versus placebo, 22 children aged 2 to 12 years were randomly assigned to receive azithromycin or placebo for a 30-day period. A trend toward reduction in AHI in the azithromycin group and an increase in AHI in the placebo group were observed (0.97 ± 2.09 vs 3.41 ± 3.01/h; $P = .23$).[47] This study showed that even though antibiotics decrease OSAS severity, they do not provide persistent relief or prevent surgical therapy.

In addition, results from a meta-analysis comparing the therapeutic effects of pharmacologic therapy on pediatric OSAS revealed that therapeutic effect of placebo was significantly poorer than that of intranasal mometasone furoate, montelukast, budesonide, and fluticasone concerning syndrome severity and, additionally, fluticasone was better than placebo concerning sleep efficiency.[48]

In conclusion, there are pharmacologic options for the treatment of OSAS in pediatric populations.

However, further research is needed to support the role of prescribed medication in improving breathing function during sleep in children with OSAS.

Nonpharmacologic Treatment

Nocturnal supplemental oxygen therapy can be used to treat children with recurrent oxygen desaturations during sleep, related to OSAS.[49] Marcus and colleagues[50] studied the effect of oxygen therapy in 23 children with OSAS aged 5 ± 3 years. In their randomized, double-blind study, oxygen was administered via nasal cannula at 1 L/min for 4 hours. Average and lowest oxygen saturation were higher when breathing supplemental oxygen. However, there was no difference in terms of number (AHI 10.9 ± 20.6/h on oxygen therapy vs 13.5 ± 19.3/h on room air; $P>.05$) and duration (14 ± 7 s on oxygen therapy vs 13 ± 5 s on room air; $P>.05$) of obstructive apneas.[50] In the same study, 2 children showed a significant increase in end-tidal carbon dioxide pressure.[50] Thus, it was concluded that supplemental oxygen does not affect obstructive events during sleep and can be suggested as a temporary solution, in view of definitive therapy, in children with hypoxemia who cannot tolerate continuous positive airway pressure, or in those cases in which surgical treatment has not been shown to be curative.[50,51] The risk of hypercapnia emphasizes the need for strict monitoring during the initiation of treatment with nocturnal supplemental oxygen in children with OSAS.

Surgical Treatment

As mentioned previously, adenotonsillectomy remains the treatment of choice because adenotonsillar hypertrophy represents the principal cause of OSAS in children.[38] However, the procedure is not free of risks and complications. Moreover, there is no consensus on the cutoff of OSAS severity for adenotonsillectomy, and it is usually reserved for children with moderate-to-severe disease.[38]

Management of Parasomnias in Children

Parasomnias are defined as undesirable physical events or experiences that occur during entry into sleep, within sleep, or during arousal from sleep. Basically, they are a temporary unstable state of dissociation. Parasomnias are divided into 2 main categories: those arising from NREM sleep (mainly confusion arousal, sleep tremor, and sleepwalking) and those of rapid eye movement (REM) sleep (mainly nightmares, sleep paralysis, and REM sleep behavior disorder). At times, NREM and REM parasomnias coexist (overlap parasomnia).[10] Arousal parasomnias are very frequent in childhood. In a large population study, the prevalence of any kind of parasomnia occurring at least once in children aged between 2 and 6 years was 84%.[52] NREM parasomnias affect 1% to 4% of the adult population.[53,54] They have characteristics of both sleep and wake states, and they usually occur in deep sleep (NREM stage 3). NREM parasomnias are more prominent during the first half of the night, because of the prominence of NREM 3, whereas REM parasomnias are more frequent during the second half of the night (more REM sleep). Sleepwalking, for example, therefore usually occurs early in the night, whereas nightmares more often at the end of the night. During an event, children may have a varied and complex clinical phenomenology, and, if they get awakened, they seem confused and disorientated.[55] There are several triggers for arousal disorders: sleep deprivation, sleep disturbing stimuli (either external [ie, noises] or internal [ie, OSAS, RLS]), and stress (emotional and/or physical). As far as the treatment is concerned, usually nonpharmacologic approaches are sufficient but, if not, drug therapy is provided in order to avoid mainly hazardous consequences.

Pharmacologic Treatment

As mentioned before, in pediatric parasomnias, medication is prescribed in cases of frequent and possibly hazardous episodes, unresponsive to conservative measures. As for insomnia, no FDA drug approval exists for pediatric parasomnias.[10,56] Given that NREM parasomnias occur mainly during deep sleep (SWS or N3), SWS suppressants are recommended, such as benzodiazepines or tricyclic antidepressants.[56,57] More specifically, the recommended tricyclic anti-depressant is imipramine (in a low dose), and recommended benzodiazepine is clonazepam (0.125–0.5 at bedtime).[56,57] Therapy is indicated for a short period (3–6 months) and slow tapering should follow. The maximum plasma concentration of clonazepam is 1 to 4 hours after ingestion, and its half-life is 30 to 40 hours (half-life is longer in adults).[27]

Nonpharmacologic Treatment

This is the first-line treatment and comprises reassurance and keeping the child and surrounding individuals (eg, siblings) safe. Moreover, safety measures should also be implemented in the sleep environment (alarms on doors, windows, removal of sharp or breakable objects from the child's room or from its common pathways).

Parasomnia triggers, which may be other primary sleep disorders (OSAS, RLS) should be, if present, addressed first. Other behavioral strategies include scheduled awakenings but these are not recommended if the child is already in N3 because they may act as parasomnia triggers.[58,59] Management of nightmares should also comprise avoiding TV a couple of hours before bedtime, having a dim light in the room, and other cognitive-behavioral techniques.[55,60,61]

Management of Narcolepsy in Children

Narcolepsy is a chronic neurologic disorder characterized by a tetrad of clinical symptoms: EDS and 3 symptoms related to REM sleep; hypnagogic/hypnopompic hallucinations, sleep paralysis, and cataplexy. Cataplexy is found in more than half of patients with narcolepsy and helps distinguishing between narcolepsy type 1 (narcolepsy with cataplexy) and narcolepsy type 2 (narcolepsy without cataplexy).[10] Other symptoms of narcolepsy (especially in children) may include disrupted nocturnal sleep, obesity, automatic behavior (ie, sloppy handwriting in children) and complex movement disorders (ie, chorea).[62–65] Narcolepsy is rare. Its prevalence in the general population is 0.025% to 0.05%, with a major incidence between 10 and 19 years.[66,67] All major symptoms of the narcoleptic tetrad, except EDS, result from intrusion of fragments of REM sleep into wakefulness. The deficiency of hypocretin (orexin), which is a wake-promoting/stabilizing neuropeptide, plays a cardinal role in the phenomenon mentioned earlier.[68,69] Narcolepsy may also present secondary to lesions of the posterior hypothalamus provoked by stroke, tumor, head injury, neuroinflammatory processes, and so forth.[70–73] In practice, the management of narcolepsy is symptomatic. The treatment should first address the most troublesome symptom, and then address less disturbing symptoms because some patients describe mostly EDS, whereas others describe cataplexy. There are both behavioral and lifestyle changes along with drug treatment.

Pharmacologic Treatment

Excessive daytime sleepiness

At present there are no approved drugs for treating EDS in the pediatric population, thus the common pharmacotherapy is off label. Treatment options for EDS include mainly central nervous system stimulants (salts of amphetamines and methylphenidate) and wake-promoting agents, such as modafinil or armodafinil[7,74]; a selective norepinephrine reuptake inhibitor (SNRI; atomoxetine) may be an adjuvant therapy, whereas lately a histamine H3 receptor antagonist (pitolisant) has been approved in the European Union with an orphan drug designation in the United States.[75–78] Amphetamines and methylphenidate have similar mechanisms of action because they are both dopamine and norepinephrine agonists. Amphetamines have a long half-life (11–30 hours), but nevertheless drug administration twice a day is preferable (dextroamphetamine 5–30 mg, dextroamphetamine-amphetamine 2.5–20 mg). Methylphenidate has a much shorter half-life (3 hours) and is again recommended twice a day (10–40 mg). Common side effects of stimulants include headache, anorexia, nervosity, insomnia, tics, and weight loss, whereas a red flag warning is heart failure.[79,80] In addition, prolonged use of amphetamines has a high risk of tolerance and addiction (FDA warning).[80,81] Modafinil and armodafinil have an unknown mechanism of action, which acts by enhancing the aminergic system (histamines and catecholamines) in the hypothalamus. Therefore, cortical arousal is promoted.[82] Both drugs are neither FDA nor European Medicines Agency approved for children aged younger than 17 years.[83] Half-lives are 4 and 15 hours for modafinil and armodafinil (which is more potent), respectively.[84] Recommended dosages are 50 to 400 mg/d divided in 2. Common side effects include nausea, vomiting, headache, and (more rarely) Stevens-Johnson syndrome. Atomoxetine may help in the management of EDS and its potential side effects include headache, increase of blood pressure, tachycardia, and weight loss.[75,76] Pitolisant is a histaminergic H3-receptor antagonist. The histaminergic neurons project widely to the cerebral cortex and facilitate arousal. H3 receptors have an inhibiting role on the histamine-secreting neurons, thus promoting sleep. Pitolisant blocks this loop and consequently promotes wakefulness by enhancing the histaminergic system, in an efficient way but still less powerful than modafinil. However, pitolisant has not been approved for children.[77,78,85]

Cataplexy

No drug has been formally approved by the FDA for the treatment of cataplexy in children. Given that REM sleep and consequently REM intrusions, which play an important role in the cataplexy mechanism, are cholinergic driven, tricyclic antidepressants with their potent anticholinergic action have been used historically for treating cataplexy, although their action is modest.[86] Tricyclic agents used are imipramine and clomipramine but, as mentioned in the earlier, these drugs have serious side effects. Dosages are 10 to 100 mg/d and 10 to 150 mg/d for imipramine and clomipramine, respectively. Except for tricyclic agents, other antidepressants (selective serotonin reuptake inhibitors [SSRIs]; eg, fluoxetine 10–30 mg/d) and SNRIs (venlafaxine 37.5–75 mg/d) have been used for cataplexy treatment.[87,88] Sodium oxybate (gamma-hydroxybutyrate) has an FDA indication for the treatment of narcolepsy with cataplexy, for both EDS and cataplexy. Its mechanism of action (it has GABAtype B receptor agonist properties) is not clear but it is considered to consolidate the sleep architecture by reducing awakenings and by increasing SWS. Thus, there is a benefit to daytime alertness with fewer REM intrusion episodes.[89–92] Sodium oxybate is an oral solution (0.5 g/mL) with a short half-life. Hence, the first dose is taken at bedtime and a second one approximately 2.5 to 3 hours later. The recommended dose is 2 to 8 g twice a day. Its side effects include somnambulism and enuresis, aggravation of sleep-disordered breathing, constipation, and tremor. Retrospective data on case series studies showed significant improvement of EDS and cataplexy with the use of sodium oxybate.[75,93,94]

Nonpharmacologic Treatment

Behavioral and lifestyle changes are also important in the management of narcolepsy. Good sleep hygiene with regular and sufficient sleep and wake times are necessary. Scheduled brief naps are highly recommended for EDS. Sleep benefits also from exercise.[95] As far as cataplexy is concerned, patient and parental education about the triggers and the nature of the episodes is important.

Management of Restless Legs Syndrome/ Periodic Leg Movements in Children

RLS, also known as Willis-Ekbom disease, is a common neurologic sleep disorder. It is characterized by an urge to move the legs, usually accompanied by uncomfortable or unpleasant sensations. The symptoms begin or worsen during rest or inactivity, are relieved by movement, and occur exclusively or predominantly in the evening or night.[10] Consensus diagnostic criteria for children were updated recently.[96,97] Periodic limb movement disorder (PLMD) is characterized by clinical sleep disturbance and by repetitive limb jerking during sleep (known as periodic limb movements of sleep) that is not better explained by another condition, medication use, or substance use.[10] Diagnosis of PLM is set by using specific polysomnographic criteria. In children, PLMD seems to be closely related to RLS, although they are distinct diagnostic entities. Nevertheless, both diseases are related to iron deficiency and have a genetic predisposition. Comorbidities commonly associated with RLS and PLMD are ADHD, anxiety, and depression.[98,99] The prevalence of RLS in the pediatric population is between 2% and 4%, whereas the moderate-to-severe type occurs in between 0.5% and 1%. The known predominance of female gender in adults occurs only in the midteens to late teens.[100–102] As far as the pathophysiology of RLS/PLMD is concerned, this seems to be multifactorial, comprising genetics and iron and dopamine deficiency.[103,104]

Pharmacologic Treatment

For mild cases of pediatric RLS, nonpharmacologic interventions are preferred, whereas drug therapy is reserved for chronic, moderate-to-severe cases. The FDA has approved no medications for pediatric RLS or PLMD.[105] For children with iron deficiency and RLS or PLMD, oral iron supplementation should be tried if ferritin levels are less than 50 mg/L or are between 50 and 75 mg/L according to newer evidence.[106,107] Besides iron supplementation, there is limited knowledge regarding other drugs in children. Case series with benzodiazepines are the most consistent in the literature on this topic; thus, clonazepam (0.25–0.5 mg) ortemazepam (7.5–22.5 mg according to age) are recommended.[99,108] In adults, dopaminergic agents or alpha-2-delta calcium channel ligands (gabapentin and pregabalin) are the treatment of choice for RLS. However, in children, these drugs must be used with skepticism. The known dopamine agonists used for RLS and for PLMD are pramipexole (0.125–0.375 mg/d) and ropinirole (0.25–0.75 mg/d). Dosages are increased in line with child's age, so these drugs should be administered 1 to 2 hours before the symptoms start. Rotigotine has no recommendation for ages less than 18 years.[99,108,109] In addition, alpha-2-delta calcium channel ligands (mainly gabapentin and pregabalin), although they do not have a specific indication for pediatric RLS pharmacotherapy, have performed well in pediatric epilepsy, which makes them safe to use.[7]

Nonpharmacologic Treatment

Before introducing drug therapy, iron and ferritin levels should be measured. Moreover, RLS or PLMD triggers, such as caffeine, nicotine, medication (SSRIs, antihistamines, dopamine blockers), insufficient and irregular sleep, or sleep apnea, should be addressed. Physical exercise has also been proved to be efficient.

DISCUSSION

Sleep disorders in children should be a matter of special attention because they are associated with developmental and cognitive deficits and with reduced learning or social skills. Of note, symptoms differ from those of the adult population and vary according to a child's age. In addition, assessment is further complicated by insufficient training in pediatric sleep medicine and the lack of guidelines and official approvals regarding pharmacotherapy.

In children, insomnia has mainly behavioral features, and pharmacotherapy should be introduced if conservative measures, such as sleep hygiene and behavioral therapies, are not sufficient. A variety of pharmaceutical agents, including melatonin, antihistaminic drugs, α-agonists, benzodiazepines and nBZRAs, antidepressants, L5-hydroxytryptophan, and CH, have been proposed. However, the lack of specific guidelines, as well as the limited amount of available data in the literature, dictates caution in the selection of drug therapy.

As mentioned previously, OSAS can occur at any age in children and the choice of treatment depends on several factors, including the child's age, polysomnogram pattern, comorbidities, and complications related to OSAS. Surgery remains the first choice, whereas nCPAP application is a valid alternative for children not eligible for surgery or in case of residual disease. Pharmacologic options are limited. Intranasal corticosteroids, leukotriene modifiers, and their combination have been proposed and are shown to reduce severity in children with mild OSAS, to whom adenotonsillectomy is contraindicated, or for mild postoperative OSAS. However, important data, such as the minimum duration of therapy for sustained benefit, are still lacking. Antibiotics, which can reduce the size of the tonsils and adenoids, do not provide persistent relief or prevent surgical therapy. In addition, nocturnal supplemental oxygen therapy does not affect obstructive events during sleep and can be suggested only as a temporary solution, in view of definitive therapy.

Pharmacologic therapy for parasomnias is necessary only when nonpharmacologic approaches, such as reassurance, safety measures, and avoidance of possible triggers, are not sufficient, in order to avoid hazardous consequences. SWS suppressants, such as benzodiazepines or tricyclic antidepressants, given for a short period followed by slow tapering, are suggested for NREM parasomnias.

For narcolepsy, treatment targets symptom relief. Central nervous system stimulants and wake-promoting agents are used for the treatment of EDS, whereas norepinephrine reuptake inhibitors and histamine H3 receptor antagonists may represent an adjuvant therapy. Tricyclic antidepressants, SSRIs, and SNRIs have also been used for cataplexy treatment. However, none of the aforementioned agents have received approval. In contrast, sodium oxybate has an indication for the treatment of narcolepsy with cataplexy, showing significant improvement of both EDS and cataplexy. Regarding nonpharmacologic therapy, good sleep hygiene combined with frequent naps is highly recommended for EDS, and education about the triggers and the nature of the episodes is important for the management of cataplexy.

In addition, for mild cases of pediatric RLS, nonpharmacologic interventions are preferred, such as physical exercise together with good sleep hygiene and trigger control, whereas drug therapy is reserved for chronic, moderate-to-severe cases. For children with iron deficiency and RLS or PLMD, oral iron supplementation is suggested. Limited data indicate benzodiazepines as an alternative therapy. Dopaminergic agents or alpha-2-delta calcium channel ligands should be used with caution in pediatric populations.

In conclusion, pharmacologic treatment of the most common pediatric sleep disorders lacks evidence, and alternative methods, which have been proved to alleviate the symptoms, are preferred in most cases. The implementation of specific guidelines is of great importance because sleep disorders in children are not rare and they can negatively affect children's development and their cognitive and social skills.

CLINICS CARE POINTS

- Data regarding pharmacologic treatment of the most common pediatric sleep disorders (namely insomnia, parasomnias, narcolepsy, restless legs syndrome) are limited.
- Non-pharmacologic methods, which have been proved to alleviate the symptoms, are preferred in most cases regarding treatment of insomnia, parasomnias, narcolepsy and restless legs syndrome in children.
- Obstructive sleep apnea syndrome in children is managed mainly surgically (with adenotonsillectomy.

REFERENCES

1. Dillon JE, Chervin RD. Attention deficit, hyperactivity, and sleep disorders. In: Sheldon SH, Ferber R, Kryger MH, et al, editors. Principles and practice of pediatric sleep medicine. 2nd edition. New York: Elsevier Saunders; 2014. p. 111.
2. Gringras P. Sleep and its disturbances in autism spectrum disorder. In: Sheldon SH, Ferber R, Kryger MH, et al, editors. Principles and practice of pediatric sleep medicine. 2nd edition. New York: Elsevier Saunders; 2014. p. 125.
3. Chervin RD, Dillon JE, Bassetti C, et al. Symptoms of sleep disorders, inattention, and hyperactivity in children. Sleep 1997;20:1185–92.
4. Owens JA, Rosen CL, Mindell JA. Medication use in the treatment of pediatric insomnia: results of a survey of community-based pediatricians. Pediatrics 2003;111:e628–35.
5. Sheldon SH, Spire JP, Levy HB. Disorders of excessive somnolence. In: Sheldon SH, Spire JP, Levy HB, editors. Pediatric sleep medicine. Philadelphia: WB Saunders; 1992. p. 91.
6. Pelayo R, Dubik M. Pediatric sleep pharmacology. Semin Pediatr Neurol 2008;15(2):79–90.
7. Troester MM, Pelayo R. Pediatric sleep pharma cology: a primer. Semin Pediatr Neurol 2015;22(2): 135–47.
8. Schnoes CJ, Kuhn BR, Workman EF, et al. Pediatric prescribing practices for clonidine and other phar macologic agents for children with sleep distur bance. Clin Pediatr (Phila) 2006;45:229–38.
9. Stojanovski SD, Rasu RS, Balkrishnan R, et al. Trends in medication prescribing for pediatric sleep difficulties in US outpatient settings. Sleep 2007;30:1013–7.
10. American Academy of Sleep Medicine. International classification of sleep disorders. 3rd edition. Darien (IL): American Academy of Sleep Medicine; 2014.
11. American Psychiatric Association. Diagnostic and statistical manual of mental disorders. 5th edition. Ar lington (VA): American Psychiatric Publishing; 2013.
12. Owens JA, Mindell JA. Pediatric insomnia. Pediatr Clin North Am 2011;58:555–69.
13. Fossum IN, Nordnes LT, Storemark SS, et al. The association between use of electronic media in bed before going to sleep and insomnia symptoms, daytime sleepiness, morningness, and chronotype. Behav Sleep Med 2014;12:343–57.
14. Shochat T, Cohen-Zion M, Tzischinsky O. Func tional consequences of inadequate sleep in ado- lescents: a systematic review. Sleep Med Rev 2014; 18:75–87.
15. Jan JE, Bax MC, Owens JA, et al. Neurophysiology of circadian rhythm sleep disorders of children with

neurodevelopmental disabilities. Eur J Paediatr Neurol 2012;16(5):403–12.
16. Honaker SM, Meltzer LJ. Bedtime problems and night wakings in young children: an update of the evidence. Paediatr Respir Rev 2014;15(4):333–9.
17. Sheldon SH, Spire JP, Levy HB. Pediatric sleep medicine. Philadelphia: WB Saunders; 1992.
18. Sivertsen B, Harvey AG, Lundervold AJ, et al. Sleep problems and depression in adolescence: results from a large population-based study of Nor wegian adolescents aged 16-18 years. Eur Child Adolesc Psychiatry 2014;23:681–9.
19. Miano S, Parisi P, Villa MP. The sleep phenotypes of attention deficit disorder, the role of arousal during sleep and implications for treatment. Med Hypoth Eses 2012;79:147–53.
20. Owens JA. Update in pediatric sleep medicine. Curr Opin Pulm Med 2012;17(6):425–30.
21. Mindell JA, Owens JA. Sleep and medication. A clinical guide to pediatric sleep: diagnosis and management of sleep problems. sleep and medication. Philadelphia: Lippincott Williams & Wilkins; 2003. p. 226–8.
22. van Geijlswijk IM, van der Heijden KB, Egberts AC, et al. Dose finding of melatonin for chronic idiopathic childhood sleep onset insomnia: an RCT. Psychopharmacology 2010;212:379–91.
23. Zee PC. Shedding light on the effectiveness of melatonin for circadian rhythm sleep disorders. Sleep 2010;33:1581–2.
24. Bruni O, Alonso-Alconada D, Besag F, et al. Cur rent role of melatonin in pediatric neurology: clinical recommendations. Eur J Paediatr Neurol 2015;19: 122–33.
25. Andersen IM, Kaczmarska J, McGrew SG, et al. Melatonin for insomnia in children with autism spectrum disorders. J Child Neurol 2008;23(5): 482–5.
26. Schwichtenberg AJ, Malow BA. Melatonin treat ment in children with developmental disabilities. Sleep Med Clin 2015;10(2):181–7.
27. Pelayo R, Yuen K. Pediatric sleep pharmacology. Child Adolesc Psychiatr Clin N Am 2012;21: 861–83.
28. Haydon RC 3rd. Are second-generation antihista mines appropriate for most children and adults? Arch Otolaryngol Head Neck Surg 2001;127: 1510–3.
29. Richardson GS, Roehrs TA, Rosenthal L, et al. Tolerance to daytime sedative effects of H1 antihis tamines. J Clin Psychopharmacol 2002;22:511–5.
30. Ingrassia A, Turk J. The use of clonidine for severe and intractable sleep problems in children with neurodevelopmental disorders—a case series. Eur Child Adolesc Psychiatry 2005;14:34–40.
31. Wilens TE, Biederman J, Spencer T. Clonidine for sleep disturbances associated with attention-deficit hyperactivity disorder. J Am Acad Child Adolesc Psychiatry 1994;33:424–6.
32. Newcorn JH, Stein MA, Childress AC, et al. Randomized, double-blind trial of guanfacine extended release in children with attention-deficit/hyperactivity disorder: morning or evening administration. J Am Acad Child Adolesc Psychiatry 2013;52:921–30.
33. Ashton H. Guidelines for the rational use of benzo diazepines. When and what to use. Drugs 1994; 48:25–40.
34. Owens JA, Rosen CL, Mindell JA, et al. Use of pharmacotherapy for insomnia in child psychiatry practice: a national survey. Sleep Med 2010;11: 692–700.
35. Pershad J, Palmisano P, Nichols M. Chloral hydrate: the good and the bad. Pediatr Emerg Care 1999;15:432–5.
36. Halal CS, Nunes ML. Education in children's sleep hygiene: which approaches are effective? A systematic review. J Pediatr (Rio J 2014;90:449–56.
37. Rosen CL, Storfer-Isser A, Taylor HG, et al. Increased behavioral morbidity in school-aged children with sleep-disordered breathing. Pediatrics 2004;114:1640–8.
38. Marcus CL, Brooks LJ, Draper KA, et al. Diagnosis and management of childhood obstructive sleep apnea syndrome. Pediatrics 2012;130:576–84.
39. Marcus CL. Sleep-disordered breathing in chil dren. Am J Respir Crit Care Med 2001;164:16–30.
40. Brouillette RT, Manoukian JJ, Ducharme FM, et al. Efficacy of fluticasone nasal spray for pediatric obstructive sleep apnea. J Pediatr 2001;138: 838–44.
41. Chan CC, Au CT, Lam HS, et al. Intranasal cortico steroids for mild childhood obstructive sleep apnea-a randomized, placebo-controlled study. Sleep Med 2015;16:358–63.
42. Kheirandish-Gozal L, Bandla HP, Gozal D. Montelukast for children with obstructive sleep apnea: results of a double-blind, randomized, placebo-controlled trial. Ann Am Thorac Soc 2016;13: 1736–41.
43. Goldbart AD, Greenberg-Dotan S, Tal A. Montelukast for children with obstructive sleep apnea: a double-blind, placebo-controlled study. Pediatrics 2012;130:e575–80.
44. Wang B, Liang J. The effect of montelukast on mild persistent OSA after adenotonsillectomy in chil dren: a preliminary study. Otolaryngol Head Neck Surg 2017;156:952–4.
45. Yang DZ, Liang J, Zhang F, et al. Clinical effect of montelukast sodium combined with inhaled corti costeroids in the treatment of OSAS children. Med Icine (Baltimore) 2017;96:e6628.
46. Kheirandish L, Goldbart AD, Gozal D. Intranasal steroids and oral leukotriene modifier therapy in

re sidual sleep-disordered breathing after tonsillec tomy and adenoidectomy in children. Pediatrics 2006;117:e61–6.
47. Don DM, Goldstein NA, Crockett DM, et al. Antimi crobial therapy for children with adenotonsillar hy pertrophy and obstructive sleep apnea: a prospective randomized trial comparing azithromy- cin vs placebo. Otolaryngol Head Neck Surg 2005;133: 562–8.
48. Zhang J, Chen J, Yin Y, et al. Therapeutic effects of different drugs on obstructive sleep apnea/hypopnea syndrome in children. World J Pediatr 2017; 13:537–43.
49. Hudgel DW, Thanakitcharu S. Pharmacologic treat ment of sleep-disordered breathing. Am J Respir Crit Care Med 1998;158:691–9.
50. Marcus CL, Carroll JL, Bamford O, et al. Supple mental oxygen during sleep in children with sleep-disordered breathing. Am J Respir Crit Care Med 1995;152:1297–301.
51. Aljadeff G, Gozal D, Bailey-Wahl SL, et al. Effects of overnight supplemental oxygen in obstructive sleep apnea in children. Am J Respir Crit Care Med 1996;153:51–5.
52. Petit D, Touchette E, Tremblay RE, et al. Dyssomnias and parasomnias in early childhood. Pediatrics 2007;119:e1016–25.
53. Bjorvatn B, Gronli J, Pallesen S. Prevalence of different parasomnias in the general population. Sleep Med 2010;11:1031–4.
54. Ohayon MM, Mahowald MW, Dauvilliers Y, et al. Prevalence and comorbidity of nocturnal wander ing in the U.S. adult general population. Neurology 2012;78:1583–9.
55. Kotagal S. Parasomnias in childhood. Sleep Med Rev 2009;13:157–68.
56. Attarian H, Zhu L. Treatment options for disorders of arousal: a case series. Int J Neurosci 2013; 123:3.
57. Provini F, Tinuper P, Bisulli F, et al. Arousal disor ders. Sleep Med 2011;12(Suppl 2):S22–6.
58. Wills L, Garcia J. Parasomnias: epidemiology and management. CNS Drugs 2002;16:803–10.
59. Frank NC, Spirito A, Stark L, et al. The use of scheduled awakenings to eliminate childhood sleepwalking. J Pediatr Psychol 1997;22:345–53.
60. Sadeh A. Cognitive behavioral treatment for child hood sleep disorders. Clin Psychol Rev 2005;25: L612–28.
61. Hauri PJ, Silber MH, Boeve BF. The treatment of parasomnias with hypnosis: a 5-year follow up study. J Clin Sleep Med 2007;3:369–73.
62. Peterson PC, Husain AM. Pediatric narcolepsy. Brain Development 2008;30:609–23.
63. Serra L, Montagna P, Mignot E, et al. Cataplexy fea tures in childhood narcolepsy. Mov Disord 2008;23: 858–65.
64. Kotagal S, Krahn LE, Slocumb N. A putative link between childhood narcolepsy and obesity. Sleep Med 2004;5:147–50.
65. Plazzi G, Pizza F, Palaia V, et al. Complex move ment disorders at disease onset in childhood nar colepsy with cataplexy. Brain 2011;134:3480–92.
66. Silber MH, Krahn LE, Olson EJ, et al. The epidemi ology of narcolepsy in Olmsted County, Minnesota: a population-based study. Sleep 2002;25: 197–202.
67. Longstreth WT Jr, Koepsell TD, Ton TG, et al. The epidemiology of narcolepsy. Sleep 2007;30:13–26.
68. Nishino S, Ripley B, Overeem S, et al. Hypocretin (orexin) deficiency in human narcolepsy. Lancet 2000;355:39.
69. Thannickal TC, Moore RY, Nienhuis R, et al. Reduced number of hypocretin neurons in human narcolepsy. Neuron 2000;27:469.
70. Arii J, Kanbayashi T, Tanabe Y, et al. A hypersomnolent girl with decreased CSF hypocretin level after removal of a hypothalamic tumor. Neurology 2001;56:1775–6.
71. Scammell TE, Nishino S, Mignot E, et al. Narcolepsy and low CSF orexin (hypocretin) concentration after a diencephalic stroke. Neurology 2001; 56:1751–3.
72. Malik S, Boeve BF, Krahn LE, et al. Narcolepsy associated with other central nervous system disor ders. Neurology 2001;57:539–41.
73. Gledhill RF, Bartel PR, Yoshida Y, et al. Narcolepsy caused by acute disseminated encephalomyelitis. Arch Neurol 2004;61:758–60.
74. Babiker MO, Prasad M. Narcolepsy in children: a diagnostic and management approach. Pediatr Neurol 2015;52(6):557–65.
75. Aran A, Einen M, Lin L, et al. Clinical and therapeu tic aspects of childhood narcolepsy-cataplexy: a retrospective study of 51 children. Sleep 2010;33: 1457–64.
76. Billiard M, Bassetti C, Dauvilliers Y, et al. EFNS guidelines on management of narcolepsy. Eur J Neurol 2006;13:1035–48.
77. Syed YY. Pitolisant: first global approval. Drugs 2016;76(13):1313–8.
78. Szakacs Z, Dauvilliers Y, Mikhaylov V, et al. Safety and efficacy of pitolisant on cataplexy in patients with narcolepsy: a randomized, double-blind, pla- cebo-controlled trial. Lancet Neurol 2017;16(3):200–7.
79. Product information: dextroamphetamine sulfate oral tablets, dextroamphetamine sulfate oral tablets. St Louis (MO): Mallinckrodt; 2007.
80. Product information: RITALIN oral tablets, methylphenidate hydrochloride oral tablets. East Hanover (NJ): Novartis; 2007.
81. Available at: https://www.fda.gov/ohrms/dockets/ac/06/briefing/2006-4202B1 _07_FDA-Tab07.pdf. Accessed March 28, 2018.

82. Thorpy MJ. Modafinil/armodafinil in the treatment of narcolepsy. In: Goswami M, Thorpy MJ, Pandi-Perumal SR, editors. Narcolepsy. A clinical guide. Switzerland: Springer International Publishing; 2016. p. 331–9.
83. Ivanenko A, Tauman R, Gozal D. Modafinil in the treatment of excessive daytime sleepiness in chil dren. Sleep Med 2003;4:579–82.
84. Harsh JR, Hayduk R, Rosenberg R, et al. The efficacy and safety of armodafinil as treatment for adults with excessive sleepiness associated with narcolepsy. Curr Med Res Opin 2006;22(4): 761–74.
85. Dauvilliers Y, Bassetti C, Lammers GJ, et al. Pitolisant versus placebo or modafinil in patients with narcolepsy: a double-blind, randomised trial. Lan-Cet Neurol 2013;12(11):1068–75.
86. Cak HT, Haliloglu G, Duzgun G, et al. Success ful treatment of cataplexy in patients with Nie- mann Pick disease type C: use of tricyclic antidepressants. Eur J Paediatr Neurol 2014;18(6):811–5.
87. Morgenthaler TI, Kapur VK, Brown T, et al. Stan dards of practice committee of the AASM. Practice parameters for the treatment of narcolepsy and other hypersomnias of central origin. Sleep 2007; 30(12):1705–11.
88. Lopez R, Dauvilliers Y. Pharmacotherapy options for cataplexy. Expert Opin Pharmacother 2013; 14(7):895–903.
89. Lammers GJ, Arends J, Declerck AC, et al. Gammahydroxybutyrate and narcolepsy: a double-blind placebo-controlled study. Sleep 1993;16: 216–20.
90. US Xyrem Multicenter Study Group. Sodium oxybate demonstrates long-term efficacy for the treat ment of cataplexy in patients with narcolepsy. Sleep Med 2004;5:119–23.
91. Black J, Houghton WC. Sodium oxybate improves excessive daytime sleepiness in narcolepsy. Sleep 2006;29:939–46.
92. Van Schie MK, Werth E, Lammers GJ, et al. Improved vigilance after sodium oxybate treatment in narcolepsy: a comparison between in-field and in laboratory measures. J Sleep Res 2016;25(4): 486–96.
93. Mansukhani M, Kotagal S. Sodium oxybate in the treatment of childhood narcolepsy-cataplexy: a retrospective study. Sleep Med 2012;13(6):606–10.
94. Lecendreux M, Poli F, Oudiette D, et al. Tolerance and efficacy of sodium oxybate in childhood narcolepsy with cataplexy: a retrospective study. Sleep 2012;35:709–11.
95. Rogers AE, Aldrich MS, Lin X. A comparison of three different sleep schedules for reducing daytime sleepiness in narcolepsy. Sleep 2001;24: 385–91.
96. Picchietti DL, Bruni O, de Weerd A, et al. Pediatric restless legs syndrome diagnostic criteria: an update by the International restless legs syndrome study group. Sleep Med 2013;14(12):1253–9.
97. Allen RP, Picchietti DL, Garcia-Borreguero D, et al. Restless legs syndrome/Willis-Ekbom disease diagnostic criteria: updated International Restless Legs Syndrome Study Group (IRLSSG) consensus criteria-history, rationale, description, and significance. Sleep Med 2014;15(8):860–73.
98. Picchietti MA, Picchietti DL. Restless legs syndrome and periodic limb movement disorder in children and adolescents. Semin Pediatr Neurol 2008;15(2):91–9.
99. Picchietti DL, Rajendran RR, Wilson MP, et al. Pediatric restless legs syndrome and periodic limb movement disorder: parent-child pairs. Sleep Med 2009;10(8):925–31.
100. Ohayon MM, O'Hara R, Vitiello MV. Epidemiology of restless legs syndrome: a synthesis of the litera ture. Sleep Med Rev 2012;16(4):283–95.
101. Picchietti D, Allen RP, Walters AS, et al. Restless legs syndrome: prevalence and impact in children and adolescents-the Peds. REST Study Pediatr 2007;120(2):253–66.
102. Zhang J, Lam SP, Li SX, et al. Restless legs symp toms in adolescents: epidemiology, heritability, and pubertal effects. J Psychosom Res 2014; 76(2):158–64.
103. Allen RP. Restless leg syndrome/Willis-Ekbom dis ease pathophysiology. Sleep Med Clin 2015; 10(3):207–14.
104. Rye DB. The molecular genetics of restless legs syndrome. Sleep Med Clin 2015;10(3):227–33.
105. Mindell JA, Emslie G, Blumer J, et al. Pharmacologic management of insomnia in children and ad- olescents: consensus statement. Pediatrics 2006;117(6):e1223–32.
106. Picchietti DL. Should oral iron be first-line therapy for pediatric restless legs syndrome and periodic limb movement disorder? Sleep Med 2017;32: 220–1.
107. Dye TJ, Jain SV, Simakajornboon N. Outcomes of long-term iron supplementation in pediatric restless legs syndrome/periodic limb movement disorder (RLS/PLMD). Sleep Med 2017;32:213–9.
108. Picchietti DL, Stevens HE. Early manifestations of restless legs syndrome in childhood and adolescence. Sleep Med 2008;9(7):770–81.
109. Walters AS, Mandelbaum DE, Lewin DS. Dopami nergic therapy in children with restless legs/periodic limb movements in sleep and ADHD. Dopaminergic Therapy Study Group. Pediatr Neurol 2000; 22(3):182–6.

9780323961653